Psychiatric Treatment: Advances in Outcome Research

Psychiatric Treatment: Advances in Outcome Research

Edited by

Steven M. Mirin, M.D.

General Director and Psychiatrist-in-Chief, McLean Hospital,
Belmont, MA; and Associate Professor of Psychiatry,
Harvard Medical School, Boston, MA

John T. Gossett, Ph.D.

Director, Psychology Department, Timberlawn Psychiatric Hospital, Inc.;
Director, Timberlawn Psychiatric Research Foundation, Inc.; and
Clinical Associate Professor of Psychology, Department of Psychiatry,
University of Texas Southwestern Medical Center at Dallas

Mollie C. Grob, M.S.W.

Director, Evaluative Service Unit, McLean Hospital, Belmont, MA; and
Associate in Psychiatry (Social Services, Administration, and Education),
Harvard Medical School, Boston, MA

American Psychiatric Press, Inc.

Washington, DC
London, England

Note: The authors have worked to ensure that all information in this book concerning drug dosages, schedules, and routes of administration is accurate as of the time of publication and consistent with standards set by the U.S. Food and Drug Administration and the general medical community. As medical research and practice advance, however, therapeutic standards may change. For this reason and because human and mechanical errors sometimes occur, we recommend that readers follow the advice of a physician who is directly involved in their care or the care of a member of their family.

Books published by the American Psychiatric Press, Inc., represent the views and opinions of the individual authors and do not necessarily represent the policies and opinions of the Press or the American Psychiatric Association.

American Psychiatric Press, Inc.
1400 K Street, N.W., Washington, DC 20005

Library of Congress Cataloging-in-Publication Data
Psychiatric treatment: Advances in outcome research / edited by
    Steven M. Mirin, John Gossett, Mollie C. Grob.
      p.   cm.
    Includes bibliographical references and index.
    ISBN 0-88048-500-0
    1. Psychiatric hospital care—United States—Evaluation.
   2. Mental illness—Treatment—Evaluation. I. Mirin, Steven M.,
   1942– . II. Gossett, John T., 1937– . III. Grob, Mollie C.
    [DNLM: 1. Outcome and Process Assessment (Health Care). 2. Mental
   Disorders—therapy. WM 400 P97344]
RC443.P77 1991
616.89'1—dc20
DNLM/DLC
for Library of Congress   91-4535
                                                                      CIP
British Cataloguing in Publication Data
A CIP record is available from the British Library.

❖   Table of Contents

Contributors ix

Introduction
Steven M. Mirin, M.D.
John T. Gossett, Ph.D.
Mollie C. Grob, M.S.W. xv

Section I. Treatment Outcome Research and the Delivery of Patient Care

1 ❖ Why Study Treatment Outcome?
Steven M. Mirin, M.D.
M. Jo Namerow, Ph.D. 1

2 ❖ Risk-Benefit Ratios in Psychiatric Treatment
John M. Kane, M.D. 15

3 ❖ Outcome of Children Treated in Psychiatric Hospitals
Ted P. Asay, Ph.D.
Thomas L. Dimperio, Ph.D. 21

4 ❖ Long-Term Treatment of the Young Adult Chronic Patient: Effect on Social Functioning and Coping
Carol L. M. Caton, Ph.D.
Alexander Gralnick, M.D. 31

5 ❖ The Effects of Inpatient Family Intervention on Treatment Outcome
John F. Clarkin, Ph.D.
Ira D. Glick, M.D.
Gretchen Haas, Ph.D.
James H. Spencer, Jr., M.D. 47

Section II. Outcome Evaluation in Specific Diagnostic Subgroups

6 ❖ Selective Review of Recent North American
Long-Term Follow-up Studies of Schizophrenia
Thomas H. McGlashan, M.D. 61

7 ❖ Effectiveness in Psychiatric Care: I. A Cross-National
Study of the Process of Treatment and Outcomes
of Major Depressive Disorder
Ira D. Glick, M.D.
Lorenzo Burti, M.D.
Koji Suzuki, M.D.
Michael Sacks, M.D. 107

8 ❖ Course and Treatment Outcome in Patients with Mania
Mauricio Tohen, M.D., Dr. P.H. 127

9 ❖ The Effectiveness of Alcoholism Treatment:
Evidence from Outcome Studies
James R. McKay, Ph.D.
Ronald T. Murphy, Ph.D.
Richard Longabaugh, Ed.D. 143

10 ❖ Outcome Studies in Patients with Eating Disorders
L. K. George Hsu, M.D. 159

11 ❖ Outcome Studies of Borderline Personality Disorder
Mary C. Zanarini, Ed.D.
Deborah L. Chauncey, A.B.
Tana A. Grady, M.D.
John G. Gunderson, M.D. 181

12 ❖ Empirical Perspectives on Narcissism
Eric M. Plakun, M.D. 195

Section III. Methodologic Issues in Outcome Research

13 ❖ Outcome Measurement: Tapping the Patient's Perspective
   Susan V. Eisen, Ph.D.
   Mollie C. Grob, M.S.W.
   Diana L. Dill, Ed.D. 213

14 ❖ Follow-up Study Methodology:
   The Menninger Project and a Proposed Ideal Study
   Lolafaye Coyne, Ph.D. 237

15 ❖ Design for a Quasi-Experimental Study to Test
   Length of Stay Prediction Hypotheses
   Herbert E. Spohn, Ph.D.
   Lolafaye Coyne, Ph.D. 255

16 ❖ Quality Assurance and Treatment Outcome:
   A Medical Perspective
   Benjamin Liptzin, M.D. 265

17 ❖ Quality Assurance and Treatment Outcome:
   A Psychiatric Nursing Perspective
   Elizabeth C. Poster, R.N., Ph.D. 279

18 ❖ Measuring Outcome:
   A Post-Discharge Assessment Model
   John W. Goethe, M.D.
   Marcia L. Gerulaitis
   Bonnie L. Szarek, R.N.
   Judith Weber, M.S.W. 293

19 ❖ Assessing the Outcome of Managing Costs:
   An Exploratory Approach
   Steven S. Sharfstein, M.D. 311

Index 321

Contributors

Ted P. Asay, Ph.D.
Clinical Psychologist, Timberlawn Psychiatric Hospital, Inc., Dallas, TX

Lorenzo Burti, M.D.
Assistant Professor of Psychiatry, Istituto di Psichiatria, Universita di
Verona, Italy

Carol L. M. Caton, Ph.D.
Associate Clinical Professor of Social Sciences in Psychiatry and Public
Health, College of Physicians and Surgeons, Columbia University, New
York, NY

Deborah L. Chauncey, A.B.
Senior Research Assistant, Psychosocial Research Program, McLean
Hospital, Belmont, MA

John F. Clarkin, Ph.D.
Director of Psychiatry, The New York Hospital, Cornell University
Medical College, Westchester Division; Professor of Clinical Psychology
in Psychiatry, Cornell Medical Center, New York, NY

Lolafaye Coyne, Ph.D.
Director, Statistical Laboratory, Associate Director, Hospital Research,
The Menninger Foundation, Topeka, KS; Adjunct Professor of
Psychology, University of Kansas, Lawrence, KS

Diana L. Dill, Ed.D.
Research Psychologist, Evaluative Service Unit, McLean Hospital,
Belmont, MA; Instructor in Psychology, Department of Psychiatry,
Harvard Medical School, Boston, MA

Thomas L. Dimperio, Ph.D.
Clinical Psychologist, Timberlawn Psychiatric Hospital, Inc., Dallas, TX

Susan V. Eisen, Ph.D.
Assistant Director, Evaluative Service Unit, McLean Hospital, Belmont, MA; Assistant Professor of Psychology, Department of Psychiatry, Harvard Medical School, Boston, MA

Marcia L. Gerulaitis
Outcome Study Coordinator, Department of Clinical Research, Institute of Living, Hartford, CT

Ira D. Glick, M.D.
Science Advisor to the Director, National Institute of Mental Health, Bethesda, MD; Professor of Psychiatry, Cornell University Medical College, The New York Hospital-Cornell Medical Center, New York, NY

John W. Goethe, M.D.
Director of Clinical Research, Institute of Living; Associate Clinical Professor of Psychiatry, Yale University School of Medicine, New Haven, CT

John T. Gossett, Ph.D.
Director, Psychology Department, Timberlawn Psychiatric Hospital, Inc.; Director, Timberlawn Psychiatric Research Foundation, Inc.; and Clinical Associate Professor of Psychology, Department of Psychiatry, University of Texas Southwestern Medical Center at Dallas

Tana A. Grady, M.D.
Medical Staff Fellow, National Institute of Mental Health, Laboratory of Clinical Science, Bethesda, MD

Alexander Gralnick, M.D.
Medical Director, High Point Hospital, Port Chester, NY

Mollie C. Grob, M.S.W.

Director, Evaluative Service Unit, McLean Hospital, Belmont, MA; and Associate in Psychiatry (Social Services, Administration, and Education), Harvard Medical School, Boston, MA

John G. Gunderson, M.D.

Director, Psychosocial Program, McLean Hospital, Belmont, MA; Associate Professor of Psychiatry, Harvard Medical School, Boston, MA

Gretchen Haas, Ph.D.

Associate Professor of Psychiatry, University of Pittsburgh School of Medicine, Pittsburgh, PA

L. K. George Hsu, M.D.

Director, Outpatient Eating Disorders Clinic, Western Psychiatric Institute and Clinic; Associate Professor of Psychiatry, University of Pittsburgh School of Medicine, Pittsburgh, PA

John M. Kane, M.D.

Professor and Chairman, Department of Psychiatry, Hillside Hospital, Long Island Jewish Medical Center, Glen Oaks, NY

Benjamin Liptzin, M.D.

Chief of Psychiatry, Baystate Medical Center, Deputy Chairman, Department of Psychiatry, Tufts Medical School, Medford, MA

Richard Longabaugh, Ed.D.

Director of Evaluation, Butler Hospital; Professor of Psychiatry and Human Behavior, Brown University, Providence, RI

Thomas H. McGlashan, M.D.

Director and Psychiatrist-in-Chief, Yale Psychiatric Institute; Professor of Psychiatry, Yale University School of Medicine, New Haven, CT

James R. McKay, Ph.D.

Investigator, Addiction Research Center, University of Pennsylvania; Research Assistant Professor of Psychology in Psychiatry, University of Pennsylvania School of Medicine, Philadelphia, PA

Steven M. Mirin, M.D.

General Director and Psychiatrist-in-Chief, McLean Hospital, Belmont, MA; and Associate Professor of Psychiatry, Harvard Medical School, Boston, MA

Ronald T. Murphy, Ph.D.

Research Fellow, Center for Alcohol and Addiction Studies, Brown University, Providence, RI

M. Jo Namerow, Ph.D.

President, Namerow & Associates, Baltimore, MD

Eric M. Plakun, M.D.

Director of Admissions, Austen Riggs Center; Member of Senior Staff, Clinical Instructor in Psychiatry, Harvard Medical School, Boston, MA

Elizabeth Poster, R.N., Ph.D.

Director of Nursing Research and Education, UCLA Neuropsychiatric Institute and Hospital; Assistant Clinical Professor, UCLA Schools of Nursing and Medicine, Los Angeles, CA

Michael Sacks, M.D.

Associate Professor of Psychiatry, Cornell University Medical College, New York, NY

Steven S. Sharfstein, M.D.

Executive Vice President and Medical Director, The Sheppard and Enoch Pratt Hospital, Baltimore, MD; Clinical Professor of Psychiatry, University of Maryland

James H. Spencer, Jr., M.D.

Clinical Associate Professor of Psychiatry, Cornell University Medical College, New York, NY; Associate Attending Psychiatrist, Payne Whitney Clinic, New York, NY

Herbert E. Spohn, Ph.D.

Director of Research, The Menninger Foundation, Topeka, KS; Adjunct Professor, Department of Psychology, University of Kansas, Lawrence, KS

Koji Suzuki, M.D.

Director of Social Psychiatry, National Institute of Mental Health, Ichikawa, Japan

Bonnie L. Szarek, R.N.

Research Nurse, Department of Clinical Research, Institute of Living, Hartford, CT

Mauricio Tohen, M.D., Dr. P.H.

Clinical Director, Psychosis Program, McLean Hospital, Belmont, MA; Instructor in Psychiatry, Harvard Medical School, Boston, MA

Judith Weber, M.S.W.

Project Coordinator, Department of Clinical Research, Institute of Living, Hartford, CT

Mary C. Zanarini, Ed.D.

Assistant Director, Psychosocial Research Program, McLean Hospital, Belmont, MA; Instructor in Psychology, Department of Psychiatry, Harvard Medical School, Boston, MA

Introduction

During the last two decades, we have witnessed enormous changes in the mental health care delivery system. Inflation, the development of new technologies, and the growing number of people defined as needing mental health treatment have all contributed to the escalating cost of care. In response, employers, third-party payers, regulatory agencies, and the federal government have all joined in the effort to contain costs. In this context, prospective payment, managed care, and increasing restrictions on insurance benefits have emerged as the principal mechanisms for controlling mental health expenditures.

With passage of the Social Security Amendments of 1983, hospital reimbursement for the care of patients insured under Medicare changed from a retrospective system based on the actual costs of care, to a prospective, fixed-fee system based on the diagnosis of the patient. However, studies carried out under the auspices of the American Psychiatric Association (APA) and the National Association of Private Psychiatric Hospitals (NAPPH) demonstrated that, for psychiatric patients, clinical diagnosis by itself was an inaccurate method of predicting hospital lengths of stay and/or the costs of hospital care and was, therefore, inappropriate as a method of determining reimbursement, prospective or otherwise. As a result, organized psychiatry was successful in obtaining a temporary exemption from prospective payment under Medicare. However, it should be noted that a growing number of hospitals and mental health care providers are now agreeing to accept predetermined, fixed fees for both inpatient and outpatient psychiatric treatment. Under such arrangements, there are substantial financial incentives for care providers to explore ways in which inpatient stays can be shortened and patients transitioned to less intense, and less expensive, treatment settings including partial hospital, community residence, and outpatient care.

Another important development in the struggle to control the cost of mental health treatment is the rapidly growing emphasis on "managing" inpatient and, to a lesser extent, outpatient care. The stated goals of managed care are to ensure that any treatment provided is both "medically necessary" and active (as opposed to custodial). However, what constitutes medical necessity is often an issue between care providers and those who are attempting to manage the care provided. Tensions arise when providers are forced to justify continuing treatment and when third-party payers and/or managed care organizations become suspicious that such justifications are driven by financial, rather than clinical, considerations. In this context, the development of mutually agreed upon, objective criteria for measuring both medical necessity and the acuity of care is an essential first step in ensuring that patients' rights to quality care are recognized and preserved.

As both the utilization and costs of mental health care have risen, some insurance carriers and employers have begun to either reduce mental health benefits or pass the increased cost of care on to consumers in the form of higher insurance premiums and/or greater use of co-insurance and deductibles. In addition, some plans have begun offering mental health care as an optional, rather than basic, benefit (at additional cost), while others preclude individuals with a known history of mental disorder from obtaining coverage at all. Finally, some third-party payers have proposed that only those treatments demonstrated to be cost-effective be reimbursed by health insurance benefit plans. In this context, neuroleptic treatment for patients with schizophrenia might be a covered service while psychotherapy with such patients might not.

In an era of increasingly scarce resources, our ability to sustain or expand desperately needed mental health services is in doubt. Increasingly, mental health policy planners and third-party payers are demanding data that demonstrate the efficacy of psychiatric care in achieving agreed-upon treatment goals if they are to consider reimbursing psychiatric care on the same basis as other potentially chronic and debilitating medical illnesses. Those who plan, pay for, or manage mental health care will also need evidence that such care is being delivered in an appropriate and timely fashion. Finally, the willingness of anyone to pay for new treatment alternatives will depend on our ability to demonstrate that such alternatives are cost-effective, in that they not only ameliorate symptoms but also increase the functional capacity of the patient and reduce the cost of subsequent psychiatric and/or medical care. In responding to these new demands, those who provide mental health care will need to know much more than we do at present about the impact of treatment on the clinical course and long-term outcome of patients. In this context, the development of reliable methods for measuring treatment outcome is an essential first step.

This volume attempts to summarize much of the work to date in the increasingly important area of treatment outcome research. The chapters in Section I provide an overview of the rationale for measuring treatment outcome as well as a sampling of outcome studies in children, adolescents, and young adults treated in inpatient settings. The impact of psychiatric treatment on social and functional adjustment within families, and in the community, is also addressed.

In Section II, the focus is on studies of both short- and long-term treatment outcome within specific diagnostic subgroups, including patients with schizophrenia, affective illness, alcoholism, eating disorders, and various types of personality disorders.

Section III addresses the host of practical and methodologic issues one faces in designing and conducting treatment outcome research. To what extent should outcome measures focus on symptom relief, functional adjustment, or the cost of subsequent care? In gathering outcome data, how do we tap the unique perspectives of patients, family members, and clinicians? How should outcome measures, and the data they generate, be integrated into ongoing systems of clinical care so as to inform clinical decision making and guide the development of more effective treatment programs? Finally, how can we ensure that all mental health disciplines are involved in the design and implementation of outcome research, as well as the clinical and programmatic changes that such studies inevitably generate?

The development and publication of this volume was supported by the Education and Research Foundation of NAPPH. Through its Clinical Research Committee and other activities, NAPPH has demonstrated a long-standing commitment to furthering psychiatric research, particularly in the area of treatment outcome. In 1982, NAPPH published its first compendium of research activities in private psychiatric hospitals (*Information on Research Activities in NAPPH Hospitals*), which was revised annually for several years. A second, expanded, monograph (*Current Research in Private Psychiatric Hospitals*) was published in 1987. The current text reflects the growing interest of NAPPH in encouraging the design and implementation of treatment outcome studies in its member hospitals and in other clinical settings. The editors are grateful to Claire Ryan and Susanne Daley for their help in the preparation of this volume. Our thanks also to Robert Thomas, Executive Director of NAPPH, and to Carol Nadelson, M.D., Editor-in-Chief, Stephanie Selice, and Carol Hennessey at the American Psychiatric Press for their support in publishing work that we hope will provide a foundation for further progress in this increasingly important area of research.

Steven M. Mirin, M.D.
John T. Gossett, Ph.D.
Mollie C. Grob, M.S.W.

❖ 1 ❖ Why Study Treatment Outcome?

Steven M. Mirin, M.D.

M. Jo Namerow, Ph.D.

Incentives for Measuring Treatment Outcome

For almost two decades, health policy movements have focused primarily on the need to contain the escalating cost of health care. In this context, various systems of prospective payment, and the development of mechanisms to "manage" care, have been the major initiatives in the cost containment struggle. In 1983, the passage of Public Law 98-21 initiated prospective reimbursement under Medicare for hospitalized patients using Diagnosis-Related Groups (DRGs), on the presumption that DRG categories would predict hospital length of stay and, therefore, the cost of treatment (Inglehard 1983). Subsequently, however, several studies (English et al. 1986; Namerow and Gibson 1988; Schumacher et al. 1986) demonstrated that DRGs were generally not useful for predicting length of stay in inpatient settings. If DRGs were to be used as the mechanism for determining reimbursement, some facilities would be overpaid for the care they actually delivered, whereas others would be grossly underpaid.

These findings support the contention that mental health care is distinct from mainstream medical-surgical care in that the relationship between a patient's diagnosis and the type, intensity, and duration of the care provided is not always straightforward. Though a temporary exemption from a DRG-based payment system was granted by Congress for both psychiatric units in general hospitals and freestanding private psychiatric hospitals, the mental health industry must now assume responsibility for developing its own cost containment strategies, lest others in the executive and legislative branches of government, as well as in the private sector, develop them independently. Furthermore, there will inevitably be closer scrutiny of the relationship between treatment services (and their associated costs) and treatment outcome.

Further incentive for examining cost-benefit ratios in mental health care has been provided by the growth of managed care organizations (Bracken et al. 1990) whose role in shortening inpatient hospital stays has had a substantial

1

impact on how mental health care is now being delivered (see Chapter 19). Increasingly, mental health providers are being forced to demonstrate that inpatient care is medically necessary and that treatment is "active" rather than custodial. In essence, third-party payers are reluctant to support inpatient treatment for all but the most acutely ill patients. In addition, there is growing incentive, for both payers and providers alike, to 1) define the characteristics of those patients who require inpatient (as opposed to outpatient) treatment, 2) agree as to what kinds of clinical problems should be addressed during a patient's hospital stay and what problems should be left for follow-up care in an ambulatory setting, and 3) determine which treatments are most useful and cost-effective in particular patient subgroups with respect to both short- and long-term outcome.

Finally, though the overriding emphasis of both health policy planners and third-party payers has been on cost containment, both providers and patients have voiced their concern that efforts at cost control not compromise the quality of care. Inherent in this wish is a basic assumption that the various players in the health care arena will be able to agree on a definition of quality and identify it when it occurs. If quality care is defined as appropriate treatment performed with good results, it follows that reliable data about the outcome(s) of care are essential. Developing methods for obtaining reliable outcome data will therefore be high on the agenda of planners, payers, providers, and patients in the coming decade.

What Should Outcome Studies Measure?

Clearly, patients are the central concern of outcome research. Not only do we seek effective treatments on their behalf, but increasingly, patients are also playing an active role in treatment design. As consumers of mental health care, patients' perceptions about treatment efficacy, and their satisfaction with the type of treatment they received and the way it was delivered, will ultimately determine which treatments they accept and which outcomes they value.

Although there is general agreement that measuring the outcome of care is desirable, there are substantial impediments to accomplishing this task. Mental health care affects the entire person—from the ability to perform basic activities of daily living to the complex cognitive and affective processes that go into making relationships. Moreover, changes in patients' symptoms, or in their functional abilities, are matters of degree along a continuum rather than absolutes. Nor is treatment outcome unidimensional in time; rather, it is an evolving process that affects many aspects of a patient's life over many years. Finally, whether or not a psychiatric patient experiences clinical symptoms, performs well at school or work, or functions appropriately with a family unit is determined not only by the treatment he or she may have received, but also by a multitude of cultural, socioeconomic, and interrelational factors.

Traditionally, treatment outcome studies have focused primarily on changes in patients' clinical status. Equally important, however, is the patient's ability to participate successfully in interpersonal relationships; function within the context of a family or social group; perform useful work; maintain an independent existence; and attend to his or her needs for self care, food, and shelter. Quality of life should also be part of the outcome equation. The common assumption that symptom relief, reduction in the frequency of illness episodes, and improvement in functional adaptation (e.g., being able to work) mean that quality of life has been enhanced may, in some cases, be unwarranted. Indeed, in some patients, these positive changes may not be accompanied by the development of meaningful interpersonal relationships, obtaining employment that they can be enthusiastic about, or being able to experience a subjective sense of satisfaction and well-being.

Outcome studies should not only assess change in the patient's primary psychiatric disorder but also any other medical and/or psychiatric disorder that may be present. For example, among the chronic mentally ill, there are a substantial number of individuals with concurrent alcohol and/or drug abuse problems (Davis 1984; Fischer et al. 1975). In these patients, remission of their primary psychiatric disorder (e.g., schizophrenia) may or may not be accompanied by a reduction in their substance abuse and its associated adverse sequelae. Remission of psychotic symptomatology is certainly a positive step, but unless the substance abuse problem is also addressed, the patient's ability to work, or to remain out of a hospital, may not be enhanced. How, then, should we assess the efficacy of treatment in these individuals? Clearly, outcome measures should encompass all extant disorders, singly and in combination. Emphasis should be not only on clinical symptomatology or pathologic behavior but also on the functional integration of the patient into his or her occupational, social, and cultural milieu. The impact of treatment on the subsequent utilization of health care and social services should also be assessed in these patients.

Finally, it should be noted that there are patients for whom treatment outcome may need to be defined in limited terms. For these patients, the positive effects of treatment on specific areas of their functioning may be minimized by the severity and/or irreversibility of their illness. For example, in a patient who develops an organic brain syndrome as a consequence of prolonged heavy drinking, maintenance of sobriety may not be accompanied by substantial functional improvement. The effects of chronic drinking on such a patient's interpersonal relationships may also be irreversible. Similarly, the chronic schizophrenic who experiences remission of positive symptoms (e.g., hallucinations/delusions) may still be left with bland affect, apathy, and inability to develop meaningful relationships. We need to define what the reasonable (and affordable) goals of treatment should be for such patients before deciding what sorts of outcome measures should be applied in assessing their treatment. By so doing, we can also shed more light on society's not-so-subtle resistance to caring for the chronic mentally ill patient. This would elevate the debate on this subject to discussions about national priorities rather than arguments about "medical necessity" or "active" treatment (Goldsmith 1983; Sharfstein 1987).

Outcome Studies From the Clinician's Perspective

The Clinician's Role in Objectifying Treatment Decisions

Just as those who pay for mental health care need outcome data to inform their decision making about resource allocation, physicians and others who provide care need outcome data to help guide their efforts. As desirable outcomes are identified and agreed upon, practice patterns will be modified. Unnecessary or ineffective treatments will be abandoned, and those that yield better results will come into more common use. Some have suggested that this may lead to a "homogenization" of treatment, with strict adherence to practice parameters developed by committees. In this Orwellian scenario, clinical innovation and discovery would be thwarted, and the "art" of medicine would be a subject discussed only by malpractice tribunals. Counterbalancing this concern are data that suggest that there is substantial diversity in how mental health practitioners diagnose psychiatric disorders (Sandifer et al. 1969; Schimel et al. 1973) as well as what they regard as the treatment of choice for any given psychiatric disorder (American Psychiatric Association 1982, 1984a, 1984b). Moreover, there is evidence that, in some instances, treatment recommendations may be influenced more by the socioeconomic status of the patient (Hollingshead and Redlich 1958) and the philosophical predilection of the treater than by a shared knowledge base (Katz et al. 1969).

Reliable outcome data are an essential first step in making treatment decisions that incorporate advances in our scientific understanding about the etiology and treatment of mental illness. It is important for clinicians to know which modalities are essential in the treatment of a given patient, which are useful adjuncts, and which are ineffective. Armed with these data, clinicians are in a better position to devise appropriate treatment regimens and negotiate their acceptance by both patients and insurers. In the absence of such data, it is increasingly difficult for all concerned to know what constitutes appropriate care and reasonable payment.

The Clinician's Role in Expanding Knowledge About Clinical Course and Long-Term Prognosis

❧Treatment outcome studies are informative, not only with respect to the efficacy of particular treatments, but also because they provide a mechanism for longitudinal follow-up of patients, many of whom have chronic relapsing illnesses. For example, as McGlashan has pointed out in this volume and elsewhere (1984, 1986a, 1986b, 1986c, 1991), treatment outcome studies unequivocally demonstrate that schizophrenia is a chronic and often disabling illness. Schizophrenic patients also have poorer outcomes than patients with schizo-affective disorder, major affective illness, or borderline personality disorder. Moreover, the illness is associated with significant comorbidity and mortality, partly because drug abuse, medical problems, and suicide are major problems in this patient population (McLellan et al. 1979; Tsuang and Woolson 1978; Tsuang et al. 1980a). As a result, male and female schizophrenics live, on average, 10 years less than nonschizophrenic controls (Tsuang et al. 1980b).

Outcome studies can also shed light on the long-term prognosis of mental disorders. For example, a number of longitudinal follow-up studies (Carpenter et al. 1987; Harding et al. 1987; McGlashan 1984) have demonstrated that schizophrenia does not invariably follow a progressive downhill course; many patients either stabilize or recover substantially from the initial manifestations of the illness. There is an extremely high rate of relapse and rehospitalization, particularly in the early phases of the disorder. But global adjustment tends to stabilize as patients learn to cope with their illness; compensate for difficulties in cognitive, interpersonal, and occupational functioning; and sustain themselves outside of a hospital setting.

Understanding more about the expected short- and long-term implications of receiving appropriate treatment, inappropriate treatment, or no treatment at all is also important in the clinician's role as consultant, advisor, and expert witness. Though it is clearly desirable that patients be active participants in determining the type of care they receive, some patients experience a level of impairment that, at least temporarily, precludes effective participation in treatment decisions. In such instances, families, guardians, and courts have generally stepped in to exercise decision-making authority; but in so doing, they rely heavily on the recommendations of care providers. This places an added responsibility on clinicians and institutions to use all available data, including treatment outcome data, in formulating treatment plans and recommendations, so as to effectively balance patient rights and the interests of families, institutions, and society.

Impediments to Collecting Useful Outcome Data

General Issues

Though outcome studies are clearly important to those who finance, provide, or consume mental health care, the collection of valid and reliable outcome data is a difficult and time-consuming task. Unlike laboratory experiments, outcome studies involve live patients with real problems. The patients' cooperation and participation must be solicited, most often by clinicians or institutions whose primary mission is delivering clinical care rather than carrying out research. Thus, outcome researchers must face a variety of daunting problems. These include recruiting adequate numbers of patients so that statistical analyses can be performed; accurately characterizing the patient population with respect to demographic and clinical characteristics; developing appropriate comparison groups; and exerting some control over the type, intensity, and duration of treatment that each patient subgroup receives. In addition, the frequency and duration of follow-up assessments must be appropriate for the questions being asked, and the reliability and validity of the assessment measures themselves must be demonstrated. Finally, there is the issue of treatment compliance and how treatment dropouts are to be handled, both clinically and experimentally.

Perhaps the biggest impediment to collecting useful outcome data is the complex nature of the mental health care delivery system itself. Mental health services are delivered in a wide variety of inpatient and outpatient settings. Moreover, even within the same institution, there may be diversity, overlap, and fragmentation among the different types of services provided, making it difficult to determine the actual amounts and types of care received by a given patient over time. In addition, the longer the time between treatment delivery and the measurement of treatment outcome, the more difficult it is to attribute outcome to the treatment(s) rendered.

The complexity and cost of outcome research limit its scope, in many cases, to single institutions. As a result, we are sometimes left wondering whether a different treater or treatment setting would have resulted in a different treatment outcome in the patients studied. Gathering outcome data at multiple sites helps to minimize sample bias and increase the generalizability of results. But institutional diversity, demographic differences in patient populations, and a host of other possible confounds dictate that study sites be carefully chosen for comparability and that treatment protocols be carefully monitored. Nationally aggregated data from many large and diverse sites is yet another approach to this problem; however, this too presents imposing methodologic problems.

Yet another barrier to conducting outcome research derives from the stigma attached to mental illness and the consequent need to maintain patient confidentiality. Unfortunately, our need to safeguard confidentiality also constitutes a major barrier to data collection efforts—ultimately to the detriment of the patients themselves. More recently, however, the proliferation of institutional review boards, the development of better procedures for enrolling subjects in research studies and obtaining informed consent (Lind 1990), and the use of improved techniques to ensure confidentiality of both patient records and research data have done much to facilitate this and other kinds of clinical research (American Psychiatric Association 1987; Meisel et al. 1977; Musto 1977).

Methodologic Issues

Patient-Related Variables

In general, outcome studies have focused on specific patient populations receiving treatment in a clinical setting (i.e., a hospital or clinic). Such studies frequently require large numbers of subjects so that statistical analysis can be used to determine whether cross-group differences in short-, intermediate-, or long-term outcome are truly significant or simply due to chance. As a result, outcome researchers do not often randomize patients into well-defined, well-controlled treatment modalities. They prefer instead to rely on studying large numbers of patients with a variety of statistical techniques to control for the effects of multiple intervening variables (e.g., life stress, medical illness) (Epstein 1990; Greenfield 1989).

Theoretically, outcome studies will enable us to better understand the relationship between patient psychopathology and the efficacy of specific treatments. This in turn will allow us to move from dogmatic assertions about the clinical superiority of one treatment or another to a more scientific approach in which patients are triaged into the most appropriate treatment modalities. However, the validity of outcome data from so-called patient-treatment matching studies rests on the accurate characterization of patients as well as the treatments they receive (Coryell et al. 1987; Frances et al. 1984).

At present, the methodology for defining patient subgroups is evolving. The simplest and most common, but least useful, method is to use patient responses to symptom checklists, rating scales, or questionnaires. Clinical diagnoses derived solely from unstructured clinical interviews are subject to substantial bias, particularly when made by clinicians from various disciplines with different levels of training (Grove et al. 1981). The use of structured clinical interviews helps to reduce such bias, because the methods for arriving at specific diagnoses are well defined and there is a shared diagnostic nomenclature (Spitzer et al. 1978). Even so, if these methods are to be reliable, certain requirements must be met. These include the training of interviewers; frequent checks of interviewer consistency; and cross-validation of diagnostic interview data with data from other sources, including family members, treatment records, and laboratory tests, where appropriate (e.g., toxic screening to confirm active alcohol or drug use) (Andreasen et al. 1981).

Of course, relying on diagnosis alone to characterize patients can also be hazardous. Patients with identical diagnoses may be quite heterogeneous in many other respects. The experience with DRGs as a predictor of length of hospitalization also suggests that diagnosis, by itself, may be a poor predictor of treatment outcome (English et al. 1986; Namerow and Gibson 1988). Indeed, even in large-scale, multisite studies involving carefully diagnosed patients, factors such as severity and chronicity of illness, presence or absence of comorbid medical or psychiatric disorders, and degree of family involvement (and whether it is positive or negative) may profoundly influence treatment outcome, regardless of the treatment(s) administered (Avison and Speechley 1987; Falloon et al. 1987). Other variables that may affect treatment response include the availability of social supports, the patient's employment history and legal status, and the level of external life stress experienced during both active treatment and any subsequent follow-up interval (Beerman et al. 1988; Miklowitz et al. 1988). Obviously, these variables should be assessed and controlled for where possible.

Treatment-Related Variables

Some of the more important methodologic issues in outcome research are related to the treatment side of the patient-treatment equation. These include establishing appropriate comparison groups and controlling for the clinical and philosophical biases of treatment programs and the treaters themselves.

Establishing experimental and control groups. As stated previously, outcome studies may be tightly controlled, with randomization of carefully matched patients into different treatment subgroups; or they may be naturalistic, observing the effects of a given treatment on a wide range of patients with varying types of psychopathology. In the absence of clearly demonstrated superiority for a specific treatment modality (e.g., antipsychotic drugs in the treatment of acute schizophrenia), random assignment of well-matched control groups to different treatments may help us reach valid conclusions about their relative efficacy for a particular psychiatric disorder. But where the efficacy of a given treatment is established without question, ethical considerations dictate that it be available to all comparison groups and that other, presumably adjunctive, treatments be regarded as the independent variables to be measured.

However, there are instances where a baseline treatment has such a powerful effect on treatment outcome that it becomes difficult to discern the incremental positive effects (if any) of other treatments. For example, it may be difficult to demonstrate the usefulness of various psychosocial treatment modalities (e.g., individual psychotherapy, group therapy) in schizophrenics being treated with antipsychotic drugs, even though the treaters themselves believe this to be the case (Gaebel and Pietzcker 1987; McGlashan 1984, 1986a). In these instances, the task is to develop outcome measures that address not only the patients' clinical symptoms but also their ability to maintain relationships, comply with medication treatment, cope with stress, and experience an improved "quality of life" (Lohr 1988).

Another variation on this theme occurs in outcome studies where the most appropriate treatment is unknown but one or more treatments have possible (as opposed to proven) efficacy. In such a case, the methodologic and ethical issue is whether to compare a group of treated patients to a group of untreated controls (Beecher 1966). Some investigators have attempted to address this problem by comparing treated patients to prospective patients who are on a waiting list but receive no formal treatment. Apart from the ethical considerations of withholding treatment, it should also be noted that being on a waiting list is not necessarily "neutral" with respect to outcome. For example, alcoholics awaiting admission to an inpatient treatment program may stop drinking in anticipation of their hospitalization, because they would prefer to experience withdrawal in a setting in which they have more control over their abstinence symptoms—or resume alcohol use. Other alcoholics in the same circumstance may binge in anticipation of entering treatment (Adelman and Weiss 1989). In either case, comparisons of treated versus "untreated" groups of patients are more complicated than they initially appear (Malia 1988).

Assessing treatment biases of patients and staff. Within treatment programs themselves, it is often difficult to avoid selection bias for specific treatments unless assignment to treatment is completely random. Most treatment staff are unable to maintain a detached view about the differential efficacy of specific treatments for specific patients, even when there may not be any scientific evidence to support their views. This problem is compounded by the fact that, with the notable exception of double-blind, placebo controlled medication trials, most treatment outcome studies are conducted on patients who know what treatment they are receiving and who have feelings about that treatment's usefulness in their particular case. Patients also develop opinions about the individuals delivering the treatment and "vote with their feet" if and when they (or staff) conclude that the treatment offered is not what they want. Thus, in any treatment protocol there is both unplanned and planned patient-treatment matching, and patients for whom the match is less than comfortable tend to drop out of treatment.

The problems inherent in patients self-selecting their treatment (i.e., agreeing with their assignments or dropping out) are sometimes compounded by the biases of treatment staff. For example, to compare the outcome of short- versus long-term hospitalization for a particular type of patient across two or more treatment programs, differences in staff attitudes and philosophy with respect to what constitutes appropriate and reasonable treatment must be assessed. Thus, staff in a short-stay institution may believe that short-term treatment produces outcomes as good, if not better, than longer term treatment for comparable patients—independent of the reasons for the program being short-term (i.e., lack of coverage for longer term treatment). The staff's confidence in their treatment approach, and their expectation that patients will respond favorably, may have an important influence on the short- and possibly long-term outcome of their patients (Moller et al. 1987).

In treatment programs where the average length of stay is relatively long, there may be a subtle denigration of short-term treatment as having limited goals or not allowing sufficient time to explore the nuances of a patient's problem or involve significant others (e.g., family members) in the treatment. In such a program, short stays may be due to patient resistance to staying longer (usually equated by staff with lack of motivation for treatment) or simply a "bad fit" between patient goals and staff expectations. In either case, unless staff biases are taken into account and controlled for, comparing short-stay patients across two programs or short- versus long-stay patients within an individual program may yield misleading conclusions about the importance of treatment duration in shaping outcome.

Dealing with treatment dropouts. It follows from this discussion that understanding what happens to treatment dropouts is crucial in assessing the impact of a particular treatment on a specific patient population (Malia 1988). Failure to do so may lead to unwarranted generalizations about the ability of clinicians to decide what treatment a patient might benefit from, the optimal duration of that treatment, and the prognosis of those who fail to comply with it. It is also important that the frequency and duration of follow-up intervals be tailored to the population and treatment modality studied. For example, in order to study the response of homeless alcoholic men to a brief treatment intervention (e.g., alcohol detoxification), a researcher might choose to assess the major outcome variable (i.e., drinking behavior) on a daily basis. In contrast, alcoholic patients with a somewhat better prognosis, who have been receiving more substantive treatment over a longer period of time, would require less frequent follow-up (defined in months and years rather than days) with more attention to intermediate- and long-term outcome.

Finally, it should be self-evident (but sometimes is not) that all treatments to be compared must be carefully defined and delivered. For example, it is insufficient to state that a patient will receive hospital-based, milieu treatment without specifically describing the type of treatment received, its intensity and duration, and the level of expertise and commitment of those who provided it. In some hospitals, the milieu is characterized by numerous highly structured and some-times mandatory activities, both psychotherapeutic and rehabilitative; in other settings, the milieu is far less structured and less intense. Parenthetically, it is also erroneous to assume that more structured, intense treatment is necessarily better for all patients. There are certainly patients for whom an active milieu program and high levels of staff/patient or patient/patient contact are extremely useful (Paul and Lentz 1977). However, there are also patients for whom numer-ous ward activities and frequent interpersonal contacts might be extremely stressful and antitherapeutic.

Conclusions

The mental health care delivery system is at a crossroads. Issues relevant to cost containment, quality of care, and therapeutic goals need to be reconciled as treatment decisions are made. Health policy planners need outcome data to determine appropriate levels of reimbursement for clinical services and to estab-lish priorities for the allocation of scarce resources (e.g., money or expensive new treatments). The managed care industry needs outcome data to determine whether existing resources (e.g., hospitals) are being used appropriately and to assess the quality and cost-effectiveness of treatments delivered by both individ-ual and institutional providers. Third-party payers need outcome data to answer the question "What are we paying for?". As such data become more available, it is reasonable to expect that these payers will take steps to differentially reim-burse health care providers based on the answers. Mental health clinicians need reliable outcome data to ensure rational decision making when assigning pa-tients to particular treatment modalities and to understand more about the rela-tionship of treatment to clinical course and prognosis.

At present, our field has made a tentative commitment to outcome research as part of a "good-faith" effort to help guide clinical practice toward the render-ing of appropriate care at a reasonable price. Unfortunately, unlike medical-sur-gical care, readily available "objective" measures (e.g., mortality rates) have relatively little applicability in assessing the outcome of mental health care. As a result, policy makers, third-party payers, and the patients themselves need to understand that measuring treatment efficacy requires a multidimensional per-spective encompassing a broad range of functional areas. Clinicians and re-searchers need to understand that research demonstrating the efficacy of mental health treatment is essential if patients, and those who care for them, are to be given the resources they so desperately need.

References

Adelman SA, Weiss RD: What is therapeutic about inpatient alcoholism treatment? Hosp Community Psychiatry 40(5):515–519, 1989

American Psychiatric Association Commission on Psychiatric Therapies: Psychotherapy Research: Methodological and Efficacy Issues. Washington, DC, American Psychiatric Association, 1982

American Psychiatric Association Commission on Psychiatric Therapies: The Psychiatric Therapies, Vol 1: Somatic Therapies. Washington, DC, American Psychiatric Association, 1984a

American Psychiatric Association Commission on Psychiatric Therapies: The Psychiatric Therapies, Vol 2: Psychosocial Therapies. Washington, DC, American Psychiatric Association, 1984b

American Psychiatric Association: Guidelines on confidentiality. Am J Psychiatry 144(11):1522–1526, 1987

Andreasen NC, Grove WM, Shapiro RW, et al: Reliability of lifetime diagnosis. Arch Gen Psychiatry 38:400–405, 1981

Avison WR, Speechley KN: The discharged psychiatric patient: a review of social, social-psychological, and psychiatric correlates of outcome. Am J Psychiatry 144(1):10–18, 1987

Beecher HK: Ethics and clinical research. N Engl J Med 274(24):1354–1360, 1966

Beerman KA, Smith MM, Hall RL: Predictors of recidivism in DUIIs. J Stud Alcohol 49(5):443–449, 1988

Bracken BW, Fox PD, Anderson SL: Psychiatric managed care: a challenge for private psychiatric hospitals. Submitted to The National Association of Private Psychiatric Hospitals. Washington, DC, by Lewin/ICF, A Health & Sciences International Company, 1990

Carpenter WT, Strauss JS, Pulver AE, et al: The prediction of outcome in schizophrenia: IV. Eleven-year follow-up of the Washington IPSS cohort. J Nerv Ment Dis (in press)

Coryell W, Grove W, Vaneerdewegh M, et al: Outcome in RDC schizo-affective depression: the importance of diagnostic subtyping. J Affective Disord 12:47–56, 1987

Davis DI: Differences in the use of substance of abuse by psychiatric patients compared with medical and surgical patients. J Nerv Ment Dis 172:654–657, 1984

English JT, Sharfstein SS, Scherl DJ, et al: Diagnosis-related groups and general hospital psychiatry: the APA study. Am J Psychiatry 143:131–139, 1986

Epstein AM: The outcomes movement: will it get us where we want to go? N Engl J Med 323(4):266–269, 1990

Falloon IRH, McGill CW, Boyd JL, et al: Family management in the prevention of morbidity of schizophrenia: social outcome of a two-year longitudinal study. Psychol Med 17:59–66, 1987

Fischer D, Halikas J, Baker J, et al: Frequency and patterns of drug abuse in psychiatric patients. Dis Nerv Syst 36:550–553, 1975

Frances A, Clarkin JF, Perry S: Differential Therapeutics: A Guide to the Art and Science of Treatment Planning in Psychiatry. New York, Brunner/Mazel, 1984

Gaebel W, Pietzcker A: Prospective study of course of illness in schizophrenia: Part III.

Treatment and outcome. Schizophr Bull 13(2):307–316, 1987

Goldsmith MF: From mental hospitals to jails: the pendulum swings. JAMA 250(22):3017–3018, 1983

Greenfield S: The state of outcome research: are we on target? N Engl J Med 320:1142–1143, 1989

Grove WM, Andreasen NC, McDonald-Scott P, et al: Reliability studies of psychiatric diagnosis. Arch Gen Psychiatry 38:408–413, 1981

Harding CM, Brooks GW, Ashikaga T, et al: The Vermont longitudinal study of persons with severe mental illness: II. Long-term outcome of subjects who retrospectively met DSM-III criteria for schizophrenia. Am J Psychiatry 144:727–735, 1987

Hollingshead AB, Redlich FC: Social Class and Mental Illness. New York, John Wiley, 1958

Inglehard JK: Medicare begins prospective payment of hospitals. N Engl J Med 308:1428–1432, 1983

Katz MM, Cole JO, Lowery HA: Studies of the diagnostic process: the influence of symptom perception, past experience, and ethnic background on diagnostic decisions. Am J Psychiatry 125(7):937–946, 1969

Lind SE: Finder's fees for research subjects. N Engl J Med 323(3):192–195, 1990

Lohr KN: Outcome measurement: concepts and questions. Inquiry 25:37–50, 1988

Malia A: An outcome study comparing refusers and acceptors of treatment for alcoholism. Canadian Journal of Psychiatry 33(3):183–187, 1988

McGlashan TH: The Chestnut Lodge follow-up study: II. Long-term outcome of schizophrenia and the affective disorders. Arch Gen Psychiatry 41:586–601, 1984

McGlashan TH: The Chestnut Lodge follow-up study: III. Long-term outcome of borderline personalities. Arch Gen Psychiatry 43:20–30, 1986a

McGlashan TH: The prediction of outcome in chronic schizophrenia: IV. The Chestnut Lodge follow-up study. Arch Gen Psychiatry 43:167–176, 1986b

McGlashan TH: Predictors of shorter-, medium-, and longer-term outcome in schizophrenia. Am J Psychiatry 143:50–55, 1986c

McGlashan T: Selective review of recent North American long-term follow-up studies of schizophrenia, in Psychiatric Treatment: Advances in Outcome Research. Edited by Mirin SM, Gossett JT, Grob MC. Washington, DC, American Psychiatric Press, 1991, pp 61–105

McLellan AT, Woody GE, O'Brien CP: Development of psychiatric disorders in drug abusers. N Engl J Med 301:1310–1314, 1979

Meisel A, Roth LH, Lidz CW: Toward a model of the legal doctrine of informed consent. Am J Psychiatry 132(3):285–288, 1977

Miklowitz DJ, Goldstein MJ, Nuechterlein KH, et al: Family factors and the course of bipolar affective disorder. Arch Gen Psychiatry 45:225–231, 1988

Moller HJ, Schmid-Bode W, Cording-Tommel C, et al: Expectancy and outcome in prescriptive vs. exploratory psychotherapy. Br J Clin Psychol 26:59–60, 1987

Musto DF: Freedom of inquiry and subjects' rights: historical perspective. Am J Psychiatry 134(8):893–898, 1977

Namerow MJ, Gibson RW: Prospective payment for private psychiatric specialty hospitals: the National Association for Private Psychiatric Hospitals prospective payment study, in Prospective Payment and Psychiatric Care. Edited by Scherl DJ, English JT, Sharfstein SS. Washington, DC, American Psychiatric Association, 1988, pp 41–54

Paul GL, Lentz RF: Psychosocial treatment of chronic mental patients: milieu versus social learning programs. Cambridge, MA, Harvard University Press, 1977

Sandifer MG, Hordern A, Timbury GC, et al: Similarities and differences in patient evaluation by U.S. and U.K. psychiatrists. Am J Psychiatry 126(2):206–212, 1969

Schimel JL, Salzman L, Chodoff P, et al: Changing styles in psychiatric syndromes: a symposium. Am J Psychiatry 130(2):146–155, 1973

Schumacher DN, Namerow MJ, Parker B, et al: Prospective payment for psychiatry: feasibility and impact. N Engl J Med 315:1331–1336, 1986

Sharfstein SS: Reimbursement resistance to treatment and support for the long-term mental patient, in Barriers to Treating the Chronic Mentally Ill. San Francisco, Jossey-Bass, 1987, pp 75–85

Spitzer RL, Endicott J, Robins E: Research diagnostic criteria. Arch Gen Psychiatry 35:773–782, 1978

Tsuang MT, Woolson RF: Excess mortality in schizophrenia and affective disorders: do suicides and accidental deaths solely account for this excess? Arch Gen Psychiatry 35:1181–1185, 1978

Tsuang MT, Woolson RF, Fleming JA: Causes of death in schizophrenia and manic-depression. Br J Psychiatry 136:239–242, 1980a

Tsuang MT, Woolson RF, Fleming JA: Premature deaths in schizophrenia and affective disorders: an analysis of survival curves and variables affecting the shortened survival. Arch Gen Psychiatry 37:979–983, 1980b

2

Risk-Benefit Ratios
in Psychiatric Treatment

John M. Kane, M.D.

Increasingly in psychiatric health care, equations are being formulated to assess benefit and risk ratios. These equations help both practitioners and health care recipients to make more reasoned decisions regarding treatment recommendations.

To measure benefit and risk accurately, a variety of considerations must be reviewed. Benefits from treatment can accrue in numerous ways to individuals, to their families, and to society as a whole. Individuals may be relieved of personal suffering or may improve psychosocial or vocational adaptation; families may have a reduced emotional burden; and society may benefit through a reduction in socially dysfunctional behavior and secondary health care and other costs, and an increase in vocational productivity.

These few examples clearly suggest the complexity of assessing potential benefit. Various psychiatric illnesses, by their very nature, have features that make these assessments of benefits even more difficult. Some illnesses may not be static but may be associated with deterioration or spontaneous improvement over time. The extent to which such deterioration can be minimized or prevented (or improvement facilitated) represents potential treatment benefit, which at first blush may not be readily apparent. This is why it is important to have a perspective on long-term outcome, both with and without appropriate treatment.

There are numerous studies that demonstrate the need for a long-term perspective in assessing treatment outcome. Some treatments may have acute effects; others may provide full benefit only if administered over long periods of time (psychotherapy being a prime example). Interactive or additive effects between different treatment modalities may also occur over time.

Therefore, it is very important when discussing benefits of treatment with a patient to be clear not only about what type of illness (or illnesses) are present and what type(s) of treatment (or treatments) are being administered, but also what the goals are for a given time frame. This issue is frequently among the most confusing to consumers who are trying to assess potential benefits of treatment.

When documenting improvement over time in order to assess benefit, it is useful to have both subjective and objective measures. If possible, the latter should be provided by various members of the treatment team and by significant others in the patient's life. The patient and his or her family should have ongoing feedback as to progress (or lack of it) so that they can continue to evaluate risks and benefits of particular treatments.

Other chapters in this book focus on the potential benefits of treatments in a variety of conditions. It may be useful here to provide an overview of some potential risks in psychiatric treatment.

Cost

With increasing efforts by consumers and third-party payers to contain health care costs, the cost of treatment becomes a factor in assessing benefit and risk. Mental health care professionals should be prepared to discuss the potential cost of treatment based on their treatment plan; and if changes in the treatment plan have significant cost implications, the patient should be informed. At the same time, the treatment of mental illness is in many situations not covered adequately by third-party payers. In some cases, clinicians are unable to offer optimal treatment because of this limitation. Clearly, educational efforts and further research supporting the cost-effectiveness of such treatment should have the highest priority in the profession.

Confidentiality and Stigma

National advocacy groups, governmental agencies, and professional organizations are making considerable progress in overcoming the stigma associated with psychiatric illness. These groups are achieving results by increasing the knowledge base regarding the causes and the biologic factors contributing to the development of mental illness. A great deal of concern about real or perceived risk can surround the issue of confidentiality. Increasing attention is being given to providing legal protection from discrimination to people with mental disabilities, but much remains to be done.

Overutilization

Some critics of mental health care have suggested that treatment creates dependency needs and perpetuates itself, or that it becomes difficult for patients to know when to stop treatment or when to reduce the frequency or intensity of specific treatment modalities. Unlike with surgery or the treatment of infectious disease, the end point in the treatment of mental illness is often not clear-cut. In some cases, improvement can be viewed on a continuum, whereas in others it may be focused on a particular symptom or symptom pattern. It is the responsibility of the clinician to establish and continually reevaluate goals and objectives in treatment, and the patient should be informed of these assessments. Transference issues and unrealistic expectations of the therapist are important foci of treatment, and the good therapist knows how to manage them.

No doubt there are therapists who are not conscientious or who maintain people in treatment to satisfy their own needs. (As in any field of endeavor, psychiatry as a whole should not be judged by the behavior of certain unethical or misguided individuals.) However, the risk of a patient's falling into the hands of such a person can be minimized. First, the patient should know the training and credentials of the person who is treating him or her. Second, the patient has a right to know the treatment plan and to have some estimate of the projected frequency, intensity, and length of treatment. Third, if the patient has concerns about how the treatment is going at some point, the clinician should be able to discuss this in a responsive fashion and should not be adverse to the patient's request for a consultation or second opinion.

Each of these issues applies equally to inpatient or outpatient treatment; but in the case of inpatients, another major question arises regarding the need for hospitalization. Just as some practitioners undoubtedly abuse their role, some psychiatric institutions may be guilty of such practices. Although third-party payers attempt to apply checks and balances to minimize this risk, frequently they are not in a position to review thoughtfully or accurately the indications or contraindications for hospitalization. In addition, in some cases, premature discharge compromises the gains made in the hospital. It is also true that with attempts to reduce reimbursement costs by decreasing the number and length of hospitalizations, the lack of parity between inpatient and outpatient treatment increases rather than decreases both patient's and provider's incentive to seek and provide inpatient treatment.

The patient and his or her family can reduce the risk of unnecessary hospitalizations by checking on the hospital and its reputation in the community; by asking for a clear rationale as to why inpatient treatment, rather than ambulatory care, is indicated; and by requesting some estimate of expected or typical length of stay for individuals with similar problems. It is also useful to ask about disposition following inpatient treatment, so that arrangements can be made as early as possible and length of stay is not increased unnecessarily. Additional questions relating to follow-up, aftercare, or outpatient treatment are particularly important. The emphasis should be on what strategies are most likely to maintain or further the gains made in the hospital, and what treatment plan is most likely to reduce the need for subsequent hospitalizations. It may also be useful to ask what the dropout rate has been in a particular clinic or aftercare program.

Misdiagnosis

A major criticism of mental health care has been the lack of reliability and validity of psychiatric diagnoses. In the last two decades, enormous progress has been made in the reliability and validity of the major diagnostic categories, when diagnoses are carefully made according to criteria in DSM-III-R (American Psychiatric Association 1987). Psychiatric diagnoses compare favorably with diagnoses in most medical specialties. Certainly, diagnosis is unclear in some situations. Even when diagnosis appears clear-cut, a continual process of reevaluation should take place; in many instances, a longitudinal approach is critical.

The risk of misdiagnosis can be minimized by having all available information, preferably from multiple sources. In some cases, information that should be provided to the clinician is lacking or misleading—for example, when covert substance abuse is contributing to a behavioral problem. Clinicians must be sensitive to such issues and ask sufficient questions to make a careful differential diagnosis. Here, too, the patient can reduce the risk of misdiagnosis by asking to be informed of the diagnosis and the basis on which it was made, and by requesting reevaluation if treatment progress is not being achieved in a reasonable amount of time.

Negative Treatment Outcome

The concept of negative treatment outcome has been used to describe a worsening in a condition that is brought about by the therapy itself. In some cases, it is difficult to distinguish a negative therapeutic effect from a deterioration associated with the illness process itself, but clearly each (or even both) are possibilities that should be considered when the patient's condition worsens. For example, it is well established that various forms of psychotherapy can increase an individual's symptoms or subjective distress, at least for some period of time. This may relate to increased awareness of previously denied or unconscious conflicts; increased recognition of painful experiences; or effects or aspects of the treatment process itself, such as deprivation, painful interpretations perceived as narcissistic injuries, and so on. Here also, the therapist's competence to achieve the desired goals is critical in minimizing the risk of transient negative effects that might result in a true negative outcome for the patient.

Most negative therapeutic outcomes are subtle. But other negative effects may be more serious, such as suicide attempts or psychotic reactions. The therapist's training, awareness, and sensitivity to the possibility of negative effects are essential in minimizing this risk.

Adverse Effects of Medication

In the case of psychotropic medications or somatic treatments in general, the possibility of adverse effects is always present. Some degree of adverse effect occurs in the majority of patients. Most such side effects are minor, but some untoward effects can be persistent or life threatening.

Anyone receiving such medication must be informed that risks are involved. Physicians must make judgments as to what side effects should be discussed with the patient, but it is not customary practice to discuss every side effect that has ever been reported as potentially associated with a particular drug. However, a side effect such as tardive dyskinesia occurs with significant frequency, and it can be of such severity as to warrant specific mention in a discussion of risk and benefit.

Adverse effects can have an important impact on treatment in various ways. First, if side effects are unpleasant or troublesome, noncompliance with the prescribed regimen can result. It is important for the clinician and the patient to talk candidly about adverse effects and their impact—for example, on such areas as sexual functioning, which may not be volunteered by the patient.

Some adverse effects may be manifested behaviorally and not immediately identified as due to medication. Examples include akathisia, which may appear to be increased anxiety and agitation; or akinesia, which may appear to be flat affect of psychomotor retardation. Clinicians must be constantly attuned to the possibility of behaviorally manifest adverse effects that may be subtle or even paradoxical (e.g., with benzodiazepines, increased anxiety or hostility).

Conclusions

In general, the benefits of appropriate psychiatric treatment far outweigh the risks, but this by no means implies that risks should be ignored or underestimated. The critical factors in reducing risks are appropriate training and accreditation of mental health professionals; appropriate education of patients (and their families, if indicated); and an ongoing process of treatment evaluation and dialogue between clinician and patient.

References

American Psychiatric Association: Diagnostic and Statistical Manual of Mental Disorders, 3rd Edition, Revised. Washington, DC, American Psychiatric Association, 1987

❖ **3** ❖ Outcome of Children
Treated in Psychiatric Hospitals

Ted P. Asay, Ph.D.
Thomas L. Dimperio, Ph.D.

Concern about the mental health needs of children has become one of the pressing issues facing our society in general and those involved in providing mental health services in particular. Recent epidemiologic data suggest that 15–19% of this country's approximately 63 million children and adolescents are in need of mental health treatment. Of this group, 3–8% suffer from serious emotional disturbances requiring intensive care, which may include hospitalization (Tuma 1989). At the same time, utilization data suggest that less than 1% of the nation's children receive mental health treatment in a hospital or residential treatment center in a given year, and only 5% are treated in outpatient settings (Taube and Barrett 1985). Thus, 70–80% of children who are in need of mental health services are not receiving appropriate care (Tuma 1989).

Although there is a clear need for psychiatric services for children, the appropriateness, clinical effectiveness, and cost efficiency of various treatment approaches have been seriously questioned. This has been especially true for hospital treatment of children, where the scrutiny from consumers, outside agencies, third-party payers, and, at times, mental health professionals has been particularly intense. In addition, there have been increasing demands for empirical documentation attesting to the effectiveness of hospital treatment.

The authors wish to acknowledge their appreciation to Mark J. Blotcky, M.D., Principal Investigator, Timberlawn Child Follow-Up Study, and Clinical Director, Timberlawn Psychiatric Hospital, Inc.; John T. Gossett, Ph.D., Consultant, Timberlawn Child Follow-Up Study, and Director, Timberlawn Psychiatric Research Foundation, Inc.; Kathy Shores-Wilson, Ph.D., Research Coordinator, Timberlawn Child Follow-Up Study, Timberlawn Psychiatric Research Foundation, Inc.; Alexandria H. Doyle, Ph.D., Clinical Psychologist, Child and Adolescent Service, Timberlawn Psychiatric Hospital, Inc., and Research Associate, Timberlawn Psychiatric Research Foundation, Inc.; Karen A. Sitterle, Ph.D., Clinical Psychologist, Timberlawn Psychiatric Hospital, Inc., and Research Associate, Timberlawn Psychiatric Research Foundation, Inc.; and Virginia Austin Phillips, Senior Research Associate, Timberlawn Psychiatric Research Foundation, Inc.

Fortunately, some clinicians have tried to empirically evaluate the effects of inpatient treatment on children. Even though not many reports have been published—primarily because of the time-consuming, expensive, and methodologically complex nature of follow-up investigations—the data generated thus far have shed important light on the question of treatment effectiveness. In addition, there appears to be an increasing interest among clinicians and researchers alike in conducting well-designed follow-up investigations of children treated in inpatient settings. These investigations are conducted to both demonstrate the effectiveness of treatment and to gather empirical data that can be used to improve existing treatment programs.

In this chapter, we will briefly review the findings of previously published follow-up studies; discuss relevant methodological issues; and present some preliminary findings from the Timberlawn Child Follow-Up Study, a long-term follow-up study of hospitalized children that is currently in progress.

Review of Previous Follow-Up Findings

The majority of studies of children treated in hospital or residential settings report improvement in patient functioning at follow-up. Although different measurement methods preclude exact comparisons between studies, improvement rates generally fall between 40% and 80% among heterogeneous samples. In their review of child follow-up studies, Blotcky and colleagues (1984) concluded that all follow-up studies reported some positive treatment outcomes. In patients who were described as primarily having personality disorders, more than 50% demonstrated positive long-term outcomes. Less than 50% of the psychotic or neurologically impaired patients were doing well at follow-up, but improvement occurred even among these patients.

Results of more recent follow-up studies also support the data attesting to the effectiveness of hospital treatment. For example, Berland and Safier (1988) conducted a follow-up study at 6 months and then at 1 year on 42 children and adolescents receiving inpatient treatment at the Children's Hospital of the Menninger Clinic. Subjects were diagnosed as having personality disorder, conduct disorder, or psychosis. Although the sample size of the study was admittedly small, the researchers reported that 29 subjects (69% of those receiving treatment) were functioning in the adaptive range at 6-month follow-up and 28 (67%) at 1-year follow-up, as measured on global ratings after telephone interviews with parents and patients.

In another recent investigation, Ney et al. (1988) obtained 1-year follow-up data on 112 children who received 5 weeks of intensive inpatient treatment and

5 weeks of post-discharge follow-up contact. Most of the children carried a diagnosis of conduct disorder. Other diagnoses included encopresis, anorexia, major depression, autism, epilepsy, and fire-setting; some children had been subjected to various types of child abuse and neglect. Follow-up questionnaires were administered to patients, parents, and teachers. The follow-up results indicated that 84% of parents felt the program was helpful, 8% felt it made no difference, and 4% felt it made their child's problem worse. All of the children were found to be significantly improved on the five parameters of the Patterson-Quay Behavior Problems Checklist (Quay et al. 1966): conduct, personality, immaturity, delinquency, and psychosis.

In a follow-up study of 42 children, 37 (88%) of whom were diagnosed as psychotic or borderline, Koret (1980) reported 25 (60%) to be functioning in the fair to excellent category 6 months to 6 years post-discharge. Patients were rated by parents along dimensions of education or employment adjustment, community adjustment, and family adjustment. In another well-designed study, Kazdin and Bass (1988) reported follow-up data from 140 children ages 5–13 who were suffering from acute disorders characterized by highly aggressive or disturbed behavior, suicidal or homicidal behavior, and family problems. Diagnoses included conduct disorder, depression, attention deficit disorder, anxiety disorder, and adjustment disorder. Patient functioning was measured at pretreatment, post-treatment, and follow-up by parents and teachers, using the Child Behavior Checklist (Achenbach and Edelbrock 1983) and the School Behavior Checklist (Miller 1977). Both parents and teachers rated the children as showing significant improvement in behavior problems and school adjustment at 1 year post-discharge.

In addition to global ratings of improvement, analyses of existing child follow-up studies have shown three groups of variables to be significantly related to the long-term adjustment of children treated in hospitals or residential treatment centers. These are patient variables (intelligence, organicity, diagnosis, and symptom patterns); family variables (parental psychopathology and family mental illness); and treatment variables (program completion and involvement in aftercare). An examination of research on patient variables suggests that patients who achieve better long-term functioning have less severe psychopathology at admission. Specifically, youngsters with less severe personality disorders fare better in adolescence and young adulthood than those who have more profound personality disorders, psychotic disorders, clear signs of neurologic dysfunction, and below-average intelligence (Berland and Safier 1988; Blotcky et al. 1984; Lawder and Nordan 1963; Parham et al. 1987). Children who exhibit antisocial or bizarre behavior also tend to have poorer outcomes (Davids and Salvatore 1976; Morris et al. 1956).

The level of family functioning has also been shown to have an important relationship to long-term post-hospital functioning. Patients returning to a competent family system typically demonstrate positive long-term adaptations. A history of mental illness in the family, severe parental psychopathology, family instability, and ongoing family conflict have been found to correlate with poor long-term functioning (Lawder and Nordan 1963; Levy 1969; Lewis et al. 1980; Stewart et al. 1978).

Treatment variables that have consistently shown a relationship to long-term outcome are completion of treatment goals and involvement in an appropriate aftercare program. In general, patients who remain in treatment for the recommended length of time are much more likely to accomplish important treatment goals and to attain positive treatment outcomes (Davids and Salvatore 1976). Patients who leave treatment early, particularly in the beginning phases, have been shown to have poor long-term adjustment (Levy 1969). The importance of patient involvement in aftercare programs in order to solidify treatment gains and avoid regressions in functioning has also been demonstrated (Doherty et al. 1987; Koret 1980).

Methodological Issues

Conducting meaningful follow-up research carries with it a substantial investment in time, human resources, and money. In addition, there are many methodological hurdles to overcome when attempting to assess complex personality and behavioral variables over a significant period of time in a uniform or standardized fashion. As a result, relatively few follow-up studies on children have been carried out, and the results of those studies that have been conducted are sometimes compromised by methodological problems. Among the most common methodological difficulties are lack of appropriate comparison groups, patient attrition, inadequate measurement methods, and poorly conceived research designs. Several researchers have discussed the methodological problems encountered in this type of research, and strategies for dealing with them (Blotcky et al. 1984; Gossett et al. 1983; Pfeiffer 1989).

Despite methodological obstacles, meaningful follow-up studies have been carried out, and others are currently in progress. Those that will ultimately provide the most useful information on long-term functioning of children will be prospective, longitudinal studies for which data are collected on a range of predictor and outcome variables at admission, during treatment, at discharge, and at follow-up. Measurement instruments that are reliable, valid, clinically meaningful, and completed by more than one source yield more generalizable and useful results.

Patient attrition, a problem that plagues follow-up research, must be minimized to prevent undue bias in the research results. The use of control groups has not been possible because of ethical constraints prohibiting the withholding or modification of treatment. However, comparison subgroups could be used that might be defined by variables such as age, gender, or diagnosis.

Preliminary Results From the Timberlawn Child Follow-up Study

The Timberlawn Child Follow-Up Study, a prospective long-term follow-up project, has two primary goals: 1) to evaluate the long-term adjustment of children treated in a psychiatric hospital; and 2) to identify patient, family, and treatment variables that are predictive of treatment outcome (Dimperio et al. 1986).

The Riedel Children's Unit at Timberlawn Psychiatric Hospital, a 20-bed coed locked unit, utilizes a multidisciplinary, multimodal treatment model and includes a structured milieu; specialized education; individual, group, and family therapies; occupational and recreational therapies; and pharmacologic treatment. The treatment orientation emphasizes a psychodynamic-developmental model, although other methods (e.g., behavior therapy) are also utilized.

The basic research design is quasi-experimental/correlational and involves the collection of data at four points: admission to the hospital, discharge from the hospital, 1 year post-discharge, and 5 years post-discharge. Data are collected on individual, family, and treatment variables at each of these points. Nearly 200 children are currently in the study. The results presented here are from information collected on the first 40 subjects at 1-year follow-up.

The first cohort of subjects consisted of 15 girls and 25 boys who had a mean age at admission of 10.5 years. The average length of stay in the hospital was 500 days and ranged from 12 days to 3 years. Most of the children were diagnosed as having conduct disorder, attention deficit disorder, or various personality disorders, although some were also diagnosed as having psychotic or major affective disorders. Most children received multiple diagnoses, and nearly three-fourths of the sample had a primary DSM-III diagnosis on Axis II (personality disorders). Approximately 40% of the subjects were discharged with maximum hospital benefit, whereas 5% were transferred to other facilities and 5% were discharged against medical advice. About 50% were discharged before completion of recommended treatment, at the request of family or for financial or personal reasons. Of the 40 subjects followed, 35 (88%) could be located whose family members agreed to participate in the study.

Data related to demographic variables (age, gender, diagnosis, socioeconomic status) and some treatment variables (length of stay, discharge status, prognosis) were obtained from medical records and/or admission questionnaires. One-year follow-up data were obtained by mailing research instruments to the family for each patient's parents to complete. If the parents did not return the forms, the instruments were administered over the telephone and completed based on parental responses. The measures used to evaluate follow-up functioning were the Progress Evaluation Scale (PES) (Ihilevich and Gleser 1982) and the Timberlawn Child Follow-Up Rating Scale (TCFURS).

Preliminary results at 1-year follow-up reveal that parents rated the majority of children (77%) as improved in their overall functioning when compared to the year prior to admission. Of these, 68% were rated as "much improved" or "greatly improved." Looking at the specific areas of peer relations, family interactions, and school or job performance, most parents also rated their children as functioning in the adaptive range. Sixty percent of children were rated as able to get along with others most of the time and having few or only occasional conflicts with friends. The majority of subjects were also judged to be functioning well in school or at a job. Seventy-nine percent were attending school regularly and passing all subjects or were holding a regular job with little or no difficulty. Only three subjects (9%) continued to have significant difficulties in school or in holding a job. Parental ratings of family functioning indicated that 17 children (49%) were able to engage in cooperative family relationships and demonstrated an appropriate degree of independence. Fifty-five percent also were rated as manageable or easily managed at home.

There were also significant correlations between patient information variables at admission and parental ratings of functioning at 1-year follow-up. A clinically meaningful finding was that a patient's diagnosis was a powerful predictor of long-term functioning after treatment. Specifically, children who received a diagnosis of depression at admission had more adaptive family interactions at follow-up. In contrast, those who had a diagnosis of schizophrenia had the poorest family interactions 1 year post-discharge. Additionally, children having mixed or atypical personality disorders had more positive peer interactions after treatment. Children who had the most difficulties in school/job performance and in peer relationships carried a diagnosis of conduct disorder or passive-aggressive personality disorder.

The level of family functioning was also shown to be an important predictor of long-term adjustment. To examine this relationship, correlations were calculated between ratings of family functioning on the Beavers-Timberlawn Family Evaluation Scale (Lewis et al. 1976) and ratings of child functioning obtained from the PES and the TCFURS. In general, children who did better in school/job performance came from families with effective parental leadership, low rates of invasive interactions, empathic awareness and responsiveness to others' feelings, and few occurrences of openly displayed criticism or resentment in family interactions. In contrast, children who came from chaotic or rigidly controlled families—characterized by invasions of personal boundaries among family members, low levels of empathic communication, and frequent critical interactions—demonstrated poorer school/job adaptation.

In addition, children who functioned more adaptively within the home came from families with closeness along with clear interpersonal boundaries and effective problem-solving skills. In these families, members took responsibility for personal thoughts or actions, and family interactions were characterized by infrequent invasions of personal boundaries, receptiveness to others' perceptions, and low rates of critical interactions. Children who were in families that exhibited behaviors such as amorphous or indistinct personal boundaries; poor problem-solving skills; frequent invasive interactions; avoidance of individual responsibility; disregard for others' perceptions; and highly critical, intrusive, or emotionally overinvolved communication patterns had less adaptive functioning in the home at 1-year follow-up.

These findings provide meaningful information on the post-hospital functioning of children, which supports previous research findings demonstrating the effectiveness and utility of hospital treatment of children with severe emotional disorders. At a time when the appropriateness of hospital treatment for children is being seriously questioned in many quarters, this information is extremely useful to be able to present to funding bodies, insurance carriers, mental health professionals, and consumers—all of whom have an important role in decisions that will ultimately determine how mental health care will be provided in the future.

The results of this study also yield important information concerning variables that predict functioning—both positive and negative—in specific areas associated with long-term adjustment. This information can be very useful in making decisions geared toward implementing more effective, individually tailored treatment programs. For example, we know that children with conduct disorders or passive-aggressive personality disorders do poorly in peer relationships and in school functioning compared to other aspects of their lives. This information may provide the basis for a more focused treatment program where these problems could be addressed more intensively. Finally, this investigation also demonstrates the feasibility of using a prospective, longitudinal research design wherein multiple measures and multiple variables are used to assess the long-term post-hospital adjustment of children. Although this study is small and lacks a comparison group, the findings are of value clinically and administratively.

Conclusions and Recommendations

The organization and implementation of high-quality follow-up research on hospitalized children is a tedious and taxing endeavor. However, well-designed follow-up studies contribute significantly to what we know about the long-term adjustment of hospitalized children. Such studies also provide important information to help us improve existing treatment programs—programs that can ultimately lead to better long-term functioning of children in their home environments after discharge from the hospital.

Another benefit of follow-up research with children is that it can significantly improve the morale of the treatment staff, who see children at their most disruptive or regressed level of functioning. To learn that the improvement of these patients continues after they leave the hospital rewards the staff's exacting efforts.

The findings of follow-up studies conducted thus far clearly demonstrate that hospital treatment of children is effective. More specific questions can be explored in future studies. For example, a comparison of differing treatment approaches, such as inpatient treatment, partial hospitalization, residential treatment, and outpatient treatment, can provide a basis for answering the important and complex question of which treatment approaches work best with which children in which settings. Also, careful follow-up assessment of treatment approaches designed for children who generally show a poorer response to hospital treatment (i.e., children diagnosed as having psychotic, neurologically impaired, or profound personality disorders with antisocial features) would allow further innovation and refinement of the methods used to treat these difficult cases. Answering such research questions can improve the quality and cost-effectiveness of hospital care with this underserved population. We can also hope to slow the growing tide of skepticism concerning inpatient treatment.

References

Achenbach TM, Edelbrock CS: Manual for the Child Behavior Checklist and Revised Child Behavior Profile. Burlington, VT, University Associates in Psychiatry, 1983

American Psychiatric Association: Diagnostic and Statistical Manual of Mental Disorders, 3rd Edition. Washington, DC, American Psychiatric Association, 1980

Berland DI, Safier EJ: One-year follow-up report on long-term hospital treatment of children and adolescents. Bull Menninger Clin 52:145–149, 1988

Blotcky MJ, Dimperio TL, Gossett JT: Follow-up of children treated in psychiatric hospitals: a review of studies. Am J Psychiatry 141:1499–1507, 1984

Davids A, Salvatore P: Residential treatment of disturbed children and adequacy of their subsequent adjustment: a follow-up study. Am J Orthopsychiatry 46:63–73, 1976

Dimperio TL, Blotcky MJ, Gossett JT, et al: The Timberlawn Child Functioning Scale: a preliminary report on reliability and validity. The Psychiatric Hospital 17:115–120, 1986

Doherty MB, Manderson M, Carter-Ake L: Time-limited psychiatric hospitalization of children: a model and 3-year outcome. Hosp Community Psychiatry 38:643–647, 1987

Gossett JT, Lewis JM, Barnhart F: To Find a Way: The Outcome of Hospital Treatment of Disturbed Adolescents. New York, Brunner/Mazel, 1983

Ihilevich D, Gleser GC: Evaluating Mental Health Programs: Progress Evaluation Scales. Lexington, MA, Lexington Books, 1982

Kazdin AE, Bass D: Parent, teacher, and hospital staff evaluations of severely disturbed children. Am J Orthopsychiatry 58:512–523, 1988

Koret S: Follow-up study on residential treatment of children ages 6 through 12. Journal of the National Association of Private Psychiatric Hospitals 11:43–47, 1980

Lawder D, Nordan R: What Have We Learned! A Report of the First 10 Years of the Astor Home: A Residential Treatment Center for Emotionally Disturbed Children. New York, Chartmakers, 1963, pp 38–52

Levy EZ: Long-term follow-up of former inpatients at the Children's Hospital of the Menninger Clinic. Am J Psychiatry 125:1633–1639, 1969

Lewis JM, Beavers WR, Gossett JT, et al: No Single Thread: Psychological Health in Family Systems. New York, Brunner/Mazel, 1976

Lewis M, Lewis DO, Shanok SS, et al: The undoing of residential treatment: follow-up study of 51 adolescents. J Am Acad Child Psychiatry 19:160–171, 1980

Miller LC: School Behavior Checklist Manual. Los Angeles, CA, Western Psychological Services, 1977

Morris HH Jr, Escoll PJ, Wexler R: Aggressive behavior disorders of childhood: A follow-up study. Am J Psychiatry 112:991–997, 1956

Ney PG, Adam RR, Hanton BR, et al: The effectiveness of a child psychiatric unit: a follow-up study. Can J Psychiatry 33:793–799, 1988

Parham C, Reid S, Hamer RM: A long-range follow-up study of former inpatients at a children's psychiatric hospital. Child Psychiatry Hum Dev 17:199–209, 1987

Pfeiffer SI: Follow-up of children and adolescents treated in psychiatric facilities: a methodology review. The Psychiatric Hospital 20:15–20, 1989

Quay HC, Sprague RL, Shulman HS, et al: Some correlates of personality disorders and conduct disorders in a child guidance clinic. Sample Psychology in the Schools 3:44–47, 1966

Stewart NA, Adams CC, Meardon J: Undersocialized aggressive boys: a follow-up study. J Clin Psychiatry 39:797–799, 1978

Taube CA, Barrett SA (eds): Mental Health, United States, 1985 (DHHS Publ No ADM-85-1378). Washington, DC, U.S. Government Printing Office, 1985

Tuma JM: Mental health services for children: the state of the art. Am Psychol 44:188–199, 1989

❖ 4 ❖ Long-Term Treatment of the Young Adult Chronic Patient: Effect on Social Functioning and Coping

Carol L. M. Caton, Ph.D.
Alexander Gralnick, M.D.

The Young Adult Chronic Patient

Mentally ill young adults have never been strangers to the psychiatric hospital, because they suffer from disorders that reach their peak in adolescence and early adulthood. It is well documented that first episodes of schizophrenia occur during this age span (Babigian 1985). Recent epidemiologic data indicate that anxiety disorders, major depression, and alcohol and drug abuse commonly begin in the 15–30 age period (Christie et al. 1988). In the past two decades, larger numbers of young adult patients have come to the attention of mental health professionals, as the post–World War II baby-boom generation has come of age (Bachrach 1982; Kramer 1977).

Significant changes in mental health policies governing the use of the psychiatric hospital have had important implications both for the patients in this age group and for mental health providers as well. Deinstitutionalization of patients in public mental health services in the United States has created an "uninstitutionalized generation" (Bachrach 1982; Pepper et al. 1981) of patients who suffer from serious disorders that become chronic and debilitating. Nonetheless, these patients spend little time, if any, within institutional walls. Typically, such patients experience a series of brief hospital stays followed by aftercare in place of long-term hospitalization. Clinicians have found that many of these patients are resistant to treatment and use mental health services only in a crisis or on a sporadic basis. Denial of illness abounds, as patients struggle to keep up with their nonpatient peers. Significantly, unlike their institutionalized predecessors, today's young chronic psychiatric patients have an excessively high prevalence of drug and alcohol abuse (Bender 1986; Caton et al. 1989; Holcomb and Ahr 1986; Schwartz and Goldfinger 1981).

The special needs of these patients have prompted clinicians to develop innovative programs targeted for them (Harris and Bergman 1987; Neffinger 1987; Pepper and Ryglewicz 1984). In other instances, patients in this age group are being treated with eclectic approaches in widespread use in established inpatient and outpatient programs. We believe that all such efforts should be carefully studied and evaluated, so as to identify program components of greatest value for the treatment of these patients. To address this need, we have focused our chapter on long-term inpatient treatment, particularly as it affects social functioning and coping skills.

There are, of course, many aspects of a person's life that could be influenced by a specific treatment, such as symptom level, functional status, work performance, or need for subsequent psychiatric care (Strauss and Carpenter 1972). Although treatment evaluation studies should probe multiple dimensions of outcome, the maintenance of social functioning and coping skills is particularly important for those suffering from serious mental illness. Social deficits, such as the inability to work effectively or to relate to others in a satisfying way, and inadequate self-care and community survival skills are the markers of chronicity. The prevention and treatment of such deficits have become as important as the identification of positive symptoms.

Moreover, young adults are struggling with the developmental challenges of becoming independent from parents, forming meaningful ties with peers, and pursuing educational and career goals. A focus on these issues can be a touchstone for reaching those reluctant to assume a patient-role identity. A recently completed study contrasting the social functioning of young chronic patients (age range 18–35) with that of older chronic patients (age range 36–84) revealed that, although both groups experienced social withdrawal, the younger group was more likely to be gainfully employed (Dozier and Franklin 1988). Indeed, maintenance of some measure of occupational functioning with the chronically mentally ill is not only good for morale but can offset the cost of disability (Weisbrod et al. 1980).

Deinstitutionalization and the Private Hospital

The deinstitutionalization era has left the public hospital with short-term wards as the locus for active treatment and long-term back wards for those in need of custodial care. Treatment goals are limited to symptom remission achieved with state-of-the-art psychopharmacological therapy. Long-term rehabilitation has been delegated to outpatient programs. Despite the funding and policy mandates that have constrained public institutions, private psychiatric hospitals have continued to provide long-term active treatment, enabling the pursuit of treatment goals that reach beyond symptom remission to include improved coping skills.

Deinstitutionalization may have had a limited direct impact on the private system, but demographic changes in private hospitals have proven significant. Our own investigation of 2,041 admissions to a long-term private psychiatric hospital over a 25-year period from 1962 to 1986 revealed that the most important shift in patient characteristics was a decline in the average age (Caton and Gralnick 1989). In 1962, the mean age of patients admitted to the hospital was 38 years. By 1986, the mean age had dropped to 25 years. Others have reported an increase in seriously disturbed young people in need of psychiatric care (Blotcky and Gossett 1989). Associated with the decline in age was an increase in the number of patients who were students (from about one-quarter in 1962 to one-half in 1986) rather than workers or homemakers, and who had not yet married (in 1962, only one-quarter of admitted patients were single, compared to three-quarters in 1986). Indeed, by the early 1980s, the hospital's atmosphere was dominated by the youth of its patient population. Diagnostic profiles revealed that concurrent drug or alcohol abuse were insignificant problems among patients admitted in the early 1960s. However, such problems were apparent in one out of three admitted in the 1980s. Cocaine, alcohol, marijuana, and poly-drug use were the most common problems reported.

Length-of-Stay Studies

The trend toward briefer hospital stays has been supported by studies of the effects of different lengths of stay on subsequent hospital use and post-hospital adjustment. Findings from these studies tend to support the practice of shortened hospital stay, particularly for chronic patients with adequate family support (Caton 1984). However, they also underscore the need for further study and evaluation of the effects of length of hospital stay on different subgroups of patients.

Even in well controlled studies, questions are raised by methods and findings. For example, studies employing random assignment of different length-of-stay groups have somewhat arbitrary definitions of "short" and "long" hospital stay. "Short" hospital stay has ranged from an average of 11 days in the studies of Herz et al. (1979) and Kennedy and Hird (1980) to 89 days in the study of Mattes et al. (1977; see Table 4–1). "Long" hospital stay has ranged from an average of about 24 days (Kennedy and Hird 1980) to 179 days (Mattes et al. 1977). Indeed, a hospital stay of 22–29 days was defined as short in three studies (Caffey et al. 1971; Glick et al. 1975; Hirsch et al. 1979) and long in two (Hirsch et al. 1979; Kennedy and Hird 1980).

Further, most studies have focused on mixed diagnostic groups (affective disorders, alcoholism, neuroses, schizophrenia), but two analyses concern only

TABLE 4–1. A summary of controlled studies of length of hospital stay

Investigator	Length of stay (days) Long	Short	Sample size	Diagnosis	Sex	Aftercare	Outcome Rehospitalization	Role function
Caffey et al. 1971	83	29	201	Schizophrenia	All males	All referred; 2 of 3 groups had Rx with inpatient staff	No difference	No difference
Glick et al. 1975 Hargreaves et al. 1977[1]	90–120	21–28	260	Mixed	Mixed	Individualized	Non-schizophrenia: No difference Schizophrenia: No difference	Non-schizophrenia: No difference Schizophrenia: good prehospitalization; function did better with LT
Herz et al. 1979	60	11	175	Mixed	Mixed	3 groups: 1) Long plus aftercare 2) Short plus aftercare 3) Short plus day	No difference	Long-stay patients had worse role/work functioning
Mattes et al. 1977	Unlimited $\overline{X}=179$	90 or less $\overline{X}=89$	173	Mixed	Mixed	Individualized	No difference	No difference
Hirsch et al. 1979	$\overline{X}=28$ Median = 17	$\overline{X}=22$ Median = 17	127	Mixed	Mixed	Individualized	No difference	No difference
Kennedy and Hird 1980	$\overline{X}=24.1$	$\overline{X}=10.8$	247	Mixed	Mixed	Individualized	Higher in short-stay groups	No difference

Source. Caton et al. 1990, p. 26.
[1] Glick and colleagues (1975) and Hargreaves and colleagues (1977) reported on the same set of data.

schizophrenic subjects (Caffey et al. 1971; Hargreaves et al. 1977). Five of six controlled studies reviewed (see Table 4–1) found no differences in rates of rehospitalization. However, Kennedy and Hird (1980) reported that short-stay (mean 10.8 days) patients in their study had a higher rate of rehospitalization than long-stay (mean 24.1 days) patients, but long-stay patients had longer durations of stay for readmission episodes.

There were no differences in role functioning in four of six studies reviewed (see Table 4–1). It is notable that Herz et al. (1979) found that their long-stay (60 days) patients had more impaired role and work functioning than short-stay (11 days) patients. Whereas Glick et al. (1975) found no differences in role functioning for nonschizophrenic patients, they noted that schizophrenics with histories of good prehospital functioning in the long-term (90–120 days) hospitalization group had better post-hospitalization role functioning than short-stay (21–28 days) patients. Thus, it appears that although a briefer hospitalization offers no marked advantage in terms of rehospitalization or role functioning, it is no worse for some patients. This overall conclusion, coupled with its economic cost advantage, has led to the widespread dissemination of brief hospitalization policies (Caton 1982; Caton and Gralnick 1987; Maxmen 1984). Yet there is mounting concern that the studies described above do not really justify their claims for patients generally, nor do they warrant disposing of long-term programs (Kleespies 1986).

None of the controlled studies of length of stay has evaluated a hospital program in which duration of stay exceeded 6 months. This is especially significant. However, naturalistic studies of patients who have received active treatment for 6 months to 2 years on specialized long-stay units have provoked interest in the patients' outcome (Gralnick 1990; McGlashan 1984a, 1984b; Plakun et al. 1985).

Long-Term Inpatient Treatment

The private sector of care in the United States offers a wide range of options for program emphasis and length of stay. It is of interest, however, that the national average length of stay at participating NAPPH inpatient programs was 30.9 days (NAPPH 1988). Although relatively brief hospitalizations have become the norm, in some instances long-term programs have been maintained to serve patients for whom short-term hospitalization has failed. However, the continued existence of such programs is threatened.

Inpatient treatment, especially for those whose illnesses are compounded by concurrent substance abuse or personality disorder, is essential if these patients are to be "brought to productive adulthood" (Blotcky and Gossett 1989). However, it is important to pursue those unanswered questions concerning the effects of hospital treatment on patients with differing types of clinical problems (Caton and Gralnick 1987). In so doing, attempts should be made to explore the many aspects of inpatient care other than length of stay that have a bearing on outcome. A study by Lehman and associates (1982) provides evidence that many aspects of hospitalization, such as decision-making styles, can exert an important effect on the results of treatment. Ours is an attempt in such a direction.

The High Point Evaluation Program

In an effort to identify characteristics of patients who respond to long-term active hospital treatment and those who do not, a research program has been established at a small, private psychiatric hospital where such treatment is usually given. First, we will describe the treatment program at this hospital, and then we will present our research efforts focused on treatment outcome.

The Hospital Treatment Program

High Point Hospital is a 45-bed intermediate- to long-term facility. The majority of patients are admitted for at least 3 months, up to a period of 6 to 12 months or more. Including the Medical Director, the medical staff consists of seven full-time board-eligible or board-certified psychiatrists. There are two social workers, an activities director, and two recreation therapists. In addition, there are approximately 7 nurses and/or aides on during each of 3 shifts (a total of 21 staff in a 24-hour period) to provide care for patients.

Using Maxmen's (1984) classifications for types of unit-wide programs (crisis intervention units, therapeutic community, token economy unit, individualized eclecticism unit, or custodial care unit), it becomes apparent that the High Point Hospital Program does not specifically fall into one category but has elements of both a therapeutic community and an individualized eclecticism unit. According to Maxmen's criteria, the High Point program has some similarities to a traditional therapeutic community in that it attempts to employ the full therapeutic resources of the entire staff. Both professional and nonprofessional staff interact therapeutically with patients to help them learn socialization skills and social responsibility. The hospital program differs from a pure therapeutic community approach in that patients are seen several times a week in individual therapy and regard their therapists, not other patients, as their primary therapeutic resource. Patients do not have the responsibility of assigning privileges to other High Point patients, and they also do not have access to psychiatric information about others as they might in a true therapeutic community.

The High Point program also shares some concepts with the individualized eclecticism–type unit in that the clinical approach to patients is both biological and psychosocial. The use of medication is common. Treatment of patients is individualized according to their needs. However, this hospital differs from a traditional individualized eclecticism unit in that a specific structure and organized group program provide a framework for determining the treatment of individual patients.

The hospital treatment program has been designed to emphasize social functioning and awareness of social responsibility. The activities program is used to emphasize social relationships to patients. Skills needed for a particular activity are minimized, but their developmental aspects are highlighted. Thus, the social substance in the activity is emphasized rather than the particular type of activity or the patient's level of skill.

The treatment program is highly structured, consisting of three groups, each with its own goals and expected levels of patient functioning. Although each doctor treats his or her own caseload, treatment decisions for all patients are dependent on the team's approval. The treatment of the patients is monitored through interdisciplinary staff conferences held for approximately 8 hours per week. Therapists interact with the patients, including their own, in other activities besides psychotherapy (individual and group), thus enhancing a team approach and ensuring that no therapist treats a patient alone.

Group One patients are maintained on the locked unit. They are believed to be either at risk to themselves or others or to be unable to handle the stimulation of being off the unit. Nevertheless, these patients are encouraged to socialize as much as possible and to participate in the activities that are held on the unit. Patients are not permitted to remain isolated in their rooms. They are closely monitored by staff and are supervised in the skills of daily living as necessary. The time a patient spends in Group One is designed to be used as a holding period to help him or her work toward accepting more responsibility in order to function better later in Group Two and Group Three.

Group Two patients are able to go off the unit to the school building and to activities. They are expected to be more organized in their self care and are able to be motivated to be more active participants in the hospital program. These patients are at a level where they are becoming aware of social interactions and the role they play with their peers. The patients use the Group Two phase to increase their social skills and to work toward functioning more independently on the open unit.

Patients in Group Three live on the open unit. They participate in a variety of activities useful to the hospital society, such as serving in the dining room and functioning on the patient committees. Each committee has a psychiatrist and a nurse advisor, thus providing additional feedback about patients' functioning in the hospital system. The committee responsibilities include the following: publishing a monthly patient newspaper, planning entertainment for the whole patient population, organizing and maintaining the hospital library, helping the housekeeping staff keep the hospital clean, planting a garden, and helping with garden maintenance. The committee experience teaches patients skills they will be able to apply to their lives outside the hospital. Patients learn how to work effectively in a group, how to delegate responsibility when necessary, and how to contribute significantly to the routine operation of the hospital and the general welfare of other patients.

The Pilot Study

In a beginning effort to explore the efficacy of the High Point program, we conducted a follow-up of discharged patients. (The pilot study reported here, including Table 4–1 and the case summaries, is taken from Caton et al. 1990.) All 71 patients under 45 years of age who had experienced at least 6 months of continuous hospitalizations and were released from the hospital between 1981 and 1983 were potential subjects for our study. Those meeting our criteria for inclusion in the study were contacted initially by mail. A letter from the hospital director explained that a follow-up of patients treated at the hospital would assist in evaluating the efficacy of inpatient programming and assured expatients that their rights with regard to confidentiality would be respected. A follow-up questionnaire and stamped, self-addressed envelope were included for those who chose to respond by mail.

In fact, very few (only about 10%) returned the questionnaire by mail. The remainder were interviewed by telephone in order to obtain information to complete the questionnaires. Respondents were either the ex-patient or a family member. We were successful in getting information on 60 out of 71 possible candidates for the study (84.5%). Seven subjects could not be located, and four refused to participate in the study.

The Follow-up Questionnaire

The follow-up questionnaire, which takes less than 10 minutes to complete, elicits information on the ex-patient's current living arrangement, employment, schooling, or primary social role, source of financial support, psychiatric hospitalizations since discharge, and use of aftercare treatment services. Subjects were also asked to comment on how they feel now compared to how they felt when they were discharged from the hospital, and they were afforded an opportunity to comment on the strengths and weaknesses of the hospital program. Data on sociodemographic variables, illness and treatment history, admission symptoms, discharge DSM-III diagnosis, and course in hospital were obtained from the clinical case record.

Sample Characteristics

The age range of study subjects was 11 to 45 years, with a mean age of 19.1 years. The youth of the study subjects is further underscored by the fact that 83% were 21 years or younger when admitted to hospital. Sixty-three percent were male. All religious backgrounds were represented, and the majority of study subjects were Caucasian. Fifty-five percent ($n = 39$) of study subjects carried a diagnosis of schizophrenia, and 15% ($n = 11$) were diagnosed as schizoaffective. Eight percent ($n = 6$) were diagnosed as having dysthymic disorder and 8% ($n = 6$) as having major depressive disorder. The remainder carried diagnoses of attention deficit disorder ($n = 2$), borderline ($n = 1$), conduct disorder ($n = 1$), identity disorder ($n = 2$), adjustment reaction ($n = 2$), opioid dependency ($n = 1$), and eating disorder ($n = 1$).

Sixteen patients experienced their first hospitalization at the time of the index episode, 10 had one previous hospitalization, and the remaining 45 had multiple previous admissions, ranging from two to eight (mean 3.29).

Status at Follow-up

Of the 60 patients for whom follow-up data could be obtained, 10 (17%) were hospitalized at the time of follow-up. Five patients had been hospitalized continuously since discharge. However, the majority of patients ($n = 50$, 83%) were living in the community. Seventy-four percent of community resident patients were living in their own apartments or were residing with family or kin. Although some patients were living in halfway houses or residential schools, such living arrangements were not the mode. It is notable that 11 patients (18%) said they were self-supporting; however, almost half of the entire group ($n = 29$, 49%) were being supported by their families. One-third ($n = 20$) were receiving Supplemental Security Income payments. Nearly two-thirds of patients living in the community ($n = 32$, 64%) were in aftercare treatment, the remainder having terminated or dropped out. Approximately 45% ($n = 27$) had not been rehospitalized in the 1- to 3-year follow-up period. The rehospitalization rate of 55% is roughly equivalent to that found in controlled studies of brief hospitalization. Some researchers (Caffey et al. 1971; Glick et al. 1975; Herz et al. 1979) have reported 2-year rehospitalization rates of approximately 60%.

In exploring outcome, categories of outcome were derived based on overall level of functioning. Disregarding rehospitalization status, patients were evaluated as functioning well if they were engaged in competitive work or were pursuing educational goals and following through with prescribed aftercare treatment. Patients were deemed to be functioning poorly if they were isolated and unemployed (had no social role) or were full-time participants in a mental health or rehabilitation program. Using these criteria, nearly half (47%) were functioning well, being either employed or in school at the time of follow-up. Included are respondents who have been rehospitalized either once or multiple times but are currently functioning in age-appropriate roles. Considering the severity of the patient's problems at the time of admission to hospital, the relative success for nearly half of the patients studied is notable. Approximately 58% of good-outcome patients had experienced at least two previous hospitalizations, and 62% had a discharge diagnosis of schizophrenia or schizoaffective disorder. Thus, good outcomes occurred in patients whose prognosis, based on treatment history and diagnosis, might be considered guarded. The following case summaries (Caton et al. 1990) illustrate outcomes.

Case Summaries

Mr. M.   Mr. M. is a 22-year-old white single Protestant student admitted to the hospital at age 19 for approximately 14 months. Mr. M. began to exhibit psychiatric problems at age 8 following his parents' divorce. His school performance deteriorated markedly over the next several years, despite his having a Full Scale IQ of 144. The patient continued to act out and began abusing drugs and alcohol. He also demonstrated antisocial behavior such as breaking windows and slashing tires. Mr. M. was in outpatient treatment on and off since age 13 with little positive results. He dropped out of twelfth grade to join the Air Force but was rejected because of his psychiatric history. At that time, the patient also lost all contact with his father, whose whereabouts remain unknown. These events caused Mr. M. to become increasingly dysfunctional. He was admitted to a psychiatric unit in July 1981 and remained there until being transferred to High Point in December 1981.

The patient had difficulty adjusting to the hospital and was resistant to treatment for a long time. He was gradually able to verbalize his negative thoughts instead of acting on them. Mr. M. was able to receive his high school equivalency in the hospital and began taking college courses a few months before his discharge. His final diagnosis was paranoid schizophrenia, with depressive features.

Mr. M. appears to have done very well since being discharged in March 1983. He is currently a full-time college student and works part-time in a computer store. He has not been rehospitalized, and he feels that he is able to handle his responsibilities adequately.

Ms. L. Ms. L. is a 20-year-old white single Catholic unemployed female who was admitted to High Point Hospital at age 17 for 13 months. Ms. L. was allegedly functioning well until a year and a half before admission when she become involved with a heroin addict. She subsequently dropped out of school and began to prostitute herself to support her own heroin addiction. Her parents tried to get Ms. L. involved in drug rehabilitation programs, but she was resistant to treatment. The patient and her boyfriend were arrested after they held up a grocery store. The patient was put on probation as a youthful offender. Her behavior continued to deteriorate, and her parents arranged for her admission at High Point.

The patient was initially very angry at being hospitalized. She continued to be hostile and inappropriate for some time. Ms. L. manifested sociopathic behavior on the unit and was resistant to limit setting. She was depressed and negativistic for much of her hospitalization. Ms. L. gradually improved and became less depressed. She began attending Alcoholics Anonymous and Narcotics Anonymous meetings and stated she was motivated to stay drug free. Her final diagnosis was recurrent major depression, multiple drug dependence (opioids), and antisocial personality disorder.

Ms. L. was able to remain drug free after being discharged from the hospital. She was again arrested for prostitution and was remanded to a residential drug rehabilitation program, where she has been for the last 9 months.

Ms. E. Ms. E. is a 19-year-old white Protestant female student who was admitted to High Point Hospital at age 16 for 18 months. The patient began exhibiting psychiatric problems at age 12. She had been found to be dyslexic in the second grade. She began to be increasingly anxious and unable to concentrate. At age 13, Ms. E. began outpatient therapy after she manifested self-destructive behavior. She showed no improvement. At age 15, the patient became extremely depressed and had loss of appetite, command suicidal hallucinations, temper tantrums, and episodes of self-mutilation. She became aggressive with family members and attempted to suffocate her younger sister. The patient was hospitalized at that time for 3 months. She continued to show self-mutilation after discharge and was seen as an outpatient for several months, while her behavior continued to deteriorate. Hospitalization at High Point was then arranged.

The patient had a difficult adjustment to her hospitalization and remained psychotic for several months. She often refused to eat or would force herself to vomit. Ms. E. began to improve after about 7 months. She was able to gain insight into her problems and could concentrate on academics more than before. Her eating patterns also stabilized to a large extent, and she was noticeably less depressed. Her diagnosis at time of discharge was schizoaffective disorder.

Ms. E. went directly to a residential school after her discharge from High

Point. She has been doing well academically there and has not been rehospitalized. She continues in outpatient therapy at the residential school. She feels that she is able to cope with her problems and responsibilities most of the time.

The Prospective Study

Findings from the pilot study reported previously are provocative. Many of the patients we studied were suffering from major functional disorders and had histories of previous psychiatric hospitalizations. Considering the severity of their illnesses and their multiple deficits, the relatively good social adjustment outcome for half the patients studied is notable. Various investigators have observed that psychotherapeutic interventions require considerably more time to take effect than physical modes of treatment, but such interventions can positively influence the fate of even the most seriously disturbed patients (Hogarty et al. 1974).

The research to date indicates that more work is needed to further specify the clinical and social characteristics of patients who respond best to long-term active inpatient treatment (Hargreaves et al. 1977). Toward this end, we are currently conducting a longitudinal prospective study of patients in our treatment system—an approach that will yield more systematic data on the hospital treatment experience. In the prospective study, all adolescent and young adult patients admitted from October 1985 to April 1989 are being studied. Within one or two weeks after admission, patients were given the Schedule for Affective Disorders and Schizophrenia (SADS) (Endicott and Spitzer 1978), a research diagnostic interview administered by a trained rater. The interview yields current and lifetime psychiatric diagnoses, including drug and alcohol abuse, with ages of onset. Family, social, and illness history data were obtained from clinical notes and through interviews with the subjects themselves. A community follow-up of this cohort is planned for 1990–1991.

In a preliminary analysis, we explored the prevalence of substance abuse in 100 consecutive admissions to the Prospective Study. Data from the diagnostic research interviews revealed that half had concurrent diagnoses of psychiatric disorder and substance abuse (Caton et al. 1989). One-third of the dual diagnosis patients began using substances before the onset of diagnosable psychiatric disorder. Polydrug abuse was common. In our research agenda for a community follow-up of the larger cohort, we will carefully evaluate the status of both psychiatric and substance abuse problems and their relationship to social functioning and coping skills.

Conclusions

Long-term hospital treatment does assist seriously ill young people in making the best use of their personal resources. The potential value of this intervention demands that a systematic knowledge base be created to facilitate its optimal use by those who can most benefit from it. It is our view that the private psychiatric hospital can contribute significantly to this effort.

For those interested in treatment evaluation studies, we want to emphasize that our research procedure was set up so as not to interfere with the clinical functions of the hospital. Data were collected by a specially trained research staff using standardized approaches when possible, to guarantee objectivity. Clinicians were not burdened with additional paperwork but were able to share relevant information with the research staff when necessary. Collaboration among researchers and clinicians can facilitate the provision of comprehensive descriptions of treatment programs. This is done by quantifying treatment variables when possible (number of sessions, hours of treatment, days of hospitalization, etc.) to help in interpretation of results and generalizability of findings.

We are aware that the naturalistic study design implemented in our setting lacks random assignment to treatment and a control group. Despite this methodologic handicap, we will be able to compare and contrast a patient's life situation in before- and after-treatment phases, explore differences in patient subgroups, and monitor the natural history of psychiatric disorder. It is our contention that the inability to conduct a controlled trial should not be a deterrent to getting involved in outcome research. We encourage our colleagues in long-term treatment settings to contribute to a greater pool of information on treatment efficacy and outcome.

References

Babigian HM: Schizophrenia: Epidemiology, in Comprehensive Textbook of Psychiatry, Vol IV. Edited by Kaplan HI, Sadock BJ. Baltimore, Williams and Wilkins, 1985, p 644

Bachrach LL: Young adult chronic patients: an analytical review of the literature. Hosp and Community Psychiatry 33:189–197, 1982

Bender MG: Young adult chronic patients: visibility and style of interaction in treatment. Hosp Community Psychiatry 37:265–268, 1986

Blotcky MJ, Gossett JT: Psychiatric inpatient treatment for adolescents. The Psychiatric Hospital 20:85–93, 1989

Caffey EM, Galbrecht CR, Klett CJ: Brief hospitalization and aftercare in the treatment of schizophrenia. Arch Gen Psychiatry 24:81, 1971

Caton CLM: Effect of length of inpatient treatment for chronic schizophrenia. Am J Psychiatry 139:856, 1982

Caton CLM: Length of hospitalization, in The Chronic Mental Patient: Five Years Later. Edited by Talbot JA. New York, Grune & Stratton, 1984, pp 159–164

Caton CLM, Gralnick A: A review of issues surrounding length of psychiatric hospitalization. Hosp Community Psychiatry 38:858–863, 1987

Caton CLM, Gralnick A: The changing role of the long-term private hospital. Paper presented at the annual meeting of the American Society for Adolescent Psychiatry, San Francisco, CA, May 1989

Caton CLM, Gralnick A, Bender S, et al: Young chronic patients and substance abuse. Hosp Community Psychiatry 40:1037–1040, 1989

Caton CLM, Mayers L, Gralnick A: The long-term hospital treatment of the young chronic patient: follow-up findings. The Psychiatric Hospital 21:25–30, 1990

Christie KA, Burke JD, Regier DA, et al: Epidemiologic evidence of early onset of mental disorders and higher risk of drug abuse in young adults. Am J Psychiatry 145:971–975, 1988

Dozier M, Franklin JL: Social disability in the young adult mentally ill. Am J Orthopsychiatry 58:613–617, 1988

Endicott J, Spitzer RL: A diagnostic interview: the schedule of affective disorders and schizophrenia. Arch Gen Psychiatry 35:837–844, 1978

Glick ID, Hargreaves WA, Raskin M, et al: Short versus long hospitalization: a prospective controlled study. II: Results for schizophrenic patients. Am J Psychiatry 132:385, 1975

Gralnick A: Observations on In-hospital Psychiatric Treatment. Port Chester, NY, High Point Hospital (unpublished research), 1990

Hargreaves WA, Glick IA, Drues J, et al: Short vs. long hospitalization: a prospective controlled study. Arch Gen Psychiatry 34:305–311, 1977

Harris M, Bergman HC: Differential treatment planning for young adult chronic patients. Hosp Community Psychiatry 38:638–643, 1987

Herz MI, Endicott J, Gibbon M: Brief hospitalization: two year follow-up. Arch Gen Psychiatry 36:701, 1979

Hirsch SR, Platt S, Knight A, et al: Shortening hospital stay for psychiatric care: Effect on patients and their families. British Medical Journal 1:442–446, 1979

Hogarty GE, Goldberg SC, Schooler NR, et al: Drugs and sociotherapy in the aftercare of schizophrenic patients. I: two year relapse rates. Arch Gen Psychiatry 31:603, 1974

Holcomb WR, Ahr PR: Clinicians' assessments of the service needs of young adult patients in public mental health care. Hosp Community Psychiatry 37:908–913, 1986

Kennedy P, Hird F: Description and evaluation of a short-stay admission ward. Br J Psychiatry 136:205–215, 1980

Kleespies PM: Hospital milieu treatment and optimal length of stay. Hosp Community Psychiatry 37:509–510, 1986

Kramer M: Psychiatric Services and the Changing Institutional Scene, 1950–1985. Rockville, MD, National Institute of Mental Health, 1977

Lehman AF, Strauss JS, Ritzler BA, et al: First admission psychiatric ward milieu. Arch Gen Psychiatry 39:1293–1298, 1982

Mattes JA, Rosen B, Klein DF: Comparison of the clinical effectiveness of "short" versus "long" stay psychiatric hospitalization. J Nerv Ment Dis 165:387–392, 1977

Maxmen JS: Hospital treatment, in Management of Chronic Schizophrenia. Edited by Caton C. New York, Oxford University Press, 1984, pp 55–74

McGlashan TH: The Chestnut Lodge follow-up study, I: follow-up methodology and study sample. Arch Gen Psychiatry 41:573–585, 1984a

McGlashan TH: The Chestnut Lodge follow-up study, II: long-term outcome of schizophrenia and the affective disorders. Arch Gen Psychiatry 41:586–601, 1984b

National Association of Private Psychiatric Hospitals: The Annual Survey, 1988. Washington, DC, National Association of Private Psychiatric Hospitals, 1988

Neffinger GG: The partial-hospital treatment of the young adult chronic patient. International Journal of Partial Hospitalization 4:117–125, 1987

Pepper B, Kirschner MC, Ryglewicz H: The young adult chronic patient: overview of a population. Hosp Community Psychiatry 32:463–469, 1981

Pepper B, Ryglewicz H: Treating the young adult chronic patient: an update. New Dir Ment Health Serv 21:5–15, 1984

Plakun EM, Burkhardt PE, Muller JP: 14-year follow-up of borderline and schizotypal personality disorders. Compr Psychiatry 26:448–455, 1985

Schwartz SR, Goldfinger SM: The new chronic patient: clinical characteristics of an emerging subgroup. Hosp Community Psychiatry 32:470–474, 1981

Strauss JS, Carpenter WT: The prediction of outcome in schizophrenia, I: characteristics of outcome. Arch Gen Psychiatry 27:739–746, 1972

Weisbrod BA, Test MA, Stein LI: Alternative to mental hospital treatment, II: economic benefit-cost analysis. Arch Gen Psychiatry 37:400–405, 1980

❖ 5 ❖

The Effects of Inpatient Family Intervention on Treatment Outcome

John F. Clarkin, Ph.D.
Ira D. Glick, M.D.
Gretchen Haas, Ph.D.
James H. Spencer, Jr., M.D.

Although the use of family therapy on inpatient units has gained wide acceptance and has been used extensively, there are few research programs that have investigated the effectiveness of this utilization of effort and manpower. Because we were concerned by the lack of research information and convinced of the importance of treating the patient with the family in the inpatient setting, we have investigated the effects of an inpatient family intervention package for patients with major affective disorder, schizophrenia, and other major psychiatric disorders. The focus of this chapter is on the design and outcome of a clinical trial of this inpatient family intervention (IFI).

We had very little prior literature to draw upon in the construction of a family intervention with patients hospitalized with serious psychiatric disorders. Prior to our research, there had been no single controlled study of family intervention on an inpatient service. Of the two relevant inpatient studies, one was not well controlled and was limited to adolescents (Wellisch et al. 1976), and the other involved the family as a minor component in a social skills training program for schizophrenics (Wallace and Liberman 1985). In nonrandomized designs, Gossett and colleagues at Timberlawn Hospital have described the course and outcome of inpatient family work with adolescent patients (Gossett et al. 1983).

Models of Serious Psychiatric Disorders and the Family Context

The prevailing models of serious psychiatric disorders include psychosocial variables in the etiology and course of the disorder (e.g., Billings and Moos 1985; Brown and Harris 1978; Haas et al. 1985) and give credence to the development of family intervention models. These models are explicated elsewhere, but the essential points can be summarized as follows:

1. Many schizophrenic, bipolar, and depressed patients are difficult to treat, often denying the need for medication or acknowledging only the biological aspects of the disorder that can be treated with a pill. The episodes of illness are often characterized by alienated and destructive interpersonal behavior, especially within the family system (Davenport and Adland 1988).

2. Family stress is associated with a poor course of the disorder in schizophrenic and depressed patients. We do not know if the influence of high family expressed emotion (EE) is diagnosis specific, but we assume until proven otherwise that such toxic effects are probably operative in all serious psychiatric conditions.

3. Marital and family functioning is seriously affected by pathology in a family member, especially pathology involving depressive episodes. There is less problem-solving behavior and less self-disclosure in couples with a depressed member (Biglan et al. 1985). Interpersonal friction, poor communication, and diminished sexual satisfaction characterize marriages in which one spouse is depressed (Rounsaville et al. 1979; Weissman and Paykel 1974).

4. High levels of stress are associated with low social support in those who experience depression. Depressed individuals seek more social support than others and perceive themselves as receiving less (Coyne et al. 1981; Schaefer et al. 1981).

5. The coping styles of depressed individuals are characterized by poor effectiveness, seeking of emotional or informational support, wishful thinking, and negative self-preoccupation (Coyne et al. 1981; Folkman and Lazarus 1986).

Specific Aims of Family Intervention

Given the association between family environmental stress and serious psychiatric disorders, coupled with the growing evidence that family intervention can be helpful in the course of a major psychiatric condition such as schizophrenia (e.g., Falloon et al. 1982), we hypothesized that a brief IFI would be clinically useful for patients with a range of psychiatric disorders. We formulated hypotheses concerning the mechanism of action and the role of specific treatment and final goals of intervention. The accomplishment of the specific targeted treatment goals of IFI was expected to lead to improved family attitudes toward the patient and to optimal utilization of mental health services following discharge. In addition, we hypothesized that positive family attitudes toward treatment would promote patient compliance with aftercare.

In designing an inpatient family intervention, we had only modest goals in mind. We were using a brief family intervention, limited to the hospitalization phase, with no control over outpatient follow-up. We were treating patients whose pathology was severe enough to warrant a psychiatric hospitalization. The pathology was caused in varying degrees by biological factors not under the direct influence of the family nor of family intervention.

It is difficult to demonstrate an incremental effect of a specific treatment added (in this case, IFI) to a range of treatments for patients hospitalized with an acute disorder. Inpatients often show substantial improvement related to the change of environment, medication, various psychosocial interventions, and passage of time. Because both groups (IFI and non-IFI) received extensive hospital treatment, simply adding IFI might not show a robust incremental effect. Despite these difficulties, we decided to utilize this constructive (i.e., add-on) design as it reflected typical clinical practice. Many hospitals have added brief family intervention to the array of interventions typically used. The practical question at these sites concerns the effectiveness of adding a family intervention module.

Description of the Family Treatment Model

Some would argue that family intervention is almost always indicated—emotional difficulties and psychiatric disorders can be conceptualized as the result of the impact of systems malfunction on the part of the family, and the symptoms are simply expressed by one family member. Although such a rationale may be appropriate for less severe conditions, such as adolescent acting-out and marital strife, serious psychiatric conditions such as schizophrenia and major affective disorders can hardly be explained by family interactions. As our knowledge is becoming more specialized and precise, we have learned that the family appears to play a major role in the course of disorders such as schizophrenia and major depression, and that family support for the patient's medication and psychosocial treatments is probably important, if not necessary.

Our own approach evolved out of daily inpatient work with severely dis-turbed patients and their families. IFI is a brief, psychoeducational and problem-focused family intervention structured to assist the patient and family in coping with the hospitalization of a family member. This is a family "intervention" rather than family "therapy," because our assumptions are that there is only one patient with a major disorder and that the family is not in treatment but is collaborating with us to cope with the patient's condition.

Assumptions

Our family treatment model assumes that the illness is not caused by family environment or family communication problems but possibly is exacerbated by these conditions. Although greatly influenced by psychosocial factors, these dis-orders are partly biological in nature. Thus, we do not assume that the manic or depressive symptoms are under exclusive or even predominant control of the repetitive family interaction patterns. Furthermore, we cannot infer that the family interaction patterns seen at the time of the hospitalization are typical, or that such patterns of interaction caused or even maintained the symptomatic behavior in the identified patient. More often than not, family members are doing what they perceive as necessary to cope with the situation. Reducing attitudes of blame toward the family assists the clinician in establishing an alliance with the family.

We believe that providing information about the psychiatric disorder will enable the family to use its own strengths in coping with the patient's condition. The process itself can be instrumental in building a therapeutic alliance with the family and in working through basic maladaptive attitudes toward the family member who is the patient. This process can also promote more effective utiliza-tion of the mental health treatment system during and following hospitalization. Some families will not be reached by such a straightforward process, but the attempt will further differential therapeutics by testing the limits of such an approach.

It is assumed that the crisis period of hospitalization is not the time to exam-ine and rehash long-standing family and marital conflicts. These conflicts may or may not be related to the illness episode. Therefore, focusing on these issues is not the first priority. Rather, the first priority is for the clinician to take an active role in directing the dialogue away from intense emotional turmoil and long-standing family conflict or blame for the patient's episode. The focus is on immediate issues and matters at hand: what crises and/or difficulties im-mediately preceded the hospitalization? What is the family's understanding of the nature and prognosis of affective disorder? What treatment will be needed upon discharge from the hospital? Will the family—and the patient—accept this?

Treatment Goals

Six treatment goals define and guide the orientation of IFI:

1. Helping patient and family to accept the reality of the disorder and to develop an understanding of the current episode;
2. Identification of possible precipitating stresses relevant to the current episode;
3. Identification of likely future stresses both within and outside of the family;
4. Elucidation of the family interaction sequences that produce stress on the identified patient;
5. Planning strategies to manage or minimize future stresses; and
6. Educating the patient and family regarding the nature of the treatment and the need for continued treatment following discharge from the hospital.

The six goals of IFI were pursued differentially, depending upon the existing problems and the specific needs of each family case. The family therapist and the supervisor set the goals for each case at the beginning of treatment, and at time of discharge the family therapist rated the extent to which each goal was achieved.

Therapeutic Strategies

The treatment strategies of IFI involved 1) psychoeducation, 2) exploration and clarification about specific family stressors on the patient, 3) problem solving around managing the stressors, and 4) planning for aftercare. This was not behavioral family therapy, in the sense that we did not role-play or practice family communication skills and problem-solving behavior. There was not enough time to accomplish such labor-intensive behavioral rehearsal strategies. Furthermore, there was less emphasis on psychodynamic or structural family therapy strategies. These strategies were seen as too invasive for a brief intervention in the context of hospitalization for a severely debilitating disorder. The research that seemed relevant and congruent with our orientation was that reported by Goldstein and colleagues (1978) with schizophrenics and their families in an outpatient setting. Likewise, our strategies were akin to those of interpersonal therapy (IPT) (Klerman et al. 1984). For example, the patient was viewed as occupying the "sick role" (by virtue of being hospitalized); there was assessment and discussion of stress and conflict in the family environment. Disposition planning for families in need of more extensive behavioral and/or structural family treatment included referrals for outpatient family therapy.

The family clinicians in our study were social workers who had had previous family therapy experience with inpatients and their families. The social workers were often accompanied in the sessions by second-year psychiatric residents and first-year psychology interns who also served as primary therapists for the patients. The family clinicians were comfortable with the goals and strategies of IFI, and they helped formulate the specific interventions. Cases were presented periodically for group discussion and supervision, and many families were interviewed in a group setting to begin the focus of IFI.

Empirical Investigation of IFI

Patients and Their Families

Patients with DSM-III schizophrenic, major affective, and other disorders admitted consecutively to a metropolitan psychiatric hospital were screened for admission to the study using the following criteria: 1) a minimum age of 18; 2) availability of family or significant others for family intervention; and 3) an anticipated length of stay sufficient for a minimum of six sessions of family intervention.

Within the first week of admission to the hospital, all patients (and families) who satisfied the selection criteria and consented to participate in the study were randomly assigned to either multimodal hospital treatment with IFI or multimodal hospital treatment without IFI (the "comparison treatment" condition). The standard hospital treatment included medication (when indicated), individual sessions with a primary therapist, and group and milieu treatment.

Assessment and Statistical Analysis Procedures

The study design included three independent variables: treatment assignment (hospitalization with IFI, or hospitalization without IFI); diagnosis (schizophrenia, unipolar or bipolar affective disorder); and sex. There were three dependent patient variables (global outcome, symptomatology, and role functioning) and a dependent family variable (family attitude toward the patient, treatment, family burden, and openness to social support).

Patients were assessed at admission, at discharge, 6 months after discharge, and 18 months after discharge. A number of instruments were used to assess the dependent variables (see Glick et al. 1985 and Haas et al. 1988 for additional details). These included ratings of patient global functioning (Global Assessment Scale [GAS] ratings by independent rater); symptomatology (Psychiatric Evaluation Form [PEF] by independent rater); role functioning (PEF by independent rater); Role Performance and Treatment Scale [RPTS] (RPTS ratings by independent rater); treatment compliance (RPTS ratings by independent rater); and family attitudes toward the patient, toward treatment for the patient, and toward the burden the patient exerts on the family (self-report by significant family members on the Family Attitude Scale [FAS]). There were also ratings of the accomplishment of the family treatment goals by the family therapists.

Because Type 1 errors may occur when multiple tests of significance are performed on multiple outcome measures, a principal components analysis was utilized to reduce the individual measures to composite outcome scores. We will report here on the two patient composite scores and the two family composite scores that emerged from the data. The patient composite scores were global functioning and symptoms (PCOMP1) and role functioning (PCOMP2). PCOMP1 was a composite score generated by GAS, PEF-OS (PEF-Overall Severity), and PEF summary scales of grandiosity, disorganization, withdrawal, and subjective distress. PCOMP2 was a composite score from the RPTS role functioning scales concerning primary role and family, social, and leisure activities. The two family composite scores were attitude to treatment/social support (FCOMP1) and attitude to patient/family burden (FCOMP2). FCOMP1 was a composite score from the FAS Factor 2, attitude toward treatment, and FAS Factor 5, openness to social support. FCOMP2 was composed of FAS Factor 1, attitude toward the patient, and FAS Factor 4, family burden.

Outcome for All Patients

There were a total of 169 patients in the study (Spencer et al. 1988). The sample was almost evenly divided between females (54%) and males (46%). The mean age for the IFI group was 30.2 years, almost exactly that of 31.3 years for the Comparison group. The group was predominantly single (64%), with a substantial minority (25%) being married. The remainder were divorced, separated, or widowed. As for living situation, 30% were single and lived alone or with children; 44% lived with family of origin; and another 25% lived with a spouse. Seventy-three percent of the patients were Caucasian, and 17% were Black. The mean GAS score for the group as a whole upon admission was 28.2.

At 6 months, there was a main effect of treatment on the global functioning/symptoms composite score. This effect favored those patients with family treatment, and the effect was greater and more consistent in female patients. There was also a treatment-by-sex-by-diagnosis effect indicating that female patients in both schizophrenic and affective disorder groups had a better out-come with IFI.

There was no main effect of treatment on the role functioning composite measure at 6 months. However, there was a treatment-by-sex-by-diagnosis effect; that is, female patients in the poorer functioning schizophrenic group did better with family treatment.

There was a treatment main effect favoring family treatment on a composite measure of family attitude toward treatment/openness to social support at 6 months. There was also a treatment-by-sex effect on the patient rejection/family burden composite measure favoring families of females who receive IFI, as well as a treatment-by-diagnosis effect showing that family treatment was somewhat better for families of patients with a major psychosis.

There is growing recognition these days of the importance of clinical as opposed to statistical outcome. In order to assess clinical significance, we used a cutoff of 60 on the GAS to divide the entire sample into clinically significant and nonsignificant outcome groups. Results indicated that a higher proportion of patients who had family treatment than of comparison patients were in the better outcome group at 6 months ($P < .02$), which was somewhat attenuated at 18 months ($P < .07$).

At 18 months, there were no main effects of treatment. There was a treat-ment-by-sex effect, and it was once again the females in the IFI group who showed a positive effect on composite mean. There was a treatment-by-sex-by-diagnosis effect indicating that female patients with schizophrenia or affective disorder did better with IFI, whereas female patients with other diagnoses had a worse outcome with family treatment. At 18 months, there was no significant treatment effect on role functioning; the only treatment effect on patient rejec-tion/family burden was a treatment by diagnosis interaction similar to the inter-action at 6 months.

Outcome for All Affective Disorder Patients

We will provide data on 50 patients with affective disorder, 29 of whom are unipolar and 21 bipolar (Clarkin et al. 1990). The bipolar patients were predom-inantly white (81%) and female (67%), with a mean age of 32. Marital status was quite varied (52% single, 33% married, and 14% divorced). Forty-eight percent had no previous hospitalizations, and 33% had no previous episodes of illness. There was a more seriously disturbed subgroup (14%) with three or more previous hospitalizations, and 19% with three or more previous bipolar episodes. The unipolar patients were predominantly white (62%), with almost equal dis-tribution of males (45%) and females (55%). The mean age was 38. Thirty-one percent of the patients were single, 52% married, and 17% divorced or separated. Sixty-two percent of the patients had no previous hospitalizations, and 48% had no previous episodes. In contrast, 14% had experienced three or more previous hospitalizations and three or more previous episodes.

Female affective disorder patients with IFI were doing significantly better on the composite symptomatology/global outcome measure (PCOMP1) than those in the comparison group at discharge; on the other hand, affective disorder males were little affected. Role functioning (PCOMP2) was not measured at discharge, because the patients had not yet returned to family and community roles. Family attitude toward treatment was significantly better in IFI females than in comparison females, whereas family attitude toward the patient was significantly better in males who received the *comparison* treatment than in males who received IFI.

At both 6- and 18-month follow-up points, PCOMP1 and PCOMP2 did not show a main effect of treatment for all affective disorder patients. Likewise, there were no main effects of treatment on either of the two family composite measures for the total affective group.

IFI had a significant beneficial effect on bipolar patients but had a negative effect on unipolar patients. At both 6- and 18-month follow-ups, bipolar patients showed better outcome with IFI, whereas unipolar patients did better without it. On PCOMP1, there was a treatment by subdiagnosis trend that became significant at 18 months. It is clear from inspection of composite means that the bipolar patients did better with IFI, whereas unipolar patients did better with the comparison treatment. The bipolar treatment effect was due to female patients only, whereas the negative effect on unipolar patients appeared in both sexes. On PCOMP2, there was a significant interaction of treatment with subdiagnosis at both 6- and 18-month follow-ups. Again, the bipolar patients did better with IFI, and the unipolar patients did better with the comparison treatment.

On FCOMP2, attitude to patient/burden, there was a treatment by subdiagnosis interaction effect at 6-month follow-up, again favoring the IFI bipolar patients.

Outcome for Schizophrenic Patients

The schizophrenic patient sample was divided up into patients with good prehospital functioning and patients with poor prehospital functioning. We will provide data on 92 schizophrenic patients, 38 in the higher functioning group (13 IFI and 25 comparison) and 54 in the lower functioning group (24 IFI and 30 comparison) (Glick et al., in press). The schizophrenic patients were predominantly single (79%), with the remaining patients either married, divorced, or separated. Sixty-one percent were single and living with family of origin, whereas 23% were single and living alone.

At 18 months, poorer functioning schizophrenic patients who are female showed a positive response to IFI on both global functioning/symptomatology and role functioning. Male patients were unaffected by the treatment or did a little worse.

Among the total sample of families of schizophrenic patients, the families with female patients who received IFI showed a more positive attitude to the patients at both 6 months and 18 months. In the poorer functioning group, the families of both male and female patients who received IFI showed a more positive attitude toward the patients at 18 months.

A Process Model

Although it is most important to examine the results of the IFI at discharge and at follow-up, it is also clinically useful to examine the process of the treatment and its impact on the patients and family. Most important is an examination of the mediating goals of the IFI—that is, the achievement of the hypothesized effects that should lead to better patient functioning.

In our investigation, the identification and measurement of mediating goals included 1) post-hospital medication compliance; 2) post-hospital psychosocial treatment compliance; and 3) family rejection of the patient. Our results (Glick et al., in press) indicated robust correlations between the mediating variables and outcome for all diagnostic subgroups. In addition, the effects of the mediating variables on outcome were significantly enhanced by IFI, although this was not a direct effect. There is also the suggestion of moderator effects on the treatment by sex and diagnosis, as these results were seen most clearly in the total sample and for subgroups of female patients and poor prehospital functioning females with schizophrenia.

Discussion and Conclusions

In summary, it seems clear that brief family intervention during an inpatient treatment episode is advantageous and effective. However, there are some differential treatment suggestions above and beyond this general statement. Bipolar patients and their families responded best to the treatment, followed by schizophrenic patients. Unipolar patients did not respond positively to the family treatment. In terms of the sex of the patient, female patients did better in the family treatment.

In an effort to help future research efforts, we will briefly discuss problems in the design of the current study and methods of improving similar study designs

in the future. In this study, we were not able to monitor the therapeutic intervention consistently. Optimally, this would have been done by videotaping a
sample of the therapy sessions. Ratings of the videotaped sessions would have
been instrumental in ensuring consistency and competency in the delivery of
the treatment. We are impressed with the recent literature that suggests substantial variance among individual therapists (e.g., Luborsky et al. 1986) and a
decrement in therapist competence when faced with patients (and, probably
more so, with families) who are hostile toward the therapist or the therapy itself.

There is tremendous heterogeneity of the patients who met DSM-III criteria
for schizophrenia and major affective disorder. While the patients were homogeneous to Axis I criteria, they were heterogeneous to Axis II, IV, and V and other
nondiagnostic patient variables. Unfortunately, we did not have a reliable diagnosis of the Axis II pathology for the patients (or family members) included in
this study. Prior research suggests that an affective disorder group would have a
substantial number of individuals with coexisting personality pathology. It is our
impression that the personality disorders of both patient and family members
heavily influenced both the receptivity to and the issues raised by the IFI sessions.

To further complicate the issues, the heterogeneity of the families of the
patients must be recognized. This was a heterogeneity that existed on many
levels. Family composition (e.g., single parent, parents and sibs) and developmental stage (e.g., young adult with parents, patient and spouse) were variable.
There was also wide variation in the personal adjustment of the individual
family members. GAS scores on all family members could conceivably produce a
range of scores as wide as that of the range of scores for the patients themselves.
And more directly, there was wide variation both between and within families
along dimensions of acceptance-rejection of the patient, denial-acceptance of
the mental disorder, and low to high perceived burden in relation to the patient
and the illness. There is some documentation of this variability in the range of
family attitude scores (on the FAS scale) toward the patient, his or her disorder,
and the need for treatment.

In future studies, there will be a need for greater specification and measurement of these important family variables, all of which singly and collectively
could contribute to the course of the patient's disorder and recovery. Other
important nondiagnostic patient and family variables may influence or modify
patient and family outcome. These include prior treatment compliance, sex of
the identified patient, sex of therapist, socioeconomic status, religion, and race.

What would have been the results if inpatient family intervention (IFI) had
been followed up with some outpatient family sessions? Future studies need to
assess the impact of "booster" outpatient sessions that build on a positive response to family work during the inpatient phase. It may be possible to differen-

tiate between those families that need little or no post-discharge intervention and those that need further family intervention (because of such factors as family denial of illness or long-standing conflict and lack of support for the patient). A next step in systematic research on IFI would be to test the incremental benefits of continuing such treatment into the post-hospital recovery phase.

It is clear from the outcome for the entire sample that IFI is an effective treatment. Thus, it is reassuring to know that the resources that we are expending in providing family intervention in the hospital setting produce positive effects. However, this study has not demonstrated that IFI is effective for everyone.

The data suggest that IFI has good efficacy for female patients with schizophrenia or bipolar disorder. Our results do not show efficacy for males, nor does IFI appear to be advantageous in unipolar disorder.

Because this is a single study with the limitations described, we would not recommend that family intervention be withheld from patients with unipolar disorder or from male patients. However, our differential findings should be considered by clinicians working with limited resources and those who are trying to evaluate the results of their own inpatient family work.

IFI is helpful for the families of males and females with schizophrenia and with bipolar disorder. This latter point raises a dilemma for hospitals in terms of how much of their resources they may wish to devote to the families of seriously disturbed patients when there may be no immediate benefits for the patient. As to the group of patients with personality disorders and/or substance abuse problems (a large and ever-growing segment of the hospital population), further studies with larger samples are needed to replicate these and our other findings.

References

Biglan A, Hops H, Sherman L, et al: Problem-solving interactions of depressed women and their spouses. Behav Ther 16:431–451, 1985

Billings AG, Moos R: Psychological stressors, coping, and depression, in Handbook of Depression: Treatment, Assessment and Research. Edited by Beckham E, Leber W. Homewood, IL, Dorsey Press, 1985, pp 940–974

Brown GW, Harris TO: Social Origins of Depression: A Study of Psychiatric Disorder in Women. New York, Free Press, 1978

Clarkin JF, Glick ID, Haas G, et al: A randomized clinical trial of inpatient family intervention: V. Results for affective disorders. J Affective Disord 18:17–28, 1990

Coyne JC, Aldwin C, Lazarus RS: Depression and coping in stressful episodes. J Abnorm Psychol 90:439–447, 1981

Davenport YB, Adland ML: Family therapy intervention in the management of manic episodes, in Affective Disorders and Family Intervention. Edited by Clarkin JF, Haas

G, Glick ID. New York, Guilford, 1988, pp 173–195

Falloon IRH, Boyd JL, McGill CW, et al: Family management in the prevention of exacerbations of schizophrenia: A controlled study. New Engl J Med 306:1437–1440, 1982

Folkman S, Lazarus RS: Stress processes and depressive symptomatology. J Abnorm Psychol 95:107–113, 1986

Glick ID, Clarkin JF, Haas G, et al: A randomized clinical trial of inpatient family intervention: VI. Mediating variables and outcome. Fam Process (in press)

Glick ID, Clarkin JF, Spencer JH, et al: A controlled evaluation of inpatient family intervention. Arch Gen Psychiatry 42:882–886, 1985

Goldstein MJ, Rodnick EH, Evans JR, et al: Drug and family therapy in the aftercare treatment of acute schizophrenics. Arch Gen Psychiatry 35:1169–1177, 1978

Gossett JT, Lewis JM, Barnhart RD: To Find a Way: The Outcome of Hospital Treatment of Adolescents. New York, Brunner/Mazel, 1983

Haas G, Clarkin JF, Glick ID: Marital and family treatment of depression, in Handbook of Depression: Treatment, Assessment, and Research. Edited by Beckham E, Leber W. Homewood, IL, Dorsey Press, 1985, pp 151–184

Haas GL, Glick ID, Clarkin JF, et al: Inpatient family intervention: A controlled study. II. Results at discharge. Arch Gen Psychiatry 45:217–224, 1988

Klerman GL, Weissman MM, Rounsaville BJ, et al: Interpersonal Psychotherapy of Depression. New York, Basic Books, 1984

Luborsky L, Crits-Christoph P, McLellan AT, et al: Do therapists vary much in their success? Findings from four outcomes studies. Am J Orthopsychiatry 56(4):501–512, 1986

Rounsaville BJ, Weissman MW, Prusoff BA, et al: Marital disputes and treatment outcome in depressive women. Compr Psychiatry 20:483–490, 1979

Schaefer C, Coyne JC, Lazarus RS: The health-related functions of social support. J Behav Med 4:381–406, 1981

Spencer JH, Glick ID, Haas G, et al: A randomized clinical trial of inpatient family intervention: III. Effects at 6-month and 18-month followups. Am J Psychiatry 145:1115–1121, 1988

Wallace CJ, Liberman RP: Social skills training for patients with schizophrenia: A controlled clinical trial. Psychiatry Res 15:239–247, 1985

Weissman MM, Paykel E: The Depressed Woman: A Study of Social Relationships. Chicago, University of Chicago Press, 1974

Wellisch DD, Vincent J, RoTrock G: Family therapy versus individual therapy: A study of adolescents and their parents, in Treating Relationships. Edited by Olson D. Lake Mills, IA, Graphic Publishing Co., 1976, pp 275–302

❖ 6 ❖   Selective Review of Recent North American Long-Term Follow-up Studies of Schizophrenia

Thomas H. McGlashan, M.D.

It appears to me a most excellent thing for the physician to cultivate Prognosis; for by foreseeing and foretelling, in the presence of the sick, the present, the past, and the future, and explaining the omissions which patients have been guilty of, he will be the more readily believed to be acquainted with the circumstances of the sick; so that men will have confidence to intrust themselves to such a physician. And he will manage the cure best who has foreseen what is to happen from the present state of matters. For it is impossible to make all the sick well; this, indeed, would have been better than to be able to foretell what is going to happen; but since men die, some even before calling the physician, from the violence of the disease, and some die immediately after calling him, having lived, perhaps, only one day or a little longer, and before the physician could bring his art to counteract the disease; it therefore becomes necessary to know the nature of such affections, how far they are above the powers of the constitution; and, moreover, if there be anything divine in the disease, and to learn a foreknowledge of this also.

Hippocrates (1929 translation)

Introduction

The pathogenesis and diathesis of schizophrenia often tend to be chronic. Therefore, follow-up studies provide valuable guidelines for clinical and research purposes. Because of our ignorance concerning etiology, the dimension of longitudinal course plays a key role in defining and validating discrete psychiatric syndromes. Furthermore, data about natural history are central to evaluating the efficacy of treatment efforts, because gains made in therapy depend upon natural prognostic potential and need to be evaluated against estimates of likely lifetime

This article appeared originally in *Schizophrenia Bulletin* 14:515–542, 1988.

outcomes without treatment. For these and other reasons (estimating disability, allocating resources, etc.), the follow-up study has been, and remains, a central investigative tool.

This chapter focuses upon the long-term follow-up studies of schizophrenia from North America. It begins with an outline of the study selection criteria. The studies are then described in some detail, with special attention to sample characteristics. The major findings are summarized under three thematic headings: natural history, prognosis, and nosology.

Follow-up Study Selection Criteria

The following criteria were used to select the follow-up studies for review. The studies are North American. They are recent, meaning within the past 30 years, when major methodological advances began to be introduced. They are follow-up studies of schizophrenia, especially schizophrenia by operationalized diagnostic criteria. Not included are follow-up studies of atypical schizophrenia (by Feighner criteria; Feighner et al. 1972), brief reactive psychosis or schizophreniform psychosis (by DSM-III criteria; American Psychiatric Association 1980), or schizoaffective disorder (by any criteria). The latter cohort is considered by Samson and colleagues (1988). Included are follow-up studies beginning with an identified schizophrenic patient. Not included are the so-called "follow-back" studies, which attempt to identify premorbid clues marking a child who is vulnerable to developing schizophrenia. "Long-term" is defined as a minimum average follow-up of 10 years. Studies selected focus on the long-term course and outcome of the schizophrenic proband; excluded are studies that focus on the schizophrenic patients' families and first-degree relatives. Finally, studies are included if they introduced or incorporated any of the following methodological advances:

1. Independence of index (baseline) and outcome assessment;
2. Diagnosis using operationalized criteria and multiple systems to assess comorbidity;
3. Extensive description of the samples demographically and prognostically;
4. Outcome checked for veracity and assessed by multidimensional, operationalized ratings that can be case calibrated and translated across sites;
5. Reliability training and testing for all measures;
6. Explicit accounting for missing subjects and missing information; and
7. Testing for any sampling biases introduced by such attrition (McGlashan et al. 1988).

Ten studies or groups of studies met these criteria. These studies summarized in Table 6–1 are described below.

Description of the Follow-up Studies

The Massachusetts Mental Health Center Follow-up Studies

Vaillant conducted two long-term follow-up studies out of the Massachusetts Mental Health Center, a state-supported university teaching hospital in Boston. The first study (Vaillant 1964b) was retrospective in design. The hospital records of 72 schizophrenic patients consecutively admitted between 1947 and 1950 were assessed in 1962. The patients were given a clinical diagnosis based on Bleulerian concepts (autism, ambivalence, loose associations and/or flat, inappropriate affect as primary symptoms; hallucinations and/or delusions as secondary symptoms). They were included in the study if they retained this diagnosis during their entire hospital stay. The charts were rated by Vaillant for the presence/absence of seven prognostic criteria. Items not mentioned in the chart were scored as absent.

Six to 12 months later, Vaillant followed up the cohort. First, he consulted the central files of the Massachusetts Department of Mental Health to determine whether any of the patients had required further hospitalization. Subsequent charts were then gathered for clinical information. Efforts were made to contact next of kin on those patients for whom definitive follow-up information could not be obtained from subsequent hospital admissions. For this, telephone contacts or personal interviews were used. Outcome was specified on the dimensions: hospitalization, work, and independence. It was rated on a five-point scale as follows: 1 = 10 or more years residence in a mental hospital; 2 = 3 or more years in a hospital and inability to work or manage a household more than 50% of the time spent in the community; 3 = less than 3 years hospitalized with inability to work more than 50% of the time spent in the community; 4 = ability to work more than 50% of the time, but unable to live independently of parents or siblings; 5 = able to work full-time or to manage a household effectively and to live independently of family of origin. Patients in follow-up categories 4 and 5 were considered long-term social remissions.

Of the original 72 patients, 97% could be followed reliably for at least 2 years, 89% for at least 8 years, and 63% for a full 12–15 years after admission. The average follow-up period was not reported. The outcomes reported were as follows: 1, 28%; 2, 6%; 3, 25%; 4, 15%; 5, 26%. Collapsing categories, 41% could be classed as social remissions (4 + 5), and 59% were "essentially invalid" (1 + 2 + 3). Outcome correlated with predicted prognosis based upon the seven criteria. Finally, the author noted that reliable long-term follow-up proved more

TABLE 6–1. Selective review of North American follow-up studies

Study	Investigators	Schizophrenic N at baseline/ n follow-up	Follow-up average length/range	Sample drawn from	Diagnostic criteria	Comparison groups	Data source(s) Baseline	Follow-up
Massachusetts Mental Health Center 1 (MMHC)	Vaillant 1964b	72/ 97%—2 yrs 98%—8 yrs 63%—12–15 yrs	No average/ 2–15 yrs	Schizophrenic patients admitted to MMHC 1947–1950	Clinical diagnosis based on Bleulerian criteria	None	Hospital records	Primary hospital records
Massachusetts Mental Health Center 2	Vaillant 1978	56/51	10 yrs/ 4–16 yrs	Schizophrenic patients admitted to MMHC and remitted between 1959 and 1962	Clinical diagnosis based on Bleulerian criteria	None	Hospital records and prior studies	Hospital records and personal interview
Phipps Clinic	Stephens et al. 1963 Stephens 1978	472/143	12 yrs/ 10–16 yrs	Schizophrenic patients admitted to Phipps Clinic between 1948 and 1959	Clinical diagnosis, criteria?	None	Hospital records	Potpourri (see text)
Iowa 500	Tsuang et al. 1979	200/186	No average/ 30–40 yrs	Patients admitted to Iowa Psychopathic Hospital between 1934 and 1944	Operational criteria, Feighner et al. system	Mania ($n = 100$) Unipolar dep. ($n = 225$) Surgical controls ($n = 160$)	Hospital records	Structured personal interview
Alberta 1	Bland et al. 1976	92/88	10 yrs/ no range	First admission schizophrenic patients to Alberta Hospital in 1963	Consensus diagnosis based on DSM–II criteria	None	Hospital records	Personal interview
Alberta 2	Bland et al. 1978	45/43	14 yrs/ no range	Same as 1976 sample	At least one (1) first rank symptom, (2) New Haven Schizophrenia Index, (3) Feighner definite, (4) Feighner probable	None	Hospital records	Personal interview

TABLE 6-1. (continued)

Study	Methodology checklist[1]																		Sample distinction	Outcome or natural history for schizophrenia	
	1	2a	2b	3a	3b	3c	3d	4a	4b	4c	5a	5b	5c	5d	5e					
Massachusetts Mental Health Center 1		x	x						x		x		x			NI	Poor	1–	28%	
																		2–	6%	
																		3–	25%	
																		4–	15%	
																	Good	5–	26%	
Massachusetts Mental Health Center 2									x		x		x			Remitted patients	Remitted		61%	
																	Chronic		39%	
Phipps Clinic	x		x						x							First admissions	Recovered		24%	
																	Improved		46%	
																	Unimproved		30%	
Iowa 500	x		x	x				x	x		x		x		x	85% ill 1 year; rural	Schizophrenia worst			
																	Mania and depression better			
																	Surgical control best			
																	Schizophrenia suicide rate		10%	
Alberta 1			x					x			x		x		x	First admissions	Recovered		58%	
																	Periodic mild		9%	
																	Periodic severe		9%	
																	Chronic mild		7%	
																	Chronic severe deficit		9%	
																	Chronic hospitalized		8%	
																	Suicide		2.3%	
Alberta 2			x	x	x						x		x		x	First admissions	Recovered		21%	
																	Periodic mild		30%	
																	Periodic severe		21%	
																	Chronic mild		12%	
																	Chronic severe deficit		14%	
																	Chronic hospitalized		2%	

TABLE 6–1. Selective review of North American follow-up studies (*continued*)

Study	Investigators	Schizophrenic N at baseline/ n follow-up	Follow-up average length/range	Sample drawn from	Diagnostic criteria	Comparison groups	Data source(s) Baseline	Follow-up
New York City Outpatient Clinic	Engelhardt et al. 1982	670/646	No average/ 15–20 yrs	Schizophrenic patients admitted to outpatient research clinic between 1958 and 1962	Clinical diagnosis based on DSM-II	None	Hospital and study records	State and hospital records
Boston State Hospital	Gardos et al. 1982a, 1982b	124/90	12 yrs/ no range	Schizophrenic patients admitted to hospital drug study in 1965	Clinical diagnosis	None	Hospital and study records	Personal interview
Chestnut Lodge	McGlashan 1983a, 1984b	188/163	15 yrs/ 2–32 yrs	Patients discharged from the hospital between 1950 and 1975	Operational criteria, several systems including DSM-III	BI ($n = 33$) UNI ($n = 58$) SA ($n = 87$) BPD ($n = 93$) SPD ($n = 33$)	Hospital record abstracts	Semistructured personal interview
Vermont State Hospital	Harding et al. 1987a, 1987b	118/82	20 yrs/ 20–25 yrs	Inpatients referred to rehabilitation program at Vermont State Hospital between 1955 and 1960	DSM-III operational criteria, DSM-I	DSM-III non-schizophrenia ($n = 71$) DSM-I schizophrenia ($n = 149$)	Hospital records	Structured personal interview

TABLE 6-1. (continued)

Study	Methodology checklist[1]															Sample distinctions	Outcome or natural history for schizophrenia	
	1	2a	2b	3a	3b	3c	3d	4a	4b	4c	5a	5b	5c	5d	5e			
New York City Outpatient Clinic								x				x				Outpatients, largely institutionally chronic	Eventually hospitalized	63%
																	Number hospitalizations	2.7
																	Total length of hospitalization per patient	44 mos
Boston State Hospital			x					x	x		x		x		x	Biologically and institutionally chronic; urban, low SES	Structured living situation	97%
																	Nonsheltered employment	6%
																	GAS Score	40
																	IMPS global severity score (markedly ill)	4.8
Chestnut Lodge	x	x	x	x	x	x	x	x	x	x	x		x	x	x	Biologically and institutionally chronic; upper SES	Structured living situation	49%
																	Nonsheltered employment	41%
																	In year before follow-up:	
																	Not in hospital	54%
																	Few or no symptoms	21%
																	Social network	29%
																	Health-sickness rating score	37
																	Global outcome distribution:	
																	Recovered	6%
																	Good	8%
																	Moderate	23%
																	Marginal	23%
																	Continuously incapacitated	41%
																	Outcome stable over the long term	
																	Suicide rate	8%
Vermont State Hospital	x	x	x				x	x	x	x	x	x	x		x	Institutionally chronic; rural low SES	In year before follow-up:	
																	Not in hospital	82%
																	Employed	40%
																	Few or no symptoms	68%
																	Social network	61%
																	GAS score distribution:	
																	Fair (31–60)	40%
																	Good (> 61)	60%
																	Schizophrenia and nonschizophrenia outcome no different	
																	DSM-III schizophrenia and DSM-I schizophrenia no different	

TABLE 6–1. Selective review of North American follow-up studies (*continued*)

Study	Investigators	Schizophrenic N at baseline/ n follow-up	Follow-up average length/range	Sample drawn from	Diagnostic criteria	Comparison groups	Data source(s) Baseline	Follow-up
Washington International Pilot Study of Schizophrenia	Carpenter and Strauss, 1991	?/40	11 yrs/ no range	Patients admitted to psychiatric units in general hospitals, Prince George's County, MD, in 1968–1969	Clinical diagnosis based on DSM-II and ICD-9	Nonschizophrenic patients (*n* = 13)	Structured personal interview	Structured personal interview
Columbia-Psychiatric Institute	Stone 1986	99/94	No average/ 10–23 yrs	Patients admitted to a long-term (average 1 yr) academic unit in NYC between 1963 and 1976	DSM-III operational criteria	SA (*n* = 64) M-D (*n* = 39) BPD (*n* = 205)	Hospital records	Semistructured personal interview

Abbreviations: BI = bipolar affective disorder; UNI = unipolar affective disorder; SA = schizoaffective psychosis; BPD = borderline personality disorder; SPD = schizotypal personality disorder; M-D = manic-depressive psychosis; GAS = Global Assessment Scale; SES = socioeconomic status; IMPS = Inpatient Multidimensional Psychiatric Scale.

[1] = independence of assessment; 2a = data, missing information; 2b = data, missing subjects; 3a = diagnosis, operationalized criteria; 3b = diagnosis, multiple systems; 3c = diagnosis, comorbidity; 3d = diagnosis, reliability; 4a = sample description, demography; 4b = sample description, predictors; 4c = sample description, reliability; 5a = outcome, multidimensional; 5b = outcome, veracity check; 5c = outcome, operational scales; 5d = outcome, case calibration; 5e = outcome, reliability.

TABLE 6–1. *(continued)*

Study	Methodology checklist[1]															Sample distinctions	Outcome or natural history for schizophrenia
	1	2a	2b	3a	3b	3c	3d	4a	4b	4c	5a	5b	5c	5d	5e		
Washington International Pilot Study of Schizophrenia	x	x	x					x	x	x	x		x			Acute to subchronic manifest illness	Schizophrenia worse than nonschizophrenia on all dimensions Outcome was level between 5 and 11 years
Columbia-Psychiatric Institute				x				x			x		x			Acute to subacute manifest illness; middle class	GAS score 39 Ever married 13% Suicide 10% Schizophrenia outcome worse than comparison groups

difficult among patients who appeared to do well. All patients with less than 8 years of follow-up fell into groups 4 and 5. This was perhaps the first suggestion that missing subjects in follow-up studies constituted a healthier group of patients.

The second follow-up study (Vaillant 1978) from the 1970s was basically prospective in design. Between 1970 and 1975, Vaillant obtained follow-up information on 51 of 56 schizophrenic patients from the Massachusetts Mental Health Center who had achieved complete remission during 1959–1962. Remission was judged either retrospectively by the patients' doctors at the time (Vaillant 1962) or was ascertained prospectively in a short-term follow-up study conducted at that time (Vaillant 1964a). The diagnosis of schizophrenia was clinical and based on Bleuler's primary symptoms. The patients had to have been hospitalized at least 2 months, with a discharge diagnosis of schizophrenia. Records were scored for prognostic factors as in the earlier follow-up study. Patients were followed up through hospital records or interview 4 to 16 years later (average 10 years).

Presence or absence of remission constituted the outcome measure. Remission was a multidimensional concept, and its rating required that five conditions be met: 1) the patient had been free from psychotic symptoms for 1 year; 2) the patient had been free from Bleuler's primary symptoms for 1 year; 3) the patient had reattained his or her best level of premorbid adjustment; 4) the patient was not on phenothiazines; and 5) the patient had at least one friend. According to these criteria, 61% of the patients sustained their remissions, whereas 39% did not and went on to follow a "chronic" course. The latter was not characterized beyond number and length of subsequent hospitalizations. Scores on the prognostic variables did not discriminate outcome groups, leading Vaillant to conclude that remitted schizophrenia is not necessarily a discrete subtype requiring a fresh label or nosologic reassignment to the affective disorders.

The Phipps Clinic Follow-up Study

Stephens and coworkers conducted a large retrospective follow-up study of 472 schizophrenic patients discharged from the Phipps Clinic in Baltimore, Maryland, between 1948 and 1959 (Stephens 1970, 1978; Stephens and Astrup 1963, 1965). Patients were first admissions, hospitalized for at least 3 weeks, who received a discharge clinical diagnosis of schizophrenia (criteria not specified). Their charts were independently classified according to specified process and nonprocess categories (Stephens and Astrup 1963), and later the charts were also independently scored for the presence or absence of 43 prognostic variables (Stephens et al. 1966, 1967).

Follow-ups of from 5 to 16 years duration were obtained on 78% of the sample based on "letters, telephone conversations, and personal contacts with the patients, their relatives, and hospitals" (Stephens and Astrup 1965). Missing subjects did not differ from included subjects vis-à-vis discharge status or process/reactive classification. Outcome was described in three categories:

1. "Recovered" meant *complete* recovery without evidence of residual pathology. It excluded patients with frequent exacerbations and remissions.
2. "Improved" included patients who may have appeared recovered at follow-up but who had repeated exacerbations and hospitalizations, as well as patients with residual symptoms.
3. "Unimproved" referred to active, chronic psychosis. Most of these patients remained hospitalized for most of the follow-up period.

Of the total follow-up cohort, 143 patients were assessed 10 years or more after baseline (average 12 years, range 10–16 years). Their outcomes distributed as follows: recovered, 24%; improved, 46%; unimproved, 30%. Outcome clearly correlated with the process/non-process category and with the prognostic variables in the directions expected.

The Iowa 500 Follow-up Study

The Iowa 500 follow-up study has been massively innovative as well as massive in scope (Clancy et al. 1974; Morrison et al. 1972; Tsuang and Winokur 1975; Tsuang et al. 1979, 1980). It introduced specified diagnostic criteria for the selection of subjects, the use of psychiatric and nonpsychiatric comparison groups, detailed description of samples, and independence of diagnostic and outcome assessments, among other innovations.

The study was retrospective and based on patients admitted between 1934 and 1944 to the Iowa State Psychiatric Hospital, a 60-bed short-term treatment facility serving the entire state of Iowa. Roughly 370 patients were admitted each year, and over 3,800 records were accumulated. Among these patients, 13% received a chart diagnosis of schizophrenia and 19% a chart diagnosis of manic-depressive psychosis or involutional melancholia. Their records (874 in all) were selected for evaluation. Although no missing data rate was reported, the records sound very complete as described (Morrison et al. 1972). Records were screened diagnostically using the Feighner criteria for schizophrenia and affective disorders (Feighner et al. 1972). These criteria were purposefully stringent to reduce heterogeneity—especially for schizophrenia. One-fourth of the affective disordered patients' records and two-thirds of the schizophrenic patients' records were excluded. Schizophrenic patients' charts ($n = 315$) were excluded mostly for episodic course and/or short duration. This process resulted in the selection of three samples—200 patients with schizophrenia, 100 patients with mania, and 225 patients with unipolar depression. To this the investigators added a nonpsychiatric comparison group ($n = 160$) drawn from surgical patients (appendectomy and herniorrhaphy) hospitalized at the University of Iowa over the same time period. The study also evaluated the first degree relatives of study patients ($n = 2,055$), but this will not be elaborated here.

Follow-up data were collected between 1972 and 1976, roughly 30–40 years after index admission. The mean age of the schizophrenic patients at follow-up was 64 years. Field work was conducted blind to the original study diagnoses by trained personnel: psychiatric residents, medical students, and "other personnel" (Clancy et al. 1974). Patients who were alive and willing to be interviewed were given a face-to-face or telephone structured interview (Tsuang et al. 1980) designed to evaluate normality, psychopathology, and multiple domains of functioning. Outcome for deceased subjects was approximated by giving this structured interview to a first degree relative of the deceased. Other sources of information came from state hospital records, death certificates, and sundry medical records.

The team was able to trace and rate 95% of the original schizophrenic cohort. Follow-up diagnoses were assigned by consensus after review of the structured interview by up to four psychiatrists (Tsuang 1978a). Functional outcome was operationalized according to four dimensions: marital, residential, occupational, and symptomatic, and each rated on a 3-point scale: poor, fair, or good. Missing information was incorporated into the outcome ratings in specified ways (Tsuang and Winokur 1975; Tsuang et al. 1979).

This study sample of 200 Feighner criteria schizophrenic patients had the following characteristics: male—52%; married—20%; poor premorbid adjustment and work—50%; high school graduate—28%; precipitating factors—11%; age of onset (median)—26 years; age at admission (median)—27 years; ill more than 1 year before admission—85%. The population was predominantly rural and relatively nonmobile, because they were hospitalized during the Depression years. They were also hospitalized in the era prior to ECT, drugs, or outpatient treatment networks. Return to the community, therefore, depended entirely upon improvement in mental status. Of the 200 schizophrenic patients from this sample, 26% were discharged to the community following index hospitalization. This sample comes the closest of all the North American follow-up studies of approximating natural history of schizophrenia unperturbed by modern treatments.

Outcome was dichotomized into good and fair/poor for each dimension. Results demonstrated unequivocally—on all dimensions—that schizophrenic patients had the poorest outcome. Surgical control patients did the best, and affectively disordered patients were in between. The best scores among the schizophrenic cohort on the four dimensions of outcome were distributed as follows: 1) marital status—21% married; 2) residential status—34% at home or relatives' residence; 3) occupational status—35% employed, retired, housewife, or student; and 4) symptomatic status—20% no symptoms.

The Alberta Follow-up Studies

Bland and coworkers conducted two follow-up studies of schizophrenic patients in the 1970s, the first of a broadly defined, first admission cohort (Bland et al. 1976) and the second of a "narrowly" defined subsample (Bland and Orn 1978). The samples were selected from patients hospitalized in 1963 at Alberta Hospital, an inpatient psychiatric unit serving the southern half of the province of Alberta. Since this was virtually the only such facility in the area at the time, the admission rate approximated the incidence of schizophrenia over the entire provincial population served.

In the first study (1976), the files of newly admitted patients with a chart diagnosis of schizophrenia were examined. Selected were 92 cases with adequate data for diagnosis that met DSM-II criteria (American Psychiatric Association 1968) for schizophrenia as agreed upon by two psychiatrists. Follow-up was conducted by interviewing patients and significant others (family and/or professional) in 1974 and 1975, 10 years after admission. It was successful in 88 (96%) of the cases. Deceased patients were included. Outcome was multidimensional and assessed social adjustment, marital stability, work productivity, institutional treatment, subsequent care/medicines, and a global estimate of psychiatric condition. The latter consisted of 6 levels: 1) recovered, no social or intellectual deficit; 2) periodic mild social and/or intellectual deficit; 3) periodic severe social and/or intellectual deficits; 4) mild chronic social and/or intellectual deficits; 5) chronic severe social and/or intellectual deficit; and 6) chronic unremitting institutionalization.

Of the 88 patients followed up, 48 were male. Their average age at index admission (which was their first psychiatric hospital admission) was 34 years (range 14–66 years). Fifty-one percent of the cohort was single. Outcome proved to be better than Bland and colleagues expected. The global rating broke down as follows: 1, 58%; 2, 9%; 3, 9%; 4, 7%; 5, 9%; 6, 8%. Regarding further care, the authors noted that of the 51 recovered patients, 45% had discontinued their medications within 10 months of discharge, and only 39% continued medications for 5 years or more.

The second follow-up study (1978) began with the same baseline cohort from the first study. This time, however, the sample was constructed by the application of "stricter" criteria to the charts. Nearly one-half of the original sample was excluded for psychotic affective disorder, organic brain syndrome, alcoholism, mental deficiency, or another diagnosis sufficient to explain the clinical picture. Five additional subjects were dropped, because it was learned that they were not first admissions. Included were 45 subjects meeting one or more of the following operationalized diagnostic criteria: 1) Schneider's first rank symptoms (Schneider 1959) minus somatic passivity; 2) the New Haven Schizophrenia Index (Astrachan et al. 1972) using the recommended cut-off score; and 3) the Feighner et al. (1972) criteria, both definite and "probable" cases. The latter patients were defined as those meeting all criteria except the duration item, which requires "a chronic illness with at least 6 months of symptoms prior to the index evaluation, without return to the premorbid level of psychosocial adjustment." Follow-up was conducted as in the first study, but in 1977, 14 years after admission. Forty-three patients were traced. Deceased subjects were included. Outcome was assessed using the same multidimensional ratings.

The final follow-up sample of 43 broke down by diagnostic criteria as follows: 1) first rank symptoms: positive in 38 subjects; 2) New Haven Schizophrenia Index: met by 42 subjects; and 3) Feighner criteria: 20 probable and 20 definite cases. Demographically, the sample consisted of 22 males, and 53% of the sample was single at admission. The mean age at index admission (which was their first psychiatric hospitalization) was 33 years. Although the sample was undoubtedly defined by more explicit criteria than the 1976 sample, these criteria were not necessarily more narrow, as the authors contend. Schneider's first-rank symptoms and the New Haven Schizophrenia Index are often broadly encompassing systems (see section on nosology), and less than half of the sample met the strictly defined Feighner criteria. The resultant sample was more like the 1976 sample than different—largely acute, first admission schizophrenic patients.

Outcome, although not as good as the 1976 sample, was not much worse. Global ratings broke down as follows: 1, 21%; 2, 30%; 3, 21%; 4, 12%; 5, 14%; 6, 2%. Seventy-nine percent of patients had an average of 2.7 further hospitalizations averaging 15% of the follow-up period. Fifty-one percent of the sample remained on neuroleptic medications for a mean of 7 years.

The New York City Outpatient Clinic Follow-up Study

In 1982, Engelhardt and co-workers reported a 15-year follow-up of schizophrenic patients who had participated in a Brooklyn-based outpatient clinic drug study of maintenance phenothiazines (Engelhardt et al. 1982). The label "outpatient clinic" is attached here to highlight its unique character as the only North American long-term follow-up starting with outpatients rather than with inpatients. As noted by the authors, " . . . less than one-half of the individuals carrying a diagnosis of schizophrenia are likely to be represented in 'classical' follow-up studies originating in-hospital" (p. 502). Furthermore, 21% of their sample had no prior history of hospitalization, and such a cohort is totally unrepresented in follow-up studies. The authors state that only by studying schizophrenics who have not yet experienced hospitalization can one obtain the maximum heterogeneity possible in order to develop an adequate data base of course and prognosis.

The study was retrospective in design. The sample consisted of 670 schizophrenic outpatients who participated in a federally funded study of ataractic drugs that began in 1958. Patients were between 18 and 45 years old, had a primary diagnosis of schizophrenia based on DSM-II criteria, and gave evidence of mental illness of at least 1 year's duration. More than one-half of the sample showed signs of mental illness for 10 years or more. Hospitalization experience prior to the clinic admission varied. As mentioned, 21% had no previous history of psychiatric hospitalization. Twenty-two percent experienced exclusively "crisis" admissions in a municipal hospital, and the remainder (57%) had at least one admission to a long-term psychiatric facility.

Outcome was unidimensional and consisted of cumulative hospitalization rates for each follow-up year from the patient's entry into the study (1958–1962) through December 31, 1977. This made the minimum follow-up 15 years (range 15–20 years). Hospitalization data were collected from the records of the New York State Department of Mental Hygiene and the Kings County Psychiatric Hospital. Information on deceased patients and those hospitalized out of New York State was excluded.

At baseline, the sample had a mean age of 30 years. Fifty-four percent were male. Sixty-eight percent were white, 28% were black, and 4% were Hispanic. Three-fourths of the patients were in the lower two socioeconomic classes (Hollingshead and Redlich 1958). Forty-seven percent were single. Slightly more than one-third were either self-supporting or supported by a spouse. Forty-five percent were supported by relatives, and 19% received public assistance. Only 27% had fairly regular employment, 21% worked sporadically, and 52% had rarely or never been employed.

Results.   Three hundred eighty patients were eventually hospitalized at least once, giving a 59% cumulative hospitalization rate by 15 years. The average number of hospitalizations was 2.7, and the average length of a single hospitalization was 16 months. The average length of total hospitalization per patient was 44 months (range 1–174 months). Interestingly, the proportion of patients residing in hospitals per year went from a high of 35% at year 2 of the follow-up to a low of 12% by year 15. Such a trend could reflect a diminution in psychopathology; it could also be secondary to the deinstitutionalization movement, which was in full swing at the time. The majority (63%) of patients eventually returning to hospitals did so within the first 2 years of follow-up. Engelhardt and colleagues (1982) cite this as evidence that schizophrenia is not a disease of slow, progressive deterioration; after approximately the first 5 years, the average patient's course either plateaued or improved gradually.

The Boston State Hospital Follow-up Study

Gardos and coworkers conducted a 12-year follow-up study of 124 chronic schizophrenic patients hospitalized at Boston State Hospital in Boston, Massachusetts (Gardos et al. 1982a, 1982b). The study was retrospective in design. Subjects had participated as the Boston State Hospital cohort of a federally funded multihospital collaborative study of chlorpromazine in 1965. The drug study had required a primary diagnosis of schizophrenia and at least 2 years of continuous hospitalization.

Because of their involvement in the drug study, subjects had been assessed repeatedly, and considerable data existed regarding their psychopathology and social adjustment. Following the drug study, this cohort continued to receive usual treatment consisting of neuroleptics, milieu therapy, and vocational rehabilitation. Additionally, in the late 1960s and 1970s they were part of the deinstitutionalization movement.

Follow-up was conducted in 1977, 12 years after admission to the drug study, by a psychiatrist and psychiatric nurse. The hospital records of each patient were examined from 1965 until follow-up or until discharge. Then each patient was personally interviewed. Outcome was assessed multidimensionally. Complete follow-up data were gathered on 90 patients or 73% of the sample. Seventeen patients (14%) were deceased; analysis revealed them to have been a sicker cohort. Seventeen patients (14%) were not located or refused participation; analysis of existing data (e.g., post study hospital course) revealed them to be significantly healthier than the assessed cohort.

The sample fits the profile of the early onset, drug treatment resistant, institutionalized patient. On the average, subjects were first hospitalized at age 24. They entered the study at age 41 after undergoing 13 years of hospitalization. They had all been exposed to neuroleptic medication, often in high doses. Eighty-one percent were single, and 60% had not graduated from high school. Prior to hospitalization, 33% had been skilled workers or better, 26% semiskilled, and 41% unskilled. Their global severity of illness at study entry on a 7-point scale was 5.2, or markedly ill.

At follow-up 12 years later, nearly all of the 90 patients were distributed among a variety of structured domiciles: 21 in state hospitals, 35 in nursing homes, 5 with their families of origin, 12 in family care homes, and 13 in cooperative apartments. Only four patients (3%) were living in rooms unsupervised. The mean Global Assessment Scale (Endicott et al. 1976) score of the patients was 40, corresponding to major impairment in work, relationships, communication, judgment, thinking, and mood. Their 7-point global severity of illness score at follow-up was 4.8, not much different from their score at baseline. Only 17 patients worked, 12 in hospital-based industries or sheltered workshops and 5 in competitive but menial jobs. Summarizing, the authors stated, "The overall psychosocial adjustment of the interview cohort of 90 patients was rather dismal. The typical patient at follow-up can be characterized as markedly ill, receiving high doses of antipsychotics, not employed, and showing poor social skills." (1982a, p. 21).

The Chestnut Lodge Follow-up Study

McGlashan reported a retrospective follow-up study on patients discharged over a 25-year period from Chestnut Lodge, a 90-bed private tertiary care residential treatment facility in Rockville, Maryland, near Washington, DC (McGlashan 1984b, 1984c). Patients were largely young, chronically ill treatment failures from upper socioeconomic brackets who had been referred from across the continental United States. They suffered from schizophrenia, affective disorders, or borderline states.

The study included 532 patients with an index hospitalization of at least 3 months who were discharged between 1950 and 1975. The minimal stay criterion of 3 months was established to insure the presence of adequate data in the hospital record for baseline assessments. The missing data rate turned out to be 12%. Because the hospital charts were so extensive, they were first condensed into an abstract that contained all pertinent amnestic data up to and including the first 3 months of index hospitalization. One member of the research team blind to outcome then rated each abstract on multiple demographic, predictor, and psychopathological (sign and symptom) variables. Reliability of these ratings was tested, and variables achieving poor reliability were dropped. All patients were rediagnosed by applying current operational diagnostic systems, including DSM-III, to the rated sign and symptom data. Based on this, eight study diagnostic samples were defined: schizophrenia, schizoaffective psychosis, schizophreniform psychosis, unipolar and bipolar affective disorders, schizotypal and borderline personality disorders, and "other" (undiagnosed). Although patients received a primary diagnosis for the main study, their scores on all diagnostic systems were recorded to assess the presence/effects of comorbidity.

Follow-up was conducted between 1977 and 1983 by members of the research team blind to the baseline data. Outcome was assessed an average of 15 years post-discharge (range 2–32 years) by personal interviews, in person and by telephone, with patients and/or significant others. The average age of the patients at follow-up was 47 years. Deceased subjects were included. Outcome was multidimensional in scope and included rating scales from existing follow-up studies. All measures were operationalized, tested for reliability, and case calibrated. Assessment was completed on 446 patients, or 72% of the total possible sample (N = 619). Eighty-six additional hospital records of nonlocatable and refusing subjects were abstracted and rated to test for sampling biases by comparing their baseline profiles with those of the patients completing follow-up. Such biases proved to be minimal.

For the schizophrenic cohort, baseline data were available on 188 patients and follow-up data on 163 patients. This cohort had the following baseline demographic and predictor profile: males—52%, married—23%, white—100%, socioeconomic status—1.6 (Hollingshead-Redlich 1957), age of onset—19 years, age of first hospitalization—23 years, age of index hospitalization—28 years, number of prior hospitalizations—3, length of prior hospitalizations—28 months, length of prior outpatient treatments—17 months, admission psychopathology on a 7-point scale—5.5. The sample was severely and chronically ill; 80% had been ill for more than 2 years. They were also drug treatment resistant insofar as most had been tried unsuccessfully on neuroleptic medications prior to index admission. In this way, they were similar to the schizophrenic patients in the Boston State Hospital sample.

By follow-up, this schizophrenic sample distributed as follows on a 5-point global outcome scale: recovered—6%, good—8%, moderate—23%, marginal—23%, continuously incapacitated—41%. The "marginal" anchor point meant that, on the average, the patient had spent about 25% of the follow-up period in sheltered situations, worked about 20% of the time, claimed some role-specific social contacts, and experienced symptomatic expressions of illness about 75% of the time. The entire cohort scored 37 on the Health-Sickness Rating Scale, a 100-point global scale similar to the Global Assessment Scale, placing them at a level comparable to the Boston State Hospital sample. Outcome did not change significantly with follow-up time when compared across decades. Long-term course proved to be a stable plateau with no evidence of trends toward improvement or deterioration.

The Vermont State Hospital Follow-up Study

Harding and colleagues (1987a, 1987b) reported a prospective/retrospective follow-up study based on a cohort of 269 severely ill patients from Vermont State Hospital (213 of whom had DSM-I schizophrenia; American Psychiatric Association 1952) who were referred to a rehabilitation and community placement program at this institution between 1955 and 1960. Twenty to 25 years later, 97% of the patients, most still residing in Vermont, were located and/or accounted for and received comprehensive outcome assessment based on personal interviews in their own homes. Additionally, the follow-up assessors, who were blind to the patient's baseline diagnostic and functional status, checked the veracity of each patient's outcome report with knowledgeable significant others. Outcome assessments were multidimensional and tested for reliability. The lives of the deceased patients before their deaths were evaluated, although the reports to date focus only upon the patients who were alive and personally interviewed (*n* = 168). Because virtually all patients were found and assessed, missing subjects were not an issue.

Baseline demographic, predictor, and psychopathological data from each patient's hospital record were rated using a standardized review form by investigators blind to outcome. Ratings were tested for reliability. Kappa coefficients ranged between 0.40 and 0.95. Patients were then rediagnosed according to DSM-III criteria. The reliability of this judgment was tested twice; kappa coefficients were 0.40 for first trial and 0.78 for the second trial. One hundred eighteen of the original 269 patients received a DSM-III diagnosis of schizophrenia.

The final sample, after rediagnosis, consisted of 82 live and interviewed DSM-III schizophrenic patients. Their average age at follow-up between 1980 and 1982 was 61 years. At baseline this sample had the following demographic and predictor characteristics: male—50%, single—62%, completed high school education—45%. Prior to transfer to the rehabilitation program, 45% of the cohort had been hospitalized more than 6 years, 24% between 2 and 6 years, and 31% less than 2 years.

Although undoubtedly chronic by length of hospitalization standards, the patients in this sample were unique in many respects. Fortunately, numerous additional sources of information exist about the Vermont State Hospital program and its subjects that provide clues. First, neuroleptic drugs (chlorpromazine and reserpine) were introduced to Vermont State Hospital for the first time in 1954 (Brooks 1956). Some patients improved enough to leave the hospital quickly (*n* = 178, not included in the follow-up study). A larger number of patients from the back wards improved on the medications, but had no prospect of leaving the hospital for a variety of reasons, including continual dysfunction, no family, lack of placement, absent financial resources, or "raw fear" of separating from the institution (G. W. Brooks, M.D., March 1986, personal communication). It was this group of patients for which the rehabilitation/community placement program was devised, and this group from which the initial referrals to the program were made (Brooks and Deane 1965). They were moderately drug responsive but deskilled secondary to institutionalization, not deterioration (Brooks 1960).

Second, the initial group of 25 study subjects were instrumentally functional; these patients referred to the rehabilitation program were already working at hospital jobs up to 30 hours per week (G. W. Brooks, M.D., March 1986, personal communication; Chittick et al. 1961). In fact, many of the patients were selected for the rehabilitation program by asking hospital work supervisors which patients he or she could least afford to lose (Brooks 1959)! Up until 1954, two-thirds of all work at Vermont Hospital came from unpaid patient labor. Between 1955 and 1965, the success of the rehabilitation program cut this patient-labor force in the hospital by 85% (Brooks et al. 1970). Although the remainder of the cohort was profoundly disabled (Harding et al. 1987a), all of the patients in the study were highly motivated to work because they were poor and had no prospects of income from family or public welfare (G. W. Brooks, M.D., March 1986, personal communication).

The best description of the selection process for the rehabilitation program comes from *The Vermont Story* (Chittick et al. 1961):

> Subjects for the hospital's rehabilitation program were selected from improving patients in this declining population of schizophrenics. They were considered chronic rather than acute. Our definition of chronicity requires that an individual be disabled by his illness, whether or not he had been hospitalized, for at least one year prior to his selection as a rehabilitation client. This definition permitted us to work with a few chronic patients whose hospitalizations had been relatively brief. Most had been hospitalized for some years.
>
> Patients are informally referred to the rehabilitation service by anyone in the hospital. They may be referred by an attendant, nurse, work supervisor, another patient, psychiatrist, or anyone else. This usually insures that they are well enough to arouse the interest of at least one other person.
>
> Do there appear to be guiding principles which lead personnel to select certain types of patients? We can answer this question only in the most general terms. Obviously, the person referring and those accepting a patient must feel a certain optimism about him. The reasons for this optimism are hard to express and those who are involved in the selection may not be able to state precisely why one person was chosen instead of another. On the other hand, there may be some consciously held reason for optimism. Possibly the patient is a good worker in the hospital industrial program or a cooperative patient on the ward. The patient may have undergone a sudden and dramatic change in behavior which has gained him the attention of others. It is common for staff personnel to say to the rehabilitation staff, "Can't you do something for John Doe now? He's so much better than he was two months ago." It may be that some patients are just "discovered." As one staff physician reported to one of us, "I just happened to notice Joe. He was pushing a cart up and down the tunnel. I discovered that he had been doing this for five years. I decided he needed attention and I referred him to rehab." (pp. 24–27)

Clearly, patient selection was only a partially random or arbitrary matter. The process capitalized, in fact, upon emerging signs of health and hope.

The outcome of this patient cohort is also unique. A 5-year follow-up of the entire original 268 referrals to the program was reported in 1967 (Deane and Brooks 1967). Thirty percent of the patients were in the community without readmission, and 40% were in the community but had undergone about two readmissions apiece. The remaining 30% were in the hospital, two-thirds as a result of readmission from the community. Most patients were single and used community care facilities for socializing; most replaced institutional employment with sheltered employment (e.g., cook in a nursing home with bed and board) and kept close contact with their rehabilitation program counselors. The picture was one of progress, but against strong regressive resistance with high utilization of mental health manpower and support systems.

Follow-up 20 years after the program in 1980–1982 recorded that these patients had consolidated their gains of 5 years and surpassed them beyond everyone's expectations. The DSM-III schizophrenic cohort scored as follows on several of the Strauss and Carpenter (1972) outcome dimensions: not in the hospital in the past year—82%; meets with friends every week or two—61%; employed in the last year—40%; displays slight or no symptoms—68%. On the Global Assessment Scale, 60% of the patients scored over 61, designated as good functioning. No one scored in the poor functioning category (less than 31). Of further interest is that outcome was not significantly different on any dimension between the DSM-III schizophrenic cohort and either a DSM-I schizophrenic cohort ($n = 149$) or a heterogeneous DSM-III non-schizophrenic cohort ($n = 71$). As such, the Vermont study is singular in finding no differences in long-term outcome between schizophrenia defined by different criteria (DSM-III and DSM-I) and, more strikingly, between schizophrenia and non-schizophrenia (both DSM-III).

The Washington-International Pilot Study of Schizophrenia Follow-up Study

Carpenter and Strauss (1991) completed an 11-year follow-up on a subgroup of the original Washington, DC, cohort of the International Pilot Study of Schizophrenia (IPSS; World Health Organization 1979). This follow-up is the only long-term North American follow-up study using a prospective design (i.e., following the development of the illness with serial, independent, cross-sectional assessments). The first follow-up was conducted at 2 years (Strauss and Carpenter 1972, 1974) and the second at 5 years (Hawk et al. 1975; Strauss and Carpenter 1977).

The original sample consisted of 131 patients admitted in 1968–1969 to the psychiatric units of general hospitals of Prince George's County, Maryland, a largely middle- and lower-middle-class area around Washington, DC. Patients were referred for study if they displayed at least one psychotic symptom on admission and had no organic problems or drug or alcohol abuse. Patients were assessed diagnostically and prognostically at baseline by structured interview. Ratings were tested for reliability. The diagnosis of schizophrenia was made clinically using DSM-II/ICD-9 criteria. This original cohort ranged between acute and subchronic. Subjects were screened out if they had been hospitalized for more than 2 of the previous 5 years, or if they gave evidence of continuous psychosis for longer than 3 years.

Follow-up concentrated on the 68 patients who were evaluated at the 5-year follow-up. The 11-year assessment was conducted blind to any prior information about the subjects. Fifty-three patients received complete assessment. The 15 missing subjects were compared with completed subjects on key baseline variables; no consistent biases were demonstrated. The follow-up cohort was assessed with a structured personal interview by telephone or in person. Outcome was multidimensional and operationalized (Strauss and Carpenter 1972, 1974). Forty of the follow-up cohort had an original diagnosis of schizophrenia; the remaining 13 nonschizophrenic patients carried diagnoses of manic-depressive disorder, personality disorder, or neurosis.

Follow-up found the schizophrenic patients functioning at a level inferior to the nonschizophrenic patients on all dimensions: hospitalization, work, social functioning, symptom severity, and global outcome. Outcome level did not change between the 5-year and 11-year follow-ups, findings compatible with the idea that schizophrenia tends to plateau after 5 years.

The Columbia-Psychiatric Institute Follow-up Study

In 1985–1986, Stone conducted a retrospective follow-up of patients admitted between 1963 and 1976 to a long-term (average 1 year) treatment unit of the New York State Psychiatric Institute in New York City (Stone 1986; Stone et al. 1986). The unit is an academic training center in psychiatry for Columbia University and, at the time, specialized in providing intensive, psychoanalytically oriented psychotherapy. Five hundred fifty patients were selected who were less than 40 years old at admission, who registered an IQ greater than 90, and who were hospitalized on the unit for more than 3 months. Subjects were diagnosed according to DSM-III criteria applied to their hospital records. Ninety-nine patients met the criteria for schizophrenia. Comparison groups carried the following diagnoses: schizoaffective psychosis ($n = 64$), schizophreniform psychosis ($n = 36$), manic-depressive psychosis ($n = 39$), and borderline personality disorder ($n = 205$).

The author assessed outcome nonindependently by personal interview, telephone, and face-to-face between 10 and 23 years after admission. Five hundred four patients (92% of the sample) completed outcome assessment, which included ratings of work functioning during follow-up, current living situation, and global functioning by the Global Assessment Scale.

The overall cohort at admission was 22 years old, scored an IQ of 119, and came from mid-level socioeconomic circumstances (2.7 on the Hollingshead-Redlich scale; Hollingshead and Redlich 1958). They had experienced 1 to 3 months of hospitalization prior to admission.

At outcome, 13% of the schizophrenic sample had been or were married. Their Global Assessment Scale score was 39 (range 6–81), and only 8% of the sample reached a level of "good or recovered" (greater than 61). Outcome for the schizophrenic patients was inferior to that of all comparison groups.

The relevant studies have been described and summarized. Let us now review what the principal results have confirmed and/or taught us about the natural history, prognosis, and nosology of schizophrenia.

The Natural History of Schizophrenia

1. *Schizophrenia can be a chronic disease, frequently disabling for a lifetime.* This certainly comes as no surprise to anyone touched by the disorder, but its magnitude had never really been demonstrated against a normal control group until the Iowa 500. There, the outcome of schizophrenic patients proved to be significantly poorer than the outcome of non-psychiatrically disordered surgical patients. This difference extended across all domains of functioning and across three to four decades of the adult life span.

2. *The average outcome of schizophrenia is worse than that of other major mental illnesses.* The Iowa 500 was, again, the first to demonstrate significant long-term differences between schizophrenia and other psychotic disorders, specifically mania and depression as defined by the criteria designated by Feighner and colleagues (1972). The Chestnut Lodge follow-up replicated this finding for DSM-III–defined unipolar and bipolar affective disorders. Later reports detailed that the Chestnut Lodge schizophrenic cohort also had poorer long-term outcome compared to schizoaffective psychosis (McGlashan and Williams 1987; Williams and McGlashan 1987), schizotypal personality disorder (McGlashan 1986b), and borderline personality disorder (McGlashan 1986a). The Washington-IPSS investigation found schizophrenic patients doing worse than a mixed sample of patients with affective, personality, and neurotic disorders. The Columbia-PI schizophrenic cohort had the poorest outcome in comparison to DSM-III-based schizoaffective psychosis, manic-depressive psychosis, and borderline personality disorder. The only exception to this trend was the Vermont State Hospital study, which registered no difference between schizophrenic and non-schizophrenic cohorts. Overall, however, the preponderance of evidence

upholds Kraepelin's original hypothesis bifurcating the psychoses into the affective psychoses and schizophrenia, with the latter having a more pernicious long-term course and outcome.

3. *Schizophrenia is associated with an increased risk for suicide, physical illness, and mortality.* When studied, the rates of suicide proved to be significantly higher for schizophrenia than were the rates for contrasting general populations. In the first Alberta follow-up, the suicide rate was 2.3%. In the Chestnut Lodge follow-up it was 8% (Dingman and McGlashan 1986), and in both the Iowa 500 (Tsuang 1978b) and Columbia-PI studies it was 10%. Death comes more quickly to schizophrenic patients in general (Bland et al. 1976; Tsuang and Woolson 1977), and this excess mortality cannot be accounted for solely by suicide and/or accidents (Tsuang and Woolson 1978). From the Iowa 500 sample, infection and circulatory diseases also contributed (Tsuang et al. 1980a). Shortened survival was about 10 years for the male schizophrenic patients and 9 years for the female schizophrenic patients (Tsuang et al. 1980b).

4. *The schizophrenic process, while disabling and chronic, does not get progressively worse over the long term.* The hypothesis that schizophrenia follows a relentlessly downhill course to dementia has finally been put to rest. Deterioration of functioning does characterize the disease in its early stages and has, in fact, become one of the DSM-III diagnostic criteria. At some point, however, loss of functioning appears to "bottom out" or plateau. This "point" varies widely between individuals, but occurs roughly 5 to 10 years after the manifest illness becomes unequivocally established. As mentioned, the New York City Outpatient Follow-Up found that 63% of patients returning to hospitals did so within the first 2 years of follow-up. More striking were the differences in the Vermont State Hospital cohort between their 5- and 20-year follow-up assessments. As detailed above, the 5-year point found patients struggling with disability and resisting self-sufficiency. By 20 years, however, they had consolidated earlier gains; internalized rehabilitative strategies; and progressed in a steady, measurable fashion. Somewhere between 5 and 20 years, the pressure of the disease plateaued and/or relented somewhat.

This "process plateau" in chronic schizophrenia, once established, appears to be stable. For example, the Washington-IPSS study found little to no change between schizophrenic outcome functioning from 5 to 11 years. The Chestnut Lodge follow-up study demonstrated no significant differences in schizophrenic outcome across three decades post-index hospital discharge. Within any given sample, in fact, there is a remarkable steadiness. However, this diminished variance in the overall process does not appear to represent a rigidification of disease and/or personality. The semi-independent domains of outcome remain semi-independent (Carpenter and Strauss 1991), and potential still exists for progressive rehabilitation (Harding et al. 1987a, 1987b).

5. *Among patients with schizophrenia, however defined, outcome is heterogeneous.* The above remarks about long-term plateauing apply mainly to patient samples in which the schizophrenic process has already become manifestly chronic. For many patients, the disease never gets this far. Among this larger group, *all of whom lay legitimate claim to the diagnosis of schizophrenia*, heterogeneity of outcome is the rule. The evidence resides in the final column of Table 6–1 where, depending on the sample, outcome can vary between complete recovery and continuous incapacity. Furthermore, each level on the outcome spectrum is represented by substantial numbers of patients; we are not dealing with spurious occurrences or false-positive diagnoses. As will be discussed, a great deal of this heterogeneity can be attributed to sample differences. Nevertheless, an important fact remains: a lot of patients recover from schizophrenia. The certainty of negative prognosis in schizophrenia is a myth.

6. *Much of the heterogeneity in the long-term course of schizophrenia can be linked to sample characteristics and/or differences.* How can we account for this heterogeneity? Here we leave the realm of knowledge and enter the domain of speculation. Here, however, the long-term follow-up perspective affords us a rich and perhaps unique perspective for generating some reasonable hypotheses. Close scrutiny of the outcomes in Table 6–1, *in conjunction* with the characteristics of the samples studied, suggests that heterogeneity may be linked with levels of chronicity. For example, the best outcomes were recorded for patients from the two Massachusetts Mental Health Center studies, the Phipps study, and the two Alberta studies. These results arose from samples of acute, first admission, or remitted patients (i.e., nonchronic patients who were either early into their illness course or who had demonstrated hegemony of health over psychopathology). This association of acuteness with good outcome was not absolute (e.g., the second Massachusetts Mental Health Center study), but it held on the average. Thus, the length of time over which the schizophrenic illness has been manifest—as prodrome, active positive/negative symptoms, or residual defect symptoms—may be crucial to ultimate long-term outcome. Furthermore, the chronicity threshold time period may be on the order of 6 months to 1 year. The outcome of the Iowa 500 schizophrenic cohort was decidedly worse than the cohorts just cited, and all of the Iowa 500 patients had been manifestly ill for more than 6 months, as required by the Feighner criteria, or for more than 1 year (85% of the sample), but not for much longer because the average time between onset and index hospitalization was short.

Studies of samples where the documented illness was even longer found still poorer outcomes (Boston State Hospital and Chestnut Lodge), thus supporting the validity of length of mental illness (LOMI) as an outcome-determining parameter. The Vermont State Hospital Follow-up, however, stands as a key exception. Their cohort was decidedly chronic by the LOMI criterion, but their outcome was clearly better. Assuming that the LOMI criterion is valid, this discrepancy is curious.

A closer look, however, suggests that chronicity may contain more facets than just LOMI. Table 6–2 presents three long-term follow-up studies of chronic patients with sufficient baseline and outcome data for detailed comparison. The Boston State Hospital, Chestnut Lodge, and Vermont State Hospital studies utilized many comparable (and sometimes identical) outcome measures, as recorded in Table 6–1. For comparison purposes, in the final column of Table 6–2, I have translated these into a single global outcome score based on a 5-point scale (0 = continuously incapacitated, 1 = marginal, 2 = moderate, 3 = good, 4 = recovered). Table 6–2 also compares these study samples across key demographic, premorbid, and morbid characteristics. The demographic variables are gender, marital status, socioeconomic status, and physical setting. The premorbid variables are education and premorbid work/social functioning. The morbid variables are age of onset, age of first hospitalization, age of index hospitalization, length of prior hospitalizations/treatment (a measure of LOMI), and exposure/response to neuroleptic medications.

All samples were decidedly chronic by the LOMI criterion. They were also remarkably similar with respect to gender, marital status, and premorbid work/social functioning. The Boston State Hospital and Chestnut Lodge patients, furthermore, were alike in falling ill at an earlier age and in their exposure and poor response to prior trials of neuroleptic drugs. The differences in outcome between Boston State Hospital and Chestnut Lodge, therefore, may be linked to the marked discrepancy in socioeconomic status (which probably also accounts for the differences in education). This association is supported by the fact that Chestnut Lodge outcome was superior to the Boston State Hospital cohort in the follow-up dimensions of living situation and employment but not psychopathology (i.e., in domains most likely to be influenced by economic resources).

The Vermont State Hospital patients came from socioeconomic situations comparable to the Boston State Hospital patients. There, however, further similarities end. The Vermont follow-up patients were different from the Boston State Hospital and the Chestnut Lodge patients in three domains, all of which could be linked to their better outcomes. First, they resided in a rural setting. Second, they were exposed to drugs and responded, albeit incompletely. Finally, they appeared to have a later age of illness onset, suggesting that age of onset may be a more powerful predictor of outcome within schizophrenia than heretofore demonstrated.

Leaving physical setting and socioeconomic status aside for the moment, the sampling and outcome differences among these studies imply that chronicity is multidimensional. Four suggested dimensions are listed in the penultimate columns of Table 6–2. LOMI is a central dimension. Another well-known dimension is institutionalization, or the degree to which patients remain attached to or controlled by treatment milieux. The New York City Outpatient study found, for example, that the best predictor of subsequent hospitalization was amount of prior hospitalization—not degree of psychopathology. Some patients in that study were chronic by the LOMI criterion but had never been hospitalized, and they avoided later hospitalization significantly more often than patients referred to the study from long-stay institutions. This form of chronicity was probably ubiquitous among the three samples in Table 6–2.

The introduction of powerful neuroleptic drugs into the treatment of schizophrenia over the last 30 years has established another dimension of chronicity: biological treatment resistance. This form of chronicity was definitely present in the Boston State Hospital and Chestnut Lodge samples. In the former, the follow-up cohort consisted of patients who had not responded to prior drug trials at that institution. In the latter, the follow-up cohort consisted of patients who had, by their index admission, failed to respond to prior trials of somatic treatments (insulin coma, ECT, and/or neuroleptic medications) at other institutions. The Vermont State Hospital sample, however, was hospitalized in the pre-drug era. Patients there were referred to the rehabilitation program in conjunction with initial trials of neuroleptic medication being introduced to North America in the mid-1950s. Although the program patients were unable to leave the institution without additional psychosocial interventions, they were, at least from the available anecdotal reports, drug responsive to varying degrees.

Age of onset also differentiated the Vermont State Hospital from the Boston State Hospital and Chestnut Lodge samples. Might this be another facet of chronicity, with earlier onset being linked to a more constitutionally determined pathogenesis? This remains speculative, however, in the absence of further consistent empirical evidence linking age of onset with prognosis, familial pedigree, syndromal subtype, and so on. Accordingly, it is noted as a dimension of chronicity in Table 6–2, but with a question mark.

Considering chronicity as a multivariate construct may help us at least propose reasonable hypotheses to account for the large differences in outcome among our comparative samples. It appears, for example, that the patients from Chestnut Lodge and Boston State Hospital were chronic in all four of the proposed dimensions, whereas the patients from Vermont State Hospital were chronic in only two of them. Although the validity of these constructs requires further empirical study, the implications of this comparative exercise are clear: adequate sample description in follow-up studies is vital. Without it the interpretation and generalization of findings becomes severely constricted. *Minimally*, descriptors should include the variables listed in Table 6–2. Biological treatment resistance, in particular, is a new construct that needs further attention and

TABLE 6–2. Sample characteristics of three follow-up studies

Study	Male %	Single %	Socio-economic status*	Physical setting	Education: high school graduates	% Premorbid work and social functioning	Age of onset (years)
Boston State Hospital	51	81	4 and 5	Urban	40	Poor	—
Chestnut Lodge Hospital	52	77	1 and 2	Suburban	82	Poor–Moderate	19
Vermont State Hospital	50	62	4 and 5	Rural	45	—	25.8

TABLE 6–2. (continued)

Study	Age first hospitalization (yrs)	Age study admission (yrs)	Length prior hospitalization and outpatient treatment (yrs)	Drugs	Dimensions of chronicity				
					Length manifest illness long	Institution-alization present	Biological treatment resistance present (?)	Age illness onset, early	Comparative outcome (0–4 point scale)
Boston State Hospital	24	41	13	Exposed and resistant	Yes	Yes	Yes	Yes	0—poor
Chestnut Lodge Hospital	23	28	4	Exposed and resistant	Yes	Yes	Yes	Yes	1—marginal
Vermont State Hospital	—	40+	>6 45% 2–6 24% <2 31%	Exposed and responsive	Yes	Yes	No	No	3—good

*Hollingshead-Redlich (Hollingshead and Redlich 1958).

operationalization.

Clearly, a great deal of long-term outcome variance can be accounted for by sample characteristics. As a spin-off of the North American follow-up studies, we also have a clearer notion of which characteristics may be the most important. Quantifying the amount of outcome variance accounted for by each characteristic remains a task for future follow-up investigations.

7. *Long-term follow-up studies have yet to demonstrate clearly the effects of treatment on the natural history of schizophrenia.* Valid and specific estimates of treatment effects require the presence of nontreatment and/or alternate-treatment control groups. Furthermore, all of the current treatments of schizophrenia, biological and psychosocial, are time-limited. Following treatment termination, study patients are released to the mixmaster of "doctor's choice," resulting in a complete loss of treatment homogeneity. Quantification of treatment influences, therefore, remains a matter for short-term follow-up. Long-term follow-up, in fact, may never be a proper strategy for this realm of inquiry.

Long-term follow-up can still provide useful information about treatment. It is instructive to know, for example, that many schizophrenic patients do well without maintenance medication. Of the 51 recovered patients in the first Alberta Follow-up, 45% discontinued their medicine within the first 10 months of baseline. Fourteen percent of the Chestnut Lodge schizophrenic patients achieved drug-free remission for the entire follow-up (Fenton and McGlashan 1987a). Twenty-five percent of the Vermont cohort remained on medication regularly; 25% took medication only during symptomatic exacerbations; and the remaining 50% were noncompliant (34%) or required no prescriptions (16%). Such findings establish the existence and validity of important medication-relevant subgroups, the identification (or prediction) of which has implications for treatment and for identifying subtypes within the schizophrenic syndrome.

Such findings also suggest what kinds of information about treatment can be gleaned validly from long-term follow-up. For example, *uniformly* good long-term outcome in a sample not receiving treatment "x," (e.g., neuroleptics) does suggest that treatment "x" is not necessary for that sample. It says nothing about the efficacy of treatment "x" for that sample except that the benefit to risk ratio is unlikely to be advantageous. On the other hand, *uniformly* bad long-term outcome in a sample receiving treatment "y" strongly suggests that treatment "y" does not alter the natural history of illness for that sample. Here outcome does say something about the efficacy of treatment "y"; it demonstrates a low benefit-to-risk ratio of the treatment for this sample. Such were the conclusions drawn by McGlashan (1984c) and Stone (1986) regarding the utility of intensive individual psychoanalytically oriented psychotherapy as the primary treatment for young, chronic schizophrenic inpatients.

8. *Long-term follow-up can be informative about how sociocultural factors may*

influence course. Sociocultural forces are in the nature of existential situation rather than controlled perturbations of treatment. Socioeconomic status and physical setting, for example, often last a lifetime, and can reasonably be expected to make a long-term difference. Here too, however, *demonstrating* an effect requires tracking the long-term course of at least two "captive" samples that are matched except for the characteristic under consideration. The Vermont State Hospital sample is instructive in this regard. It is a remarkable cohort, perhaps unique in American psychiatry. As detailed in *The Vermont Story* (Chittick et al. 1961), these patients were provided with virtually everything that twentieth-century psychiatry has to offer, all within *one decade* between 1947 and 1957. Furthermore, these advances were introduced in proper sequence and applied with assiduous continuity of care to a target population that remained stable and local. The effects of this are undoubtedly reflected in the cohort's long-term outcome. However, teasing apart which of the many interventions were primary requires control groups that are probably impossible to find and/or construct.

These findings are still interesting in that they challenge many long-standing notions, such as that a mutually negative interaction occurs between schizophrenia and lower socioeconomic status. The Vermont patients were unquestionably poor and uneducated. However, according to George Brooks, the program's primary engineer, their poverty was a major source of motivation; they *had* to work (G. W. Brooks, M.D., March 1986, personal communication). The socioeconomic advantage of the Chestnut Lodge schizophrenic patients, on the other hand, failed to protect them from the ravages of severe psychopathology. For many, money actually worked to their disadvantage; it allowed them to purchase isolation and freedom from the necessity for initiative. Together, the Vermont State Hospital and Chestnut Lodge studies serve as gadflies to time-honored sociological shibboleths touting a simple linear relationship between economics and illness.

Together, the Vermont State Hospital and Boston State Hospital studies suggest that physical setting may strongly influence course. Low-income inner city environments such as that around Boston State Hospital may be particularly toxic, as witnessed also by the young, chronic, homeless patients that drift from one urban center to another. In contrast, small town, rural, and nontransient environments such as that in Vermont may provide a stable foundation for needed continuity of care. These studies corroborate findings that the course of schizophrenia may be more benign in developing or third world countries than in technologically developed nations (World Health Organization 1979).

Prognosis or the Prediction of Outcome in Schizophrenia

Long-term follow-up studies have demonstrated the remarkable heterogeneity of course in schizophrenia. Many of these studies have also been instrumental in reducing this heterogeneity by identifying subgroups of schizophrenic patients with more homogeneous outcomes. The characteristics identifying these subgroups are called predictors of outcome or prognostic variables. We have already seen how outcome can be linked to sample characteristics, particularly various dimensions of chronicity. This section expands upon that discussion and reviews what the North American long-term follow-up studies have taught us about prognosis.

Prediction is the formal study of the association between measurable sample characteristics and outcome in schizophrenic patients. However, since we do not know what schizophrenia is, confusion frequently arises as to whether a given variable is a sample characteristic or one of the criteria for diagnosis. What may be a *prognostic* variable in one study (e.g., LOMI) becomes a diagnostic criterion for schizophrenia in another (e.g., the Iowa 500). Clearly, then, the diagnostic criteria used to define schizophrenia in any sample have prognostic implications. This is the Heisenberg Uncertainty Principle of predicting outcome in schizophrenia: the entity you are measuring moves simply by virtue of how you define it. The implications of this are explored in more detail in the section under nosology. The discussion in this section will focus upon what we have learned about the long-term follow-up effects of the so-called "nondiagnostic" predictors of outcome. These include, in addition to the "classical" predictors, considerations of gender, subtyping, and comorbidity.

1. *The schizophrenic process may be worse for men than for women.* A recent review of the literature on sex differences and severe psychopathology (Bardenstein and McGlashan 1990) indicates that gender differences occur frequently in schizophrenic patients and that schizophrenic women exhibit a less deteriorated course of illness. Analysis of the Chestnut Lodge Follow-up schizophrenic cohort by gender strongly endorsed this view (McGlashan and Bardenstein 1990). The women were superior to the men at baseline in their social and sexual/marital functioning. At long-term outcome, the women were significantly better than the men in these areas and in time symptomatic, substance abuse, and global functioning.

The other North American follow-up study to investigate gender effects (Lloyd et al. 1985) found that sex made no significant contribution to the explanation of outcome differences. This lack of findings, however, may be a function of their defining schizophrenia by the criteria of Feighner and colleagues (1972). Lewine and co-workers (1984) found that the Feighner system completely failed to diagnose women as schizophrenic. This may arise because of women's more frequent affective symptoms. More obviously, one of the Feighner criteria for schizophrenia requires that the patient be single. As the literature repeatedly documents, schizophrenic women are married more often than schizophrenic men. Thus, narrowly defined criteria for schizophrenia, like the Feighner criteria, may select an "atypical" population of women, such that conclusions about sex differences may not be representative of the average female schizophrenic patient.

2. *Long-term follow-up supports the validity of the paranoid/nonparanoid distinction in schizophrenia.* This conclusion comes from studies on the Iowa 500 sample. Using subtyping criteria of DSM-III (1980), RDC (Research Diagnostic Criteria; Spitzer et al. 1977), ICD-9 (1978), and Tsuang and Winokur (1974), Kendler et al. (1984) divided the Iowa 500 schizophrenic cohort into paranoid and nonparanoid subtypes. Long-term outcome was better for the paranoid subtype. The paranoid/nonparanoid differences were greatest using the Tsuang and Winokur criteria, probably because they exclude patients with thought disorder and affective deterioration.

An earlier study found that the paranoid/nonparanoid subtypes were relatively stable diagnostically over the long term, but not as stable as the diagnosis of schizophrenia itself (Tsuang et al. 1981). A change of subtype from paranoid to nonparanoid was more common than vice versa.

3. *Schizophrenia can be comorbid with other forms of psychopathology and this comorbidity can have strong prognostic implications.* These conclusions come from studies on the Chestnut Lodge Follow-up sample of largely chronic schizophrenic patients. Severe obsessive-compulsive symptoms defined a subgroup ($n = 21$) of the study's schizophrenic cohort with a uniformly poorer long-term course and outcome (Fenton and McGlashan 1986). Schizophrenia in patients with a concomitant schizotypal personality disorder had a poorer prognosis at baseline, but a better outcome than "pure," non-comorbid schizophrenia (McGlashan 1986b). Schizophrenic patients with mixed borderline and schizotypal personality features also did better than schizophrenic patients without such comorbid Axis II psychopathology (McGlashan 1983).

These findings raise interesting questions. It is not surprising that "adding" obsessive-compulsive psychopathology to schizophrenia results in a worse combination, whether that combination be considered a subtype of schizophrenia or simply the coexistence of two separate illnesses (true comorbidity). However, it is surprising that by the same model, "adding" Axis II schizotypal personality disorder and/or borderline personality disorder to schizophrenia results in a *better* combination vis-à-vis long-term course and outcome. Since the Chestnut Lodge Follow-up study is the first and, to date, the only study investigating the prognostic significance of comorbidity, knowledge in this area must be considered tentative.

4. *Many important predictors of outcome have been identified by the North American Follow-up Studies.* The long-term follow-up investigations that tested for nondiagnostic predictors of outcome were the Massachusetts Mental Health Center, Phipps, Iowa 500, Chestnut Lodge, and Washington-IPSS studies. The major predictor dimensions to emerge from these efforts are summarized in Table 6–3, along with the direction of each dimension associated with better outcome. Identified predictors came from many categories: genetics, premorbid functioning, illness onset, psychopathological signs and symptoms, and course of illness up to index admission. For the most complete assessment of prognosis, these predictors should be considered in conjunction with the additional sample characteristics discussed in the previous section: socioeconomic status, physical setting, age of onset, length of manifest illness, biological treatment resistance, and institutional chronicity.

Building upon their identified predictors, four of the investigating teams developed prognostic *scales*. These consist of several key predictor variables, each scored as present or absent, and collected together to give a total score (Carpenter and Strauss 1991; Fenton and McGlashan 1987b; Stephens 1978; Vaillant 1964b). Such scales are in keeping with the notion that prognosis is a dimensional—not a categorical—phenomenon. There are no categorically "good" prognostic schizophrenic patients versus categorically "poor" prognostic cases, but rather varying combinations along a spectrum. The scores achieved on these scales usually correlate better with outcome than the scores achieved on any single constituent predictor. The reader is referred to specific citations for details.

In addition to the idea that predictors are dimensional phenomena, the following "principles" of prediction have emerged from the North American Follow-up studies. First, cross-sectional psychopathology alone, and diagnosis based primarily on cross-sectional symptoms, have limited prognostic value. Longitudinal data have greater outcome predictive power (Carpenter and Strauss 1991). Second, predictions vary according to the outcome dimension being predicted (Carpenter and Strauss 1991; McGlashan 1986c). For example, premorbid social functioning may predict follow-up social functioning but not predict follow-up hospitalization. The latter, in turn, may be predicted by some other variable, such as LOMI. Third, "like" predicts "like." In general, each domain of outcome functioning is best predicted by its premorbid dimensional counterpart (Carpenter and Strauss 1991; McGlashan 1986c). For example, marital status at outcome is best predictable by marital status at baseline. Fourth, predictors vary according to the length of follow-up. In the Chestnut Lodge schizophrenic sample, for example, premorbid functioning variables emerged as strong predictors of outcome for the first 10 years following index discharge.

TABLE 6–3.   Predictors of outcome in schizophrenia—North American follow-up studies

Predictor category dimension	Value/direction associated with better outcome	Study
Genetics		
Family history affective disorder	Present	1, 2, 3
Family history of schizophrenia	Absent	1, 2, 4, 5, 6
Premorbid		
Schizoid personality	Absent	1, 2, 3
Loner	Absent	5, 6
Social functioning	Better	7
Heterosexual functioning	Better	7
Married	Ever	1, 2
Skills and interests	Present	5, 6
Work functioning	Better	1, 2
IQ	Higher	1, 2
Illness onset		
Acute (less than 6 months)	Present	1, 2, 3
Precipitating factors	Present	1, 2, 3
Psychopathology		
Depressive features	Present	1, 2, 3, 5, 6
Hallucinations, delusions	Present	8
	Absent	7
Disorganized thought	Absent	7, 8
Assaultiveness	Absent	5, 6
Emotional blunting	Absent	1, 2
Confusion or perplexity	Present	1, 2, 3
Concern with death	Present	3
Subjective distress	Present	7
Anxiety	Present	7
Course (prior to admission)		
Process	Absent	1
Duration of prior hospitalizations	Shorter	7, 9

[1] Stephens et al. 1966.
[2] Stephens 1978.
[3] Vaillant 1964a, 1964b.
[4] Stephens and Astrup 1963.
[5] McGlashan 1986c.
[6] Fenton and McGlashan 1987b.
[7] Carpenter et al. 1990.
[8] Tsuang et al. 1981.
[9] Engelhardt et al. 1982.

Family and manifest illness variables were important in the second follow-up decade. Genetic predisposition (family history of schizophrenia) emerged with manifest illness as central to predicting outcome at three decades and beyond (McGlashan 1986d). Finally, predictors of outcome exist even for chronic schizophrenia. In the Chestnut Lodge Follow-up study, predictors accounted for approximately one-third of the outcome variance across six outcome dimensions (McGlashan 1986c).

Schizophrenic Nosology

Since we do not know its etiology or etiologies, the diagnosis of schizophrenia rests on manifestations of the disorder. Which manifestations are chosen to define cases with the disease constitutes the discipline of diagnostics or nosology. Several factors are important in constructing any particular set or "system" of diagnostic criteria, such as reliability, concordance with established clinical use, comprehensiveness, and specificity, or overlap and concordance across diagnosis (McGlashan 1984a). The factor most relevant to follow-up, however, is predictive validity, or the degree to which a set of diagnostic criteria can predict the long-term "behavior" of its identified constituents.

An early example of long-term follow-up being used in this way comes from Vaillant (1963). He retrospectively identified 12 cases of "remitting schizophrenia" (i.e., schizophrenic patients admitted to a state hospital in the early 1900s who remitted and were discharged). Follow-up more than 50 years later revealed that some patients remained well without further hospitalization. However, 75% of them were again hospitalized at some time for psychosis, and a portion of these remained chronic after relapse. Because of this, Vaillant contended that there exists no justification for separating the remitting schizophrenics from the broader class of schizophrenic patients. He used the evidence of long-term follow-up to contest the hypothesis that schizophrenia and remitting schizophrenia were different nosologic entities.

Predictive validity is usually estimated as the degree to which a given diagnostic system can predict long-term diagnostic stability, functional outcome, or specific functional states. In schizophrenia, the latter usually refer to chronically psychotic or defect end states. Table 6–4 summarizes the various diagnostic systems that have been tested for predictive validity by data from the North American long-term follow-up studies. "System stringency" in column 3 refers to the inclusiveness of a given diagnostic system, meaning the number of patients defined as schizophrenic out of the given sample. Roughly defined, these systems are considered broad or inclusive if they identify three-fourths or more of any sample as having schizophrenia and narrow or stringent if they identify one-third or less of the same sample as having schizophrenia. In Table 6–4, the degree of stringency of each system with the given follow-up sample is estimated roughly on a scale of 5.

As demonstrated in Table 6–4, there exists a rough positive correlation between diagnostic stringency and predictive power. The Feighner definite system is clearly both the most narrow and the most predictive of long-term diagnostic stability and poor outcome. The Feighner definite system, like the RDC, DSM-III, and Feighner probable systems, excludes patients with prominent affective symptoms. Like DSM-III, it excludes patients with a LOMI of less than 6 months. Unlike any other system, its criteria include items usually regarded as poor prognostic predictors, such as family history of schizophrenia, single marital status, or poor premorbid work/social functioning. Other diagnostic systems, including DSM-III, are less stringent and accordingly demonstrate a weaker correlation with long-term outcome and diagnostic stability.

Overall, the studies in Table 6–4 do not dispute the nosologic principle that the correlation of any diagnostic system to long-term outcome/diagnostic stability is proportional to the number of prognostic variables included as criteria (McGlashan 1984a; Stephens 1978). These prognostic variables may be defined as anything other than nonaffective cross-sectional signs and symptoms. Often they consist of factors that can be regarded as post-baseline (i.e., as outcomes of the illness process itself like functional inferiority or well-established psychopathology). Such criteria maximize the homogeneity of diagnostic samples. This may be an advantage for certain kinds of research, but it also renders the test of predictive validity less applicable and more an exercise in tautology.

The Vermont State Hospital findings are unique vis-à-vis schizophrenic nosology (Harding et al. 1987a, 1987b). The finding that long-term follow-up failed to distinguish between schizophrenic and nonschizophrenic patients challenges the assumption that outcome can specify or differentiate major nosologic entities. Furthermore, the finding that long-term outcome was no different for the DSM-III and the DSM-I schizophrenic patients challenges the utility of predictive validity for testing between different definitions of the same disorder. That is, it questions the assumed advantage of operationalized diagnosis. These findings may reveal that the forces of chronicity and institutionalization, when extant with sufficient length and strength, erode nosologic differences and transform distinctive psychopathologies into a homogeneous mass that defies differentiation with existing assessment methodologies. At the least, these interesting findings question many of our cherished assumptions, such as the two psychoses hypothesis of Kraepelin, and invite us to think again.

The long-term follow-up studies reviewed here support a broad definition of schizophrenia. Stringent systems and/or those that incorporate prognostic dimensions as diagnostic criteria may select narrower and smaller samples with

TABLE 6–4. Diagnostic systems tested for predictive validity by long-term follow-up

System	Follow-up study or sample	System stringency in given sample 1 = broad 5 = narrow	Predictive validity tested			Citation
			Correlation with poor functional outcome	Correlation with defect state	Diagnostically stable over follow-up	
New Haven Schizo-phrenia Index	Alberta 2	1	weak	weak		A, B
	Phipps	1	weak			C
	Chestnut Lodge	1	weak	weak	no	D
Schneider's First Rank Symptoms	Alberta 2	1	weak			A, B
	Phipps	5	weak			C
Taylor & Abrams (1978)	Phipps	2	weak			C
Feighner Definite	Alberta	2	5	strong		A
	Phipps	5	strong			C
	Iowa 500	5	strong			E
	Iowa 500	5			yes	F
	Chestnut Lodge	5	strong	strong	yes	D
Feighner Probable (without duration criterion)	Alberta 2	1	moderate			A
Non-Feighner or Atypical Schizo-phrenia	Iowa 500	2	moderate			G
Research Diagnostic Criteria	Phipps	4	strong			C
	Chestnut Lodge	3	moderate	moderate	intermediate	D
DSM-III	Phipps	5	strong			C
	Chestnut Lodge	3	moderate	moderate	intermediate	D
	Vermont State Hospital	3	weak			H

TABLE 6–4.   Diagnostic systems tested for predictive validity by long-term follow-up *(continued)*

System	Follow-up study or sample	System stringency in given sample 1 = broad 5 = narrow	Predictive validity tested			Citation
			Correlation with poor functional outcome	Correlation with defect state	Diagnostically stable over follow-up	
Washington IPPS 12-point Flexible System	Phipps	3	moderate			C
Hospital Diagnosis: DSM-I Schizophrenia	Phipps Vermont State Hospital	1	strong			C
		1	weak			H

[A] Bland and Orn 1979.
[B] Bland and Orn 1980a, 1980b.
[C] Stephens et al. 1982.
[D] McGlashan 1984a.
[E] Tsuang et al. 1979.
[F] Tsuang et al. 1981.
[G] Tsuang and Fleming 1986.
[H] Harding et al. 1987a, 1987b.

fewer false positives. But they also exclude many who probably have the disorder. Schizophrenia is heterogeneous. Some patients with the disorder do well at follow-up and should not, for this reason alone, be regarded as misdiagnosed. Good-outcome schizophrenia is not, in reality, an affective disorder, nor should it even be recategorized as such without compelling evidence from several domains in addition to long-term course. Other patients look good at baseline—the acute, remitting, good prognosis cases. However, long-term follow-up demonstrates repeatedly that a distinct proportion of these develop a chronic remitting or chronic unremitting course. For this reason, separating these patients off into diagnostic categories other than schizophrenia and its subtypes is also premature. Overall, until significant progress is made in reducing the heterogeneity of schizophrenia, its criteria should err in the direction of inclusiveness.

Implications

In summary, the North American follow-up studies have confirmed that schizophrenia is often a chronic disease, frequently disabling for a lifetime and with an outcome generally worse than that of other major functional mental illnesses. Although schizophrenia can be lethal, especially vis-à-vis increased suicide risk, the process does not appear to be progressively dementing as originally described. On the average, functional deterioration appears to plateau and even to relent somewhat after 5 to 10 years of manifest illness. Outcome overall is heterogeneous, but much of this bewildering variance can be accounted for by sample characteristics. Many of these characteristics are linked with or are expressions of psychopathology, such as diagnostic type of schizophrenia (broad versus narrow criteria); subtype; comorbidity; or dimensions of chronicity (LOMI, biological treatment resistance, age of onset, institutionalization). Other characteristics are more orthogonal to psychopathology, such as demography (gender, marital status, socioeconomic status, physical setting) and the sample's ratings on multiple "nondiagnostic" predictor variables, especially premorbid health. The careful assessment and reporting of such sample characteristics is vital for finding meaning amidst melange.

The North American long-term follow-up studies have not answered any questions about treatment. However, they have provided some interesting observations. The common occurrence of good outcome without treatment points to the existence of heterogeneity vis-à-vis treatment need and/or response. This, coupled with the notion of biological treatment resistance, suggests that fruitful advances in understanding schizophrenia may accrue by tracking how drug responsiveness segregates out meaningful subgroups. The North American long-term follow-up studies also suggest that schizophrenia may be quite malleable to prolonged environmental/psychosocial perturbations. These have negative potential if applied too intensively or ambitiously, but positive potential if applied steadily in a supportive, rehabilitative mode in the context of stable and unlimited continuity of care.

In this chapter, I have attempted to make the point by example that the more completely samples are described, both at baseline and follow-up, the more results can be compared meaningfully across studies. Accordingly, although future follow-up studies should try to incorporate as many of the outlined elements of methodology as possible, accurate and reliable descriptions of sample, diagnosis, and outcome are essential. At the very least, sample descriptions should include those variables listed in Tables 6-2 and 6-3. Baseline data should also provide sufficient sign and symptom data so that study patients can be diagnosed by any of the systems in Table 6–4 or rediagnosed by any system for schizophrenia of the future. Because comorbidity is the rule rather than the exception, diagnostic assessment should be dimensional and inclusive, not categorical and exclusive. Finally, outcome should be recognized as a multivariate construct. As with diagnosis and prognosis, outcome requires operationalization and calibrated specification for reliable assessment by trained observers.

The North American follow-up studies have taught us a great deal about schizophrenia thus far. Most importantly, they have taught us how to construct future studies that are substantive and meaningful.

References

American Psychiatric Association: Diagnostic and Statistical Manual: Mental Disorders. Washington, DC, American Psychiatric Association, 1952

American Psychiatric Association: Diagnostic and Statistical Manual of Mental Disorders, 2nd Edition. Washington, DC, American Psychiatric Association, 1968

American Psychiatric Association: Diagnostic and Statistical Manual of Mental Disorders, 3rd Edition. Washington, DC, American Psychiatric Association, 1980

Astrachan BM, Harrow M, Adler D, et al: A checklist for the diagnosis of schizophrenia. Br J Psychiatry 121:529–539, 1972

Bardenstein KK, McGlashan TH: Gender differences in affective, schizoaffective, and schizophrenic disorders: A review. Schizophrenia Research 3:159–172, 1990

Bland RC, Orn H: 14-year outcome in early schizophrenia. Acta Psychiatr Scand 58:327–338, 1978

Bland RC, Orn H: Schizophrenia: Diagnostic criteria and outcome. Br J Psychiatry 134:34–38, 1979

Bland RC, Orn H: Schizophrenia: Schneider's first-rank symptoms and outcome. Br J Psychiatry 137:63–68, 1980a

Bland RC, Orn H: Prediction of long-term outcome from presenting symptoms in schizophrenia. J Clin Psychiatry 41:85–88, 1980b

Bland RC, Parker JH, Orn H: Prognosis in schizophrenia: A ten-year follow-up of first admissions. Arch Gen Psychiatry 33:949–954, 1976

Brooks GW: Experience with the use of chlorpromazine and reserpine in psychiatry: With especial reference to the significance and management of extrapyramidal dysfunction. N Engl J Med 254:1119–1123, 1956

Brooks GW: Opening a rehabilitation house, in Rehabilitation of the Mentally Ill: Social and Economic Aspects (Publication No. 58). Edited by Greenblatt M, Simon B. Washington, DC, American Association for the Advancement of Science, 1959, pp 127–139

Brooks GW: Rehabilitation of hospitalized chronic schizophrenic patients, in Chronic Schizophrenia. Edited by Appleby L, Scher JM, Cumming J. Glencoe, IL, Free Press, 1960, pp 248–257

Brooks GW, Deane WN: The chronic mental patient in the community. Diseases of the Nervous System 26:85–90, 1965

Brooks GW, Deane WN, Laqueur P: Fifteen years of work therapy: Its impact on a mental hospital and its community. Diseases of the Nervous System, Supplement 31:161–165, 1970

Carpenter WT, Strauss JS: The prediction of outcome in schizophrenia IV: Eleven-year follow-up of the Washington IPSS cohort. J Nerv Ment Dis (in press)

Chittick RA, Brooks GW, Irons FS, et al: The Vermont Story: Rehabilitation of Chronic Schizophrenic Patients. Burlington, VT, Queen City Printers, 1961, pp 24–27

Clancy J, Tsuang MT, Norton B, et al: The Iowa 500: A comprehensive study of mania, depression and schizophrenia. Journal of the Iowa Medical Society 4:394–398, 1974

Deane WN, Brooks GW: Five year follow-up of chronic hospitalized patients, in Report from Vermont State Hospital. Waterbury, VT, September 1967

Dingman CW, McGlashan TH: Discriminating characteristics of suicides: Chestnut Lodge follow-up sample including patients with affective disorder, schizophrenia and schizoaffective disorder. Acta Psychiatr Scand 74:91–97, 1986

Endicott J, Spitzer RL, Fleiss JL, et al: The Global Assessment Scale. Arch Gen Psychiatry 33:766–771, 1976

Engelhardt DM, Rosen B, Feldman J, et al: A 15-year followup of 646 schizophrenic outpatients. Schizophr Bull 8:493–503, 1982

Feighner JP, Robins E, Guze SB, et al: Diagnostic criteria for use in psychiatric research. Arch Gen Psychiatry 26:57–63, 1972

Fenton WS, McGlashan TH: The prognostic significance of obsessive-compulsive symptoms in schizophrenia. Am J Psychiatry, 143:437–441, 1986

Fenton WS, McGlashan TH: Sustained remission in drug-free schizophrenic patients. Am J Psychiatry 144:1306–1309, 1987a

Fenton WS, McGlashan TH: Prognostic scale for chronic schizophrenia. Schizophr Bull 13:277–286, 1987b

Gardos G, Cole JO, LaBrie RA: A twelve-year follow-up study of 124 chronic hospitalized schizophrenics: I. Current psychosocial adjustment. Unpublished manuscript, 1982a

Gardos G, Cole JO, LaBrie RA: A twelve-year follow-up study of chronic schizophrenics. Hosp Community Psychiatry 33:983–984, 1982b

Harding CM, Brooks GW, Ashikaga T, et al: The Vermont longitudinal study of persons with severe mental illness: I. Methodology, study sample, and overall status 32 years later. Am J Psychiatry 144:718–726, 1987a

Harding CM, Brooks GW, Ashikaga T, et al: The Vermont longitudinal study of persons with severe mental illness, II. Long-term outcome of subjects who retrospectively met DSM-III criteria for schizophrenia. Am J Psychiatry 144:727–735, 1987b

Hawk AB, Carpenter WT, Strauss JS: Diagnostic criteria and five-year outcome in schizophrenia: A report from the International Pilot Study of Schizophrenia. Arch Gen Psychiatry 32:343–347, 1975

Hippocrates: The Genuine Works of Hippocrates. Translated by Adams F. New York, William Wood and Company, 1929, pp 43–59

Hollingshead AB, Redlich FC: Social Class and Mental Illness. New York, John Wiley, 1958

Kendler KS, Gruenberg AM, Tsuang MT: Outcome of schizophrenic subtypes defined by four diagnostic systems. Arch Gen Psychiatry 41:149–154, 1984

Lewine R, Burbach D, Meltzer HY: Effect of diagnostic criteria on the ratio of male to female schizophrenic patients. Am J Psychiatry 141:84–87, 1984

Lloyd D, Simpson JC, Tsuang MT: Are there sex differences in the long-term outcome of schizophrenia? Comparisons with mania, depression, and surgical controls. J Nerv Ment Dis 173:643–649, 1985

McGlashan TH: The borderline syndrome: II. Is borderline a variant of schizophrenia or affective disorder? Arch Gen Psychiatry 40:1319–1323, 1983

McGlashan TH: Testing four diagnostic systems for schizophrenia. Arch Gen Psychiatry 41:141–144, 1984a

McGlashan TH: The Chestnut Lodge follow-up study: I. Follow-up methodology and study sample. Arch Gen Psychiatry 41:573–585, 1984b

McGlashan TH: The Chestnut Lodge follow-up study: II. Long-term outcome of schizophrenia and the affective disorders. Arch Gen Psychiatry 41:586–601, 1984c

McGlashan TH: The Chestnut Lodge follow-up study: III. Long-term outcome of borderline personalities. Arch Gen Psychiatry 43:20–30, 1986a

McGlashan TH: Schizotypal personality disorder. Chestnut Lodge follow-up study: VI. Long-term follow-up perspectives. Arch Gen Psychiatry 43:329–334, 1986b

McGlashan TH: The prediction of outcome in chronic schizophrenia: IV. The Chestnut Lodge follow-up study. Arch Gen Psychiatry 43:167–176, 1986c

McGlashan TH: Predictors of shorter-, medium-, and longer-term outcome in schizophrenia. Am J Psychiatry 143:50–55, 1986d

McGlashan TH, Bardenstein KK: Gender differences in affective, schizoaffective and schizophrenic disorders: Analysis of the Chestnut Lodge follow-up cohorts. Schizophr Bull 16:319–329, 1990

McGlashan TH, Williams PV: Schizoaffective psychosis: II. Manic, bipolar, and depressive subtypes. Arch Gen Psychiatry 44:138–139, 1987

McGlashan TH, Carpenter WT, Bartico JJ: Issues of design and methodology in long-term follow-up studies. Schizophr Bull 14:569–574, 1988

Morrison J, Clancy J, Crowe R, et al: The Iowa 500: I. Diagnostic validity in mania, depression, schizophrenia. Arch Gen Psychiatry 27:457–461, 1972

Samson JA, Simpson JC, Tsuang MT: Outcome studies of schizoaffective disorders. Schizophr Bull 14:543–554, 1988

Schneider L: Clinical Psychopathology. New York, Grune & Stratton, 1959

Spitzer RL, Endicott J, Robins E: Research Diagnostic Criteria, 3rd Edition. New York, New York State Psychiatric Institute, 1977

Stephens JH: Long-term course and prognosis in schizophrenia. Seminars in Psychiatry 2:464–485, 1970

Stephens JH: Long-term prognosis and followup in schizophrenia. Schizophr Bull 4:25–47, 1978

Stephens JH, Astrup C: Prognosis in "process" and "non-process" schizophrenia. Am J Psychiatry 119:945–953, 1963

Stephens JH, Astrup C: Treatment of outcome in "process" and "nonprocess" schizophrenics treated by "A" and "B" types of therapists. J Nerv Ment Dis 140:449–456, 1965

Stephens JH, Astrup C, Mangrum JC: Prognostic factors in recovered and deteriorated schizophrenics. Am J Psychiatry 122:1116–1121, 1966

Stephens JH, Astrup C, Mangrum JC: Prognosis in schizophrenia: Prognostic scales cross-validated in American and Norwegian patients. Arch Gen Psychiatry 16:693–698, 1967

Stephens JH, Astrup C, Carpenter WT, et al: A comparison of nine systems to diagnose schizophrenia. Psychiatry Res 6:127–143, 1982

Stone MH: Exploratory psychotherapy in schizophrenia-spectrum patients: A reevaluation in the light of long-term follow-up of schizophrenic and borderline patients. Bull Menninger Clin 50:287–306, 1986

Strauss JS, Carpenter WT: The prediction of outcome in schizophrenia: I, Characteristics of outcome. Arch Gen Psychiatry 27:739–746, 1972

Strauss JS, Carpenter WT: The prediction of outcome in schizophrenia: II. Relationships between predictor and outcome variables: A report from the World Health Organization International Pilot Study of Schizophrenia. Arch Gen Psychiatry 31:37–42, 1974

Strauss JS, Carpenter WT: Prediction of outcome in schizophrenia: III. Five-year outcome and its predictors. Arch Gen Psychiatry 34:159–163, 1977

Taylor MA, Gaztanaga P, Abrams R: Manic-depressive illness and acute schizophrenia: a clinical family history and treatment response study. Am J Psychiatry 131:678–682, 1974

Tsuang MT: Familial subtyping of schizophrenia and affective disorders, in Critical Issues in Psychiatric Diagnosis. Edited by Spitzer RL, Klein DF. New York, Raven, 1978a, pp 203–211

Tsuang MT: Suicide in schizophrenics, manics, depressives, and surgical controls: A comparison with general population suicide mortality. Arch Gen Psychiatry 35:153–155, 1978b

Tsuang MT, Fleming JA: Long-term outcome of atypical schizophrenia. Paper presented at the annual meeting of the American Psychiatric Association, Washington, DC, May 1986

Tsuang MT, Winokur G: Criteria for subtyping schizophrenia: Clinical differentiation of hebephrenic and paranoid schizophrenia. Arch Gen Psychiatry 31:43–47, 1974

Tsuang MT, Winokur G: The Iowa 500: Field work in a 35-year follow-up of depression, mania, and schizophrenia. Canadian Psychiatric Association Journal 20:359–365, 1975

Tsuang MT, Woolson RF: Mortality in patients with schizophrenia, mania, depression and surgical conditions: A comparison with general population mortality. Br J Psychiatry 130:162–166, 1977

Tsuang MT, Woolson RF: Excess mortality in schizophrenia and affective disorders: Do suicides and accidental deaths solely account for this excess? Arch Gen Psychiatry 35:1181–1185, 1978

Tsuang MT, Woolson RF, Fleming JA: Long-term outcome of major psychoses: I. Schizophrenia and affective disorders compared with psychiatrically symptom-free surgical conditions. Arch Gen Psychiatry 39:1295–1301, 1979

Tsuang MT, Woolson RF, Fleming JA: Causes of death in schizophrenia and manic-depression. Br J Psychiatry 136:239–242, 1980a

Tsuang MT, Woolson RF, Fleming JA: Premature deaths in schizophrenia and affective disorders: An analysis of survival curves and variables affecting the shortened survival.

Arch Gen Psychiatry 37:979–983, 1980b

Tsuang MT, Woolson RF, Simpson JC: The Iowa structured psychiatric interview. Acta Psychiatr Scand Suppl 62:283, 1980

Tsuang MT, Woolson RF, Winokur G, et al: Stability of psychiatric diagnosis: Schizophrenia and affective disorders followed up over a 30- to 40-year period. Arch Gen Psychiatry 38:535–539, 1981

Vaillant GE: The prediction of recovery in schizophrenia. J Nerv Ment Dis 135:534–542, 1962

Vaillant GE: The natural history of the remitting schizophrenias. Am J Psychiatry 120:367–375, 1963

Vaillant GE: An historical review of the remitting schizophrenias. J Nerv Ment Dis 138:48–56, 1964a

Vaillant GE: Prospective prediction of schizophrenic remission. Arch Gen Psychiatry 11:509–518, 1964b

Vaillant GE: A 10-year followup of remitting schizophrenics. Schizophr Bull 4:78–85, 1978

Williams PV, McGlashan TH: Schizoaffective psychosis: I. Comparative long-term outcome. Arch Gen Psychiatry 44:130–137, 1987

World Health Organization: Mental Disorders: Glossary and Guide to Their Classification in Accordance with the Ninth Revision of the International Classification of Diseases. Geneva, World Health Organization, 1978

World Health Organization: Schizophrenia: An International Follow-up Study. New York, John Wiley, 1979

❖ 7 ❖   Effectiveness in Psychiatric Care: A Cross-National Study of the Process of Treatment and Outcomes of Major Depressive Disorder

Ira D. Glick, M.D.
Lorenzo Burti, M.D. (Italy)
Koji Suzuki, M.D. (Japan)
Michael Sacks, M.D. (United States)

Major depressions are severe and disabling illnesses that may afflict 5.1% of the general population at any time and 8.3% of the general population over the course of a lifetime (Regier et al. 1988). Fortunately, effective treatment of severe depression is now available; unfortunately, effectiveness is not always achieved (Kupfer and Freeman 1986). The treatment package includes at least four components to achieve an ideal resolution of an episode for patients and their families (Klerman 1986): 1) medication; 2) a psychosocial treatment intervention for the patient, such as individual supportive psychotherapy; 3) a psychosocial treatment intervention for the family, such as family supportive psychotherapy (Spencer et al. 1988); and 4) psychoeducation for both patient and family (Greenberg et al. 1988).

Clinical experience, and the trials that do exist, suggest that each of the four

The authors thank (in Italy) Professor M. Tansella, Cattedra i Psycologia Medica, Istituto di Psichiatria, Universita di Verona, for access to the case register; (in Japan) Drs. T. Yamaguchi, Y. Nogami, K. Okonogi, K. Maehara, K. Minakawa, M. Shimada, M. Miamoto, and N. Moriya for help in collecting the sample; and (in the United States) the Residents and Faculty of the Payne Whitney Clinic for help in collecting the sample, Gretchen Haas, Ph.D., for statistical help, and Drs. Donald F. Klein, David Kupfer, Herbert Pardes, Felton Earls, Joe Yamamoto, and Gerald Klerman for critical review of the manuscript.

Supported in part by a Fulbright Research Grant and an appointment as a Fellow of the Japan NIMH (to Dr. Glick in Japan, January–July 1987) and the Consiglio Nazionale delle Richerche, Progetto Finalizzato Medicina Preventiva e Riabilitativa 1982–1987, contract 84-02543-56 (to Dr. Tansella), and by the University of Verona School of Medicine (to Dr. Tansella).

Reprinted from *Journal of Nervous and Mental Disease* 179:55–63, 1991, with permission.

components has an additive effect. The opportunity to study the delivery of psychiatric care on three continents offered us the unique chance to investigate whether the hypothesized relationships of treatment delivery and achievement of treatment goals to outcome could be discerned despite vast cultural differences. In this chapter, we then report the results of a hypothesis-generating study of the issues involved in psychiatric treatments and outcomes.

Methodology

Rationale and Overview

What was the best way to study the question? The obvious design was to use methodology similar to the National Study of Medical Outcomes (the MOS study; Wells et al. 1989); however, such resources were not available. More importantly, by using this methodology, one of the most crucial features of treatment might be missed—that is, a more microscopic view of what actually happens in the interaction among doctor, patient, and family.

We utilized a strategy of asking (on a case-by-case basis) four basic questions that we believed to be related to good outcome: 1) what was wrong (i.e., the diagnostic process)? 2) how was it treated? 3) did the patient take the "prescription"? and 4) what was the role of the family in the process? Finally, we asked a fifth question: 5) how did the index episode turn out 1 year or more later? After that, we tried to piece together the process (i.e., do the commonly accepted, essential features of good care actually occur?) with the outcome.

Kinds of Answers

This study was not a controlled experiment. It was a review of what naturally occurs between patients and physicians in the settings and under the circumstances they have chosen. Thus, a major strength of the study was that it linked key variables (as we see them) and other explanatory variables to outcomes of care without interfering with those relationships. However, a major tradeoff is that the study could not infer causality.

Index Condition and Criteria Map

The first issue was to pick a psychiatric tracer condition that most people would agree exists and can be defined and rated in a relatively reliable and standard way. Mood disorders are the most prevalent of psychiatric disorders; major affective disorder (MAD) is well delineated in DSM-III (American Psychiatric Association 1980).

The next issue—and a crucial one—was to agree that there is an efficacious treatment for affective disorder. In 1989, most physicians would have accepted the data that suggest that what DSM-III-R (American Psychiatric Association 1987) calls mood disorder has a biological etiology (Klein et al. 1980) *and* that it can be precipitated by psychosocial stress (broadly defined; Brown and Harris 1978). On faith, even the most biologically oriented might agree that the family or significant other plays an important role in acute and chronic management.

Accordingly, most psychiatrists would agree that effective, "ideal" treatment for full resolution of an episode—meaning long-run effects on both patient and family—requires delivery of the combination of interventions mentioned in the introduction. On the other hand, because this was a naturalistic pilot study, if we did not find that, in fact, the variables related to outcome, we would be discouraged from entering into an experimental study of the related importance of the various components. Needless to say, how and to what extent these components are delivered will vary from country to country depending on the *structure* of care and particular sociocultural context. Accordingly, the study was done in three different countries—a European setting (Italy), an Asian setting (Japan), and the United States. We believed that the common denominators would generalize across most cultures in which the structure, like the providers and the money for the system, were in place.

Setting

We reasoned that if we were to study good care, we ought to do it in what were generally considered by our colleagues to be settings of excellence. Accordingly, in Italy the cases were obtained from a case register in the Department of Psychiatry at the medical school of the University of Verona in 1986 (Jablensky and Henderson 1983). In Japan, finding cases 1 year after treatment was not so easy (as they have no case register such as the one at the South Verona Community Mental Health Center), so we used three medical schools in Tokyo—Keio, Juntendo, and Nihon in 1987. In the United States, we used the outpatient clinic in the Department of Psychiatry at the Cornell University Medical College in 1987 and 1988.

Interviewing and Instruments

The next problem was how to find out what actually happened among patient, family, and doctor over the course of treatment extending up to 18 months.

The fundamental assumption was that "the truth" was something akin to a *Rashomon* story (Kemeny et al. 1984). Accordingly, we decided to separately interview the treating doctors, then the patient, then the family—and finally all together (as necessary and appropriate) to reconcile discrepancies. Each of the first three components of the interview lasted about 30 minutes. Family was defined broadly to include significant others (SOs). If necessary, other SOs were interviewed until the story made sense.

The interviews were conducted with a bilingual academic-psychiatrist-collaborator from the host country. Ratings were made independently. The need for on-the-spot consensual validation of what we were seeing and hearing made reliability ratings (in the strict sense) infeasible.

Because the interviews were done 12–18 months after the onset of the index episode, there was no good way around the issue of retrospective distortion. We did review hospital charts to ensure that the judgments we were making were consistent. We verified what happened by consensus and did the ratings of outcome on the spot.

As to the content of the interviews, the five broad questions discussed earlier (i.e., what was wrong, how was it treated, etc.) were explored. To obtain that information in replicable form, the following instruments were used.

The Criteria for Affective Disorder Form (Bech et al. 1986). This is a 9-item scale (adapted from DSM-III) to document the presence of signs and symptoms of major affective disorder at the time of the index episode. Data were obtained from the chart, physician, and patient/family. The Diagnostic Interview Schedule was not available to us when the study began.

A Quality Care Intervention Checklist. This scale, which was developed by one of us (Dr. Glick), systematically reviewed whether the criteria map was followed. It rated whether or not the doctor had delivered the following items to *both* the patient and the family: 1) interventions were designed to build a treatment *alliance*; 2) *psychoeducation* had been delivered to both patient and family; 3) the index episode had been placed in a *family context* (i.e., their dynamics, expectations, and relationships); 4) major *family problem areas* were identified (if present), and a focus for the family was identified; 5) the concepts of treatment and their relationship to problems and goals were explained (i.e., a *formulation*); and 6) treatment was prescribed, including psychotropic medication as well as individual and family psychotherapy (both broadly defined). For this variable, we made an additional judgment of the adequacy of medication trial (Klein et al. 1980)—meaning standard duration (e.g., an antidepressant of 4–6 weeks) and an appropriate dose (Binder et al. 1987) (e.g., 300–600 mg chlorpromazine and its equivalent of antipsychotics, 200–300 mg imipramine, and 900–2100 mg lithium with blood levels of 0.6–1.5 mEq/ml). In actuality, this judgment of adequacy, or inadequacy, of medication trial was very straightforward.

This scale scored whether and to what extent (either 0, "did not occur" or 1, "did occur") the practitioner(s) performed (i.e., delivered) the criteria. The focus was on the physician.

The Achievement of Practitioner Goals Scale. This questionnaire rated how well each of the above was achieved (on a scale of 0, "not achieved," to 5, "maximally achieved") for both patient and family. In addition, the scale included items on whether goals were agreed upon and how the patient and family understood the initial episode (e.g., in biological, psychological, or other idiosyncratic terms). This scale attempted to determine whether, given the mix of patient, family, and physician, the so-called ideal criteria were achieved. Accordingly, the focus was broader than just on the physician.

Global Rating of Resolution of Index Episode. This item was developed by us. It rated (also on a 0–5 point scale) how well the index episode resolved given the ideal goals of not only patient improvement, but also patient and family psychoeducation, as well as the rarely achieved change for the better (in terms of coping) for both the patient and family postepisode. For example, a good resolution might be if the patient was asymptomatic and both patient and family were coping and well educated as to the illness. It did not focus on "satisfaction."

Global Assessment Scale. The Global Assessment Scale (GAS) (Endicott et al. 1976) is a 100-point rating scale designed for the global assessment of the patient's overall level of functioning and severity of symptoms. The rating was done only at follow-up, because baseline ratings at the time of the index episode were not available. To deal with this problem, ratings of a subsample (using the charts) indicated the GAS ratings at admission were between 20 and 30, which was consistent with previous studies with this population.

Data Analyses Strategies

Our hypothesis was that effective treatment delivery (the quality care interventions) would be positively correlated with achievement of the practitioner goals of treatment, and that both of these (good treatment and reaching the goals) would correlate with good outcome (i.e., high resolution of index episode, and perhaps good global patient outcome).

This hypothesis was tested by comparing Spearman Rank Order correlation coefficients to test the magnitude of the associations between the resolution of the index episode/patient global outcome and both delivery of treatment and achievement of treatment goals. A second approach to testing this same hypothesis was to examine outcome for patients at the tails of the distribution of the data (i.e., mean ± 1 SD were defined as "best" and "worst" outcomes). For this analysis, we used one-tailed *t*-tests comparing "best" and "worst" resolutions (and outcomes) on the measures of 1) delivery of treatment and 2) achievement of practitioner goals. We used one-tailed tests because we hypothesized that medication, individual psychotherapy, and family psychotherapy would correlate positively with outcome. The second hypothesis was that the best resolutions (and patient outcomes) would have had more adequate treatment than those who had the worst resolutions and (outcomes). Z-tests were performed comparing the proportions of best versus worst cases on three parameters: adequacy of medication, delivery of individual therapy, and delivery of family psychotherapy.

Subjects

At each site, in less than 5 months we studied between 7 and 10 cases in depth. Although this may seem like a small number, the complexity of finding the cases; getting informed consent; and arranging for the patient, family, doctor, and interviewers (let alone the chart) to all get together at the same time were formidable. We asked for a consecutive series, rather than cases that went very well or very badly. In our opinion, in each country these patients were representative of the severely depressed and hospitalized.

Inclusion criteria included the following:

1. The patient had to be between ages 15 and 65.
2. The patient must have had a major affective disorder—either unipolar or bipolar. An important issue was the extent of symptom severity and of impairment. Although Hamilton scales were not done, the degree of severity and of impairment was judged by their physicians to have been enough to require hospitalization. Careful interviewing and chart review confirmed the clinical evaluation that these patients' lives had come to a functional standstill.
3. The acute episode must have been treated between 12 and 18 months prior to this interview.
4. The patient must have had a family or SOs available at the time of the index episode.

We were able to complete 7 cases in Italy, 7 in the United States, and 10 in Japan (N = 24). This resulted in more than 75 interviews (one each for physician, patient, and family—and some "synthesis" interviews for clarification). We were not able to define the sample that was not included, but we believe that our cases were those who did well rather than poorly because most were still connected to the system.

Demographics, Diagnosis, and Prognosis

Table 7–1 describes the sample diagnoses, demographics, and a judgment of prognosis (vide infra).

TABLE 7–1. Sample diagnosis, demographics, and estimate of prognosis

Country	N	Major depressive disorder	Bipolar disorder	Other disorder	Age (SD)	Sex M F	Married	Single, divorced, separated, widowed	Good	Poor
		Primary diagnosis			Age	Sex	Marital status		Judgment of prognosis	
Italy	7	5	0	1—SAD 1—DD	49.3 (7.0)	5 2	2	5	3	4
Japan	10	8	1	1—DD	43.8 (15.4)	5 5	7	3	9	1
United States	7	4	3	0	38.6 (16.9)	4 3	1	6	6	1
Combined	24	17	4	3	43.9 (14.2)	14 10	10	14	18	6

SAD = Schizoaffective disorder. DD = Dysthymic disorder.

As for the diagnosis, although all patients were referred to the study as having major affective disorder as diagnosed by faculty, after interview and chart review we judged that one Italian patient and one Japanese patient had dysthymic disorder, and one Italian patient had a schizoaffective disorder. Although there were pros and cons regarding our decision, we kept these patients in the sample. We decided to do this because all of these patients needed similar quality case interventions (i.e., medication, psychotherapy, and so on) and this was a pilot study of effectiveness of such interventions, so there was more to be gained by including the patients than by excluding them (thereby decreasing the sample size).

As level of prehospital functioning plus diagnosis (both psychiatric and medical—e.g., alcoholism or chronic heart disease) could affect global outcome (i.e., how much change was possible), we believed it important to make a judgment of prognosis. We made a dichotomous rating of good or poor prognosis for each patient in each country (Table 7–1). We judged six patients to be rated as having "poorer prognosis"—four from Italy, one from Japan, and one from the United States. The reasons were that in addition to the affective disorder, two patients had chronic alcoholism; one early dementia; one a long-standing, dependent personality disorder; one a borderline personality disorder; and one a schizoaffective disorder.

Informed consent procedures were followed according to the standards for each country.

Results

How Well Did the Index Episode Resolve? And Did the Resolution Correlate With Delivery of Treatment and Achievement of Treatment Goals?

Table 7–2 reveals that although (as expected) most patients and families had positive resolution of the index episode from the time of hospitalization, resolution averaged only about 3 on the 5-point scale. There was little difference among countries; in fact, when the one outlier was removed from the Italian sample, the mean rating was also 3.1.

How well did the resolution correlate with the delivery of interventions? There were positive correlations of high physician delivery of treatment to patient and family with better resolution of episode ($P < .008$ for the patient, $P < .04$ for the family, and $P < .006$ for the combined score).

How well did the resolution correlate with achievement of treatment goals? Table 7–2 reveals positive correlations between better patient and family achievement of goals of treatment with greater resolution of the index episode ($P < .04$ for the patient, $P < .005$ for the family, and $P < .005$ for both combined).

These correlations can be seen more clearly in an analysis of the best and the worst resolutions, using the tails of the sample. The "worst" group (cases scoring less than 2) was composed of one patient (Italian) for whom the resolution was unchanged and four patients (one American, one Italian, and two Japanese) for whom the resolution was minimal. The best group (cases scoring 4 and above) was composed of eight maximal resolutions (two Italian, three Japanese, and three American). There was no significant difference in gender between groups, although most of both the best and worst groups were male.

Analysis of the data from the two groups (Table 7–3) revealed that the group with the worst resolutions received significantly less combined treatment ($P < .02$; both patient and family) than the "best" group (i.e., almost one-half as much treatment, or 3.3 compared to 1.8 on the 5-point scale). Furthermore, when analyzing the treatment data, for the "worst resolution" cases, it was found that although four of five patients did receive medication, none of these cases had adequate trials compared to eight of eight who received adequate trials of the "best resolution" cases ($P < .002$).

Only two of five families in the "worst" received family intervention com-

TABLE 7–2.   Association of achievement of practitioner goals with patient/family resolution of the index episode and to patient global outcome for the total sample

Country	N	Means of achievement of all 8 practitioner goals (0–5)			Resolution of index episode (0–5)	Patient global outcome (0–100)
		Patient Mean	Family Mean	Combined Mean		
Italy	7	3.3	2.1	2.7	2.7	51
Japan	10	2.9	1.9	2.4	3.1	76
United States	7	3.4	2.5	3.0	3.1	71
All countries combined	24	3.2	2.2	2.7	3.0	66

Correlation Coefficients:[a]

Achievement of goals by	Resolution of index episode		Patient global outcome	
Patient	.52	($P < .04$)	.13	(NS)
Family	.51	($P < .005$)	.31	($P < .07$)
Combined	.52	($P < .005$)	.26	(NS)

[a] Correlations are Spearman Rank-Order correlations, showing two-tailed level of significance.

pared to seven of eight in the "best" group, but the difference was not significant. And of these two families, in one case the wife wanted to separate (resulting in the patient becoming more symptomatic); and in the other, the mother was so distraught and thought-disordered herself that the therapy was useless.

What was the Patient's Global Outcome?

Table 7–2 shows that the mean global patient score was 66—about what could be expected for MAD. An analysis of the best and worst outcomes revealed a trimodal distribution. We used a cutting score on the GAS of 55 (mean −1 SD), or less for worst outcomes, and 80 (mean +1 SD) and above for best outcomes, resulting in seven cases of each.

Of note, Table 7–4 shows that there is an association of global outcome and the means of the achievement of the practitioner goals for these cases. Although there was no difference between best and worst groups in what the patients achieved (3.1 and 2.9, respectively), the families of the worst outcome patients achieved only about half of what the best did (1.5 to 2.8, $P < .10$).

Likewise, it was striking that all seven patients who had best outcomes received adequate medication trials, whereas none of the worst outcomes did ($P < .001$).

TABLE 7–3.   Association between best and worst resolutions of index episode with treatment received and achievement of practitioner goals

Resolution of index episode	N	Adequate medication prescribed[a]	Individual psychotherapy[b]	Family psychotherapy[c]	Means of achievement of all 8 practitioner goals (on scale of 0–5)		
					Pt.[d]	Fam.[e]	Combined[f] Mean
Best	8	8	8	7	3.4	3.2	3.3
Worst	5	0	5	2	2.2	1.3	1.8

Z-tests were performed comparing the proportion of best versus the proportion of worst cases receiving each of the above:

    a $Z = 2.94$; $P < .002$
    b $Z = 0.73$; NS
    c $Z = 1.14$; NS

One-tailed t-tests were performed comparing the means for best versus worst cases on measures of achievements of practitioner goals for the patient, the family, and both combined:

    d $t = 1.82$; df = 11; $P < .10$
    e $t = 2.64$; df = 11; $P < .03$
    f $t = 2.75$; df = 11; $P < .02$

TABLE 7–4.   Association between best and worst patient global outcomes with treatment received and achievement of practitioner goals

Global outcome	N	Number receiving			Means of achievement of practitioner goals (on scale of 0–5)		
		Adequate medication[a]	Individual psychotherapy[b]	Family psychotherapy[c]	Pt.[d]	Fam.[e]	Mean[f]
Best	7	7	7	4	3.1	2.8	3.0
Worst	7	0	7	3	2.9	1.5	2.2

Z-tests were performed comparing the proportion of best versus proportion of worst cases receiving each of the above:

    a $Z = 3.21$; $P < .001$
    b   NS
    c   NS

T-tests were performed comparing the means for best versus worst cases of measures of achievement of practitioner goals for the patient, the family, and both combined:

    d $t = 3.27$; df = 12, NS
    e $t = 1.80$; df = 12, $P < .10$
    f $t = 1.82$; df = 12; $P < .10$

To What Degree Were the Quality Care Interventions Delivered?

As mentioned, this questionnaire rated whether or not the practitioner actually delivered the interventions, rather than achieved success with patient and family—using a 0 (not delivered) to 1.0 (delivered) and presumed ideal rating.

For all countries combined, a mean score of the eight items for the patient was 0.67, whereas for the family it was only 0.37, for a combined mean of interventions for patient plus family of 0.52. In examining the means, we observed that the main difference across countries was that the United States delivered more treatment to both patient and family than Italy and Japan. (Statistical tests between and among countries were not performed because of small sample size; more importantly, the study was not intended to provide a controlled comparison across countries.)

Examining each of the eight "delivery" items, we can see for the *alliance* item, all countries did well with the patient, but with the families, the delivery was much lower. We will discuss *psychoeducation* in a separate publication, but for now let us say that more was done with patients (.7) and less with family (.5)—especially in Italy and Japan.

As to putting the problem in the context of the families and examining their problem and goals, this was done in a very low proportion of both patient and family cases in all countries, with Japan doing least in these areas. The case formulation item revealed that it was done moderately (.6) for the patient and less often for the family (.3). The score was pulled down by the fact that in Italy, physicians are reluctant to explain what they are doing because they believe they may be promoting patient dependency; in Japan, practitioners do not do much explaining to families because of time pressures and for cultural and other reasons, including stigma.

As to treatment delivered, virtually all cases had medication prescribed (0.92—although, as discussed, often inadequate) and individual psychotherapy, but less than half of families received family intervention. Italy made the most attempt to deliver interventions with the family.

To What Degree Were the Practitioner Goals Achieved?

This item (Table 7–5) examined how well the practitioner achieved his goals (i.e., the quality care criteria, on a scale of 0—not at all, to 5—presumed ideal). This rating involved an interaction of doctor, patient, and family.

The means for achievement was 3.2 for patients and 2.2 for families, for a combined mean of 2.7 (out of a possible 5—i.e., about 54%, which is much less than what might be considered clinically ideal). Italy and United States achieved about equal levels of care, and Japan less.

As to the individual items, first in terms of forming an alliance, the alliance achieved was almost twice as good with patients (4.1) as with families (2.3; $t = 4.01$, df = 23, $P < .001$). There was very poor achievement in helping patients or their families to understand the relation of the systems to the family context, recognizing major family problem areas (causing or resulting from the illness), or achieving psychoeducation (vide infra). There was good agreement on setting goals with patients (3.3 out of 5), but (as with the development of an "alliance") less with families (only 2.1 out of 5; $t = 3.68$, df = 23, $P < .001$). Comparing countries, the United States did most with establishing an alliance, achieving psychoeducation, and setting goals with the family.

As to treatment criteria achieved, there was better achievement of acceptance of medication—3.9 out of 5 ($t = 2.18$, df = 23, $P < .04$)—and individual psychotherapeutic intervention, 4.3 ($t = 3.71$, df = 23, $P < .001$), than family supportive intervention, 2.8. There was little difference across countries.

Discussion

What do the data mean? Some might argue that an almost two-thirds resolution of an episode is good, given the limitations of our knowledge about mental illness and the realistic, human limitations of doctors, patients, and families.

TABLE 7–5. Comparison of achievement of practitioner goals for all countries combined and across countries

Means of achievement of practitioner goals on 0 (not at all) to 5 (maximal) scale

Country	N	Patient/ family formed alliance		Patient/ family understood relation of symptoms to family context		Patient/ family recognized major family problem areas		Patient/ family understood concept of biological components of illness present (psycho-education)		Patient/ family agreed on goals		Patient accepted medication and family supported compliance		Patient/family accepted psychosocial support		Means for all items combined		
		P	F	P	F	P	F	P	F	P	F	P	F	Individual therapy	Family therapy	P	F	Both P and F
Italy	7	4.0	2.1	2.6	2.0	2.7	1.4	2.6	2.0	3.0	1.6	3.7	3.1	4.7	2.7	3.3	2.1	2.7
Japan	10	4.3	3.1	2.3	1.3	2.4	1.4	0.5	0.3	3.1	1.9	3.5	3.7	4.3	2.9	2.9	1.9	2.4
USA	7	3.9	2.7	1.7	1.3	1.9	1.1	3.7	3.1	3.9	3.0	4.7	3.6	4.0	2.9	3.4	2.5	3.0
All countries combined	24	4.1	2.3	2.2	1.5	2.3	1.3	2.0	1.6	3.3	2.1	3.9	3.5	4.3	2.8	3.2	2.2	2.7

That aside, the obvious limitations in sample selection and size, reliability, and validity, as well as the fact that a correlative study is far from an experimental study, make interpretation difficult. Nevertheless, we will examine the results across countries and then look at the contribution of practitioner, patient, and family as well as their interactions.

The data suggest that, regardless of country, *the better the delivery of treatment, the higher the achievement of treatment goals.* Such achievement is associated with better resolution of the episode for the patient and the family both in terms of current patient functioning and readiness for future contingencies. To that end, and given the limitations of the data, the treatment interventions that may need most strengthening are as follows: 1) prescribing adequate medication and providing supportive family psychotherapy; 2) examining the family context in which the illness develops and in which it (the illness) will later have important effects; 3) providing patient and family psychoeducation; 4) formulating the diagnosis and treatment plans with patient and family; and 5) forming a better alliance with the family. Conversely, poor treatment was associated with inadequate resolution and poor outcome.

Across countries, it is important to take cognizance of different cultural patterns and the histories of modern medicine in each country. For example, the most cogent issue in Italy is the fact that in 1978 there was a major restructuring of the delivery of mental health services, with a shift from inpatient to outpatient care and a lessening of the "therapeutic distance" of the physician to the patient and the family (Mosher 1983). Modern diagnostic and psychopharmacologic practices are slowly being introduced in Italy as efficacy studies provide guidelines for treatment, and the model is weighted toward psychosocial issues.

In Japan, there are well-known cultural prohibitions, especially stigma and limits of time, that work against full disclosure to patient and family of diagnosis and treatment (Ohnuki-Tierney 1984). In addition, Japanese psychiatry has been heavily influenced by German psychiatry and is weighted toward psychobiological issues.

Accordingly, although the Italians worked more with families, the treatment teams in Italy were reluctant to do psychoeducation for fear of scapegoating the patient. Both Italy and Japan delivered lower doses of medication than the United States in order to try to avoid side effects, which they believed would increase patient and family noncompliance and cause treatment dropouts. In a future publication, we will elaborate on cultural differences and describe in detail the treatment interactions among physician, patient, and family.

A Quality Treatment Equation

What this study has not disproved is that quality treatment for the kind of severe psychiatric illness for which medical intervention can alter the natural course (and, we speculate, for most chronic medical illness as well) requires a combination of ingredients. Each is necessary but by itself insufficient to achieve optimal outcome over the long run for both patient and family. The reason for this is that medical management for chronic illness in the 1990s is complicated and multimodal. It requires a coalition of doctor, patient, and family and must be fueled by the motivation to work together for goals in addition to symptom relief. A useful quality-treatment equation is optimal resolution of episode results from correct diagnosis plus appropriate treatment plus patient compliance plus family compliance. Let us examine each element of the equation.

Diagnosis

In many cases, the physician did not use standard nomenclature such as that in ICD-9 or DSM-III, but preferred sociodynamic models. If MAD was not diagnosed, then most (but not all) of necessary treatment was not prescribed. Occasionally, the wrong diagnosis was made, but part of the right treatment was prescribed as part of a "polypharmacy" prescription. In other cases, the doctor made the diagnosis but either did not communicate it or the patient or the family did not believe or accept it.

Treatment

There were a variety of reasons why treatment was not given in certain cases. Most commonly, it was because the diagnosis was not made. In other cases, it was because the doctor did not know about the treatment (usually psychoeducation), did not believe in it (medication, psychotherapy), or did not know how to deliver it. For example, depending on the country, many physicians do not believe in psychobiological treatment (Keller et al. 1986), whereas for others, working with a patient's family is almost unheard of (Glick et al. 1982). Psychoeducation, delivered in a systematic and ongoing way to both patient and family, was generally not carried out in any of the three countries—perhaps because data on its effectiveness are not yet available.

The prime example of problems in treatment delivery was psychopharmacologic practices. Polypharmacy in Italy and Japan was rampant (Binder et al. 1987). For example, unipolar depressive disorder was treated with a combination of two or sometimes three antidepressants in low doses (e.g., 100 mg imipramine as a maximal dose); an antianxiety agent; a sleeping pill; and sulpiride, a new antipsychotic.

Lack of awareness of newer treatment practices was a common problem (Hawkins 1979). In Italy and Japan, the shortages of teachers compared to the large number of residents in training placed undue reliance on the knowledge of a few dedicated professors who could not be expected to be knowledgeable in all areas (Hawkins 1979). In the United States, where there were more teachers, lack of awareness of the data in the literature or lack of motivation or resources (i.e., time or personal interest) sometimes led to nonstandard treatment practices, such as not involving the family in the patient's therapy.

Patient Compliance

It is one thing for the doctor to make the correct diagnosis and prescribe the appropriate treatment; it is quite another for the patient to comply. What was most striking (and tragic) was the lack of understanding most patients had about their illness and what to do about it. Part of the reason was the cognitive impairment associated with psychiatric illness (in marked contrast to most medical illness). But part was due to the lack of a dialogue between patient and physician in terms of case formulation, psychoeducation, or the role of the patient as a partner on the treatment team. In other cases, the family actively opposed treatment. (For example, one patient's spouse was a Jehovah's Witness who pressured the patient not to take medication.) As such, it was virtually impossible for patients to have the motivation, the discipline, or the understanding of why they should adhere to the complicated quality care regimens of combined treatments currently practiced. In other cases, psychodynamic considerations overrode medical prescription.

Family Compliance

The most striking finding from our study was that, despite general acceptance by doctors of the importance of the family during the acute phase of treatment, there was often a total lack of family involvement as partners on the treatment team. In Japan and sometimes in the United States, the family is often involved, but only in a very brief session with the physician, who assumes an authority role. The time is very limited, in part because the fee is so low and thus it is difficult to spare sufficient time for psychoeducation (J. Yamamoto, M.D., May 1989, personal communication). By way of example, in Japan, one patient's wife had a relatively good understanding of the biology and treatment of affective disorder but was afraid to discuss it with her husband. She told us she thought because she had never spoken to the treating physician, it was best not to discuss anything about her husband's illness—even though it had drastically (and negatively) affected their relationship.

In other cases, the family (for reasons specific to each system) negatively affected the treatment. For example, in a case in Italy, the family (the patient's children) told us that they had felt bullied by their father all their lives. After their mother died, they took their revenge by not involving themselves in their father's treatment, although they were continually invited by the treatment team to join in. Not only that, the patient's children discouraged his use of medications, playing into his ambivalence. On the other hand, the treatment team had filled the void left by the patient's children and had set up a very solid supportive relationship with the patient.

Summary and Disclaimers

This study has examined the process of quality medical care in three changing societies using "major depressive disorder" as the index condition and examining patient, family, and doctor encounters in those circumstances. The study's principal finding is that quality care is an ideal that is often not fully attained.

The methodological problems described certainly made the data suspect. The retrospective assessment of initial status and subsequent outcome could have been inaccurate or biased, and we did not make a systematic study of psychiatric care in any of the three countries. But the data, case syntheses, and observations of and interviews with patients, families, and doctors all suggested that the care given was uneven and was incomplete in one or another component. On the other hand, not all cases need all treatments. Differential diagnosis and treatment, rather than a shotgun approach, for a particular patient/family at a certain point in time is that to which we aspire.

By and large, our findings suggested that, for the United States, care was largely determined by how well biologic or dynamic models could be integrated. In Japan, care was clearly biologic, with little time spent "talking" to patients or their families. In Italy, there was a heavy emphasis on social psychiatry and less on medical-model psychiatry, especially in northern Italy. However, treatment in southern Italy was heavily biologic in orientation and in that respect resembled care such as that administered in Japan (Mosher 1983).

Controlled studies, including cross-cultural ones, are needed to examine these suggestive findings.

References

American Psychiatric Association: Diagnostic and Statistical Manual of Mental Disorders, 3rd Edition. Washington, DC, American Psychiatric Association, 1980

American Psychiatric Association: Diagnostic and Statistical Manual of Mental Disorders, 3rd Edition, Revised. Washington, DC, American Psychiatric Association, 1987

Bech P, Kastrup M, Rafaelsen OJ: Mini-compendium of rating scales for states of anxiety depression mania schizophrenia with corresponding DSM-III syndromes. Acta Psychiatr Scand Suppl No. 326, 7:5–37, 1986

Binder RL, Kazamatsuri H, Nishimura T, et al: Tardive dyskinesia and neuroleptic-induced parkinsonism in Japan. Am J Psychiatry 144:1494–1496, 1987

Brown WG, Harris T: Social origins of depression. A study of psychiatric disorders in women. New York, Free Press, 1978

Endicott J, Spitzer R, Fleiss J, et al: The Global Assessment Scale. Arch Gen Psychiatry 33:766–771, 1976

Glick ID, Showstack JA, Klar HM: Toward the definition and delivery of appropriate care. Am J Psychiatry 139:908–909, 1982

Greenberg L, Fine SB, Cohen C, et al: An interdisciplinary psychoeducation program for schizophrenic patients and their families in an acute care setting. Hosp Community Psychiatry 39:277–282, 1988

Hawkins DR: Impressions of psychiatric education in Western European specialty training. Arch Gen Psychiatry 36:713–717, 1979

Jablensky A, Henderson J: Report on a visit to the South Verona Community Psychiatric Service (WHO Assignment Report). Copenhagen and Geneva, World Health Organization, 1983

Keller MB, Lavori PW, Klerman GL, et al: Low levels and lack of predictors of somatotherapy and psychotherapy received by depressed patients. Arch Gen Psychiatry 43:458–466, 1986

Kemeny ME, Hargreaves WA, Gerbert B, et al: Measuring adequacy of physician performance, a preliminary comparison of four methods in ambulatory care of chronic obstructive pulmonary disease. Med Care 22:620–631, 1984

Klein DF, Gittelman R, Quitkin F, et al: Diagnosis and Drug Treatment of Psychiatric Disorders: Adults and Children, 2nd Edition. Baltimore, Williams and Wilkins, 1980, p 225

Klerman GL: Drugs and psychotherapy, in Handbook of Psychotherapy and Behavior Change, 3rd Edition. Edited by Garfield S, Bergin AE. New York, John Wiley, 1986, pp 777–818

Kupfer DJ, Freedman DX: Treatment for depression. "Standard" clinical practice as an unexamined topic. Arch Gen Psychiatry 43:509–511, 1986

Mosher LR: Recent development in the care, treatment, and rehabilitation of the chronic mentally ill in Italy. Hosp Community Psychiatry 34:947–950, 1983

Ohnuki-Tierney E: Illness and culture in contemporary Japan. Cambridge, Cambridge University Press, 1984, pp 224–225

Regier DA, Boyd JH, Burke JD, et al: One-month prevalence of mental disorders in the United States based on five epidemiologic catchment area sites. Arch Gen Psychiatry

45:977–986, 1988

Spencer JH, Glick ID, Haas GL, et al: A randomized clinical trial of inpatient family intervention: III, Overall effects on follow-up for the entire sample. Am J Psychiatry 145:1115–1121, 1988

Wells KB, Stewart A, Hays RD, et al: The functioning and well-being of depressed patients: Results from the Medical Outcomes Study. JAMA 262:914–919, 1989

❖ 8 ❖   Course and Treatment Outcome in Patients with Mania

Mauricio Tohen, M.D., Dr. P.H.

The Need for Treatment Outcome Studies

The ability to predict the most likely outcome of a psychiatric disorder is an important clinical and public health consideration. Clinicians' decisions regarding the necessity and the duration of hospital treatment are increasingly being scrutinized by utilization reviewers, third-party payers, and managed care organizations. At times, the relationship is adversarial, yet none of the parties has clear data to support its position clearly. In this context, it is desirable that studies evaluating the risks, benefits, and costs of psychiatric treatment be carried out. Understanding more about the relationship of clinical treatment to patient outcome will help mental health policy planners make informed decisions on the allocation of scarce resources. Finally, outcome measurement is now also part of the standard armamentarium of those who evaluate the quality of mental health care (Fauman 1989). The Joint Commission on Accreditation of Hospitals (Joint Commission on Accreditation of Hospitals 1986) has reemphasized the importance of outcome monitoring as an important yardstick for hospital-based quality assurance programs. This chapter will review the course and outcome of patients with mania who in the majority of cases will require long-term treatment, including repeated hospitalizations.

The Prevalence of Mania

Accurate estimation of the incidence of mania is difficult, due in part to problems inherent in obtaining person-time risk data. Most prevalence estimates of mania are obtained from treatment facilities and therefore correspond to "treated" mania (Tsuang et al. 1988). However, the National Institute of Mental Health (NIMH) Epidemiologic Catchment Area Study (ECA) (Regier et al. 1984, 1988; Robins et al. 1984) did provide true prevalence rates for mania in

127

TABLE 8–1. One-month prevalence for mania (Epidemiologic Catchment Area Study)*

	Men	Women
All ages	0.3	0.4
18–24	0.4	0.8
25–44	0.5	0.6
45–64	0.2	0.2
65+	0.0	0.0

*Source: Regier et al. 1988.
Data is provided in percentages.

the general population, stratified by age and gender (see Table 8–1). The ECA data suggests that 0.4–0.8% of the people in this country experience a manic episode at some point (Robins et al. 1984). Because the vast majority of such episodes require psychiatric hospitalization, this illness has a major impact on the health care resources of the nation.

In order to best serve the needs of this clinical population, it is important for clinicians, hospital administrators, and mental health policy planners to develop a clear understanding of the various outcomes of mania in both treated and untreated populations.

In addition, because outcome is most likely heterogeneous, it is also critical to identify those factors that predict both recovery and relapse for various subgroups of manic patients.

Natural Course of Mania

In the mid-19th century, Falret (1854) described the course and prognosis of affective disorders. In the early 1900s, Kraepelin (1904) emphasized the importance of longitudinal outcome data in differentiating the major psychoses. He described manic-depressive psychosis as characterized by an episodic course with periods of recovery and normal functioning, and a generally good prognosis. More recent studies, however, suggest a less optimistic outcome for this disorder (Bratfos and Haug 1968; Carlson et al. 1974; Cassidy et al. 1955; Fahndrich and Wirtz 1987; Hastings 1958; Shobe and Brion 1971). In explaining this discrepancy, Zis and Goodwin (1979) concluded that methodological differences most likely account for the inconsistencies across studies. Nonsystematic sampling, loss of patients to follow-up, and the lack of comparability of both diagnostic criteria and outcome measures utilized across studies are among the prominent methodological problems. Lavori and colleagues (1984) came to similar conclusions after reviewing the data for major depression.

Another problem encountered in reviewing the literature on mania has to do with the use of diagnostic terms. In the earlier literature, patients given a diagnosis of manic-depressive illness sometimes included individuals with psychotic depression who had never experienced manic episodes. In addition, diagnoses were most often established on the basis of clinical impression, as opposed to the use of structured diagnostic interviews. Nonetheless, on the basis of more recent clinical/epidemiologic data, it is estimated that 60–80% of the cases of bipolar disorder initially present with a manic episode (Goodwin and Jamison 1984). In addition, approximately 10% of patients initially diagnosed with major depression will, at some point in the course of their illness, develop a manic episode (Clayton 1981). Thus, a clear distinction between bipolar and unipolar affective disorder is difficult to make without the longitudinal follow-up or until the patient experiences a manic episode (Dunner et al. 1976). With regard to the latter, Winokur and co-workers (1969) reported that the average course of an episode of mania is about 4 months. However, recent studies suggest that functional impairment may continue long after symptomatic recovery has taken place (Dion et al. 1988).

In studies of clinical course and outcome, there are again methodologic issues to consider. In some studies, illness episodes were only considered to have occurred if hospitalization was required. Not surprisingly, in studies where the criteria for relapse did *not* include hospitalization, higher rates of relapse were reported (Angst 1968; Zis and Goodwin 1979). Another source of discrepancy in these outcome studies is related to the duration of observation. This is most evident in the percentage of patients reported to have had single episodes of mania, which ranges from zero to 58% across studies (Zis and Goodwin 1979).

In exploring the natural course of mania, Angst (1968) conducted a 20-year follow-up of patients with affective disorders at the University Clinic in Zurich, Switzerland. The sample included 95 patients with bipolar disorder who were followed from the onset of their illness. The average length of follow-up was 19 years. In this group of patients, 15% had no relapse after recovering from the initial index episode. Later age of onset was a predictor of higher rate of recurrence. The study also suggested that the number of symptom-free intervals of euthymia seem to decrease with age and with the number of previous episodes. Angst also reported that the duration of euthymic episodes tended to plateau after the fourth episode and usually lasts 8 to 12 months. He suggested that early-onset bipolar patients be treated prophylactically until age 65 and that late-onset cases be treated until age 75.

The average frequency of manic episode was one every other year. These findings are consistent with more recent studies (Keller et al. 1986; Tohen 1988;

Tohen et al. 1990a) that also suggest that bipolar illness is not always a benign, remitting illness, but rather has a variable prognosis ranging from complete recovery to functional incapacitation.

Methodologic Issues

Issues of study design. Sackett and Gent (1979) defined two types of outcome studies, the explanatory trial and the management trial. The primary goal of the explanatory trial (i.e., the randomized clinical trial) is to determine whether a specific treatment works under controlled circumstances. The management trial is an outcome study wherein outcome is measured in a clinical setting under conditions that are *not* under the investigator's control. In the explanatory trial, the inclusion of subjects is restricted to those who have agreed to participate in the study (e.g., to take the medication). As most clinicians know, this study design does not always reflect clinical reality, in that patients with poor compliance and those who require complex treatments (e.g., combinations of treatments, multiple medications, and/or psychotherapeutic techniques) are simply not represented.

Until recently, most outcome studies used cross-sectional, as opposed to longitudinal, analysis methods. Yet the latter provide higher statistical power and more continuous description of patients over an entire follow-up period. Another methodologic consideration is that most studies have looked for statistical significance, as opposed to the magnitude of association. Unfortunately, P values, as a criterion for statistical significance, may be misleading, because they are highly influenced by sample size. For example, in a study in which only a few cases are observed, results may not reach statistical significance because of Type II error. On the other hand, in a study involving hundreds of cases, a relatively minor association may be highly statistically significant.

Double-blind placebo controlled and naturalistic studies. It is often said that double-blind placebo controlled treatment studies (e.g., comparing lithium to placebo in the treatment of mania) are needed to accurately assess the efficacy of various treatments for mania. Indeed, such studies would be interesting, particularly in "first-episode" patients, because it is likely that in such a sample there would be a smaller probability of bias toward adverse selection of potentially nonresponsive chronic patients. It should be noted that double-blind clinical trials do not completely solve the problem of bias.

In some double-blind studies, patient selection criteria are not clearly spelled out, and relapse information is only provided in a cross-sectional as opposed to a longitudinal context. As Chalmers and colleagues (1981) pointed out, the comparison of two treatment modalities requires that "patients being compared resemble one another in all possible prognostically important ways, except for the treatment under comparison" (p. 31). Moreover, double-blind clinical trials are not necessarily the best way to determine the outcome of a disorder; in order to be included in such a trial, very restrictive inclusion criteria may have to be met. On the other hand, the effects of treatment in outcome are, at times, difficult to disentangle in naturalistic studies. As Keller and co-workers (1983) noted, treatment as prescribed by clinicians in response to the patient's condition sometimes becomes an outcome in itself.

Lithium.   The effects of treatment on the outcome of mania have thus far focused primarily on the efficacy of medication in the following instances: 1) lessening of symptoms in manic patients; 2) usefulness of drug treatment, particularly lithium carbonate, in shortening the length of the manic episode; and 3) use of drugs such as lithium in preventing relapse. As suggested by Dion and co-workers (1988), the efficacy of pharmacologic treatment in improving *functional* outcome is less clear.

Data from Drug Treatment Studies

The vast majority of the literature focuses on the use of lithium carbonate, with evidence that it reduces manic symptoms and shortens the length of manic episodes (Kukopulos et al. 1980). In addition, a number of studies have compared the prophylactic benefit of lithium compared to placebo (Baastrup et al. 1970; Coppen et al. 1971; Cundall et al. 1972; Prien et al. 1973; Stallone et al. 1973). In Table 8–2, relapse rates have ranged from zero (Baastrup et al. 1970)

TABLE 8–2.   Lithium maintenance placebo-controlled studies

	Follow-up (months)	*n*		% Relapse	Risk Ratio*	*P* value
Baastrup et al. 1970	5	lithium	28	0	17.68	$P < .001$
		placebo	22	12		
Coppen et al. 1971	14	lithium	16	3	8.0	$P = .001$
		placebo	22	21		
Cundall et al. 1972	6	lithium	12	4	2.8	$P = .05$
		placebo	12	10		
Stallone et al. 1973	24	lithium	19	5	2.8	$P < .005$
		placebo	23	21		
Prien et al. 1973	24	lithium	84	23	6.1	$P < .001$
		placebo	65	42		

* Mantel Haenszel pooled risk ratio = 9.48, $P < .05$ (Rothman 1986).

to 23% (Prien et al. 1973) for patients treated with lithium and from 10% (Cundall et al. 1972) to 42% (Prien et al. 1973) for those receiving placebo. After reviewing the literature on this subject, Davis (1976) concluded that the efficacy of lithium in the prevention of manic-depressive episodes was well established. Additional investigations of the efficacy of lithium in the prophylactic treatment of mania comes from the work of Prien and colleagues (1973), who published the only randomized, double-blind study of lithium versus placebo that specified the probability of remaining in remission at different time intervals. In Prien's study, 32% of patients on placebo continued in remission for at least 1 year, and 23% remained in remission for at least 2 years. In contrast, 64% of patients on lithium who remained in remission for 1 year and 73% of those still being followed were well after 2 years.

Another important but now well-studied question concerns the use of preventive drug treatment after just one manic episode. Zarin and Pass (1987) reviewed this subject using a Markov model to study the trade-off between costs (exposure to lithium) and benefits (i.e., preventing a relapse). Such studies are of utmost importance in evaluating the risk-benefit ratio of all treatment modalities (see also Chapter 2).

Anticonvulsants. Although lithium is clearly superior to placebo in the treatment of bipolar patients, it should be noted that many patients do not benefit from its use. As a result, there has been growing interest in the use of other drugs, primarily anticonvulsants, in the prophylaxis of recurrent mania. In a review, Post and colleagues (1983) cited a number of studies that have found that use of carbamazepine alone, or in combination with other drugs (e.g. lithium), may reduce the frequency of relapse in manic-depressive illness (MDI). There are also studies indicating that patients with mixed dysphoric states have a better response to anticonvulsant drugs than to lithium carbonate (Post et al. 1989). However, double-blind studies of the efficacy of carbamazepine in the long-term maintenance treatment of MDI are still to be done.

The same is true with respect to valproic acid and clonazepam, drugs that also have anticonvulsant properties and have been used in the treatment of manic patients.

Antidepressants. Because patients with MDI often present with depression rather than mania, many patients have been treated, at least initially, with antidepressant drugs. Some investigators have specifically addressed the effects of antidepressant treatment on the course of manic-depressive illness (Kukopulos 1980). There are data to suggest that antidepressants may precipitate mania and that the frequency of manic recurrences (i.e., rapid cycling) increases in patients maintained on antidepressants. Parenthetically, Kukopulos and colleagues (1980) also suggested that the use of neuroleptics (i.e., to control manic symptoms) accentuates the depression that often follows such episodes.

Recovery from Acute Mania

The prediction of recovery from a manic episode is obviously of major import-ance in the treatment planning for such patients. However, thus far the defini-tion of recovery has been inconsistent, and with few exceptions (Keller et al. 1986; Tohen et al. 1990a), clear operational criteria for recovery are not speci-fied. For example, in some studies, depression following a manic episode is con-sidered to be part of the index episode. In others, it is considered a new episode.

Data provided by the NIMH Collaborative Study (Keller et al. 1986) suggest that the polarity of the index episode may predict speed of recovery, in that patients who presented with mania recovered at a faster rate than patients who presented with a depressive or mixed (i.e., manic/depressed) state. The probabil-ity of *not recovering* for at least 1 year was 7% for the "pure" manic group compared to 32% for the mixed-cycling group. Recovery estimates for bipolar patients presenting with a depressive episode fell between the pure manic and mixed-cycling groups. Keller and colleagues (1986) also pointed out that these differences in recovery rates could be explained by availability of more effective treatments for pure mania than for mixed-cycling episodes. Thus, the median time needed for recovery was 5 weeks in their pure manic group, 9 weeks for the pure depressive group, and 14 weeks for the mixed-cycling group. A history of previous major affective episodes also predicted delayed recovery. These investi-gators emphasized the importance of preventing a purely depressed or purely manic patient from developing a mixed-cycling condition.

Predictors of Relapse in Mania

Another major area of interest in outcome studies of bipolar disorder has been in the prediction of relapse. The literature, however, has been inconsistent and many different predictor variables have been identified. For example, Fahndrich and Wirtz (1987) found that later age and lower occupational status at illness onset predicted a more recurrent course, whereas Winokur and colleagues (1969) and Morgan (1972) identified symptoms of depression as a predictor of relapse. Goodnick and co-workers (1987) found that inter-episode symptoms predicted relapse and suggested that these were indications of unstable mood. Thus, even mild affective symptoms should alert the clinician about the possibil-ity of relapse and hospitalization.

In other studies, the presence of mixed affective states has been identified as a predictor of relapse (Himmeloch et al. 1976; Kotin and Goodwin 1972; Nunn 1979). More recently, Post and colleagues (1989) reported that in manic pa-tients who experienced severe degrees of depression and anxiety (i.e., dysphoric mania), the severity of the dysphoria was correlated with the number of previous hospitalizations for MDI. Rosenthal and co-workers (1979) found that the presence of psychotic features during mania was associated with good response to lithium maintenance. On the other hand, in the McLean cohort (Tohen et al. 1990a), psychotic features during the index episode predicted a shorter time in remission. The discrepancy of these results could be explained by the fact that Rosenthal's population was recruited from an outpatient clinic, suggesting they were probably less severely ill than the McLean population, which was recruited from an inpatient setting.

The presence of comorbidity (i.e., concurrent psychiatric illness) has also been proposed as a predictor of poor outcome in bipolar disorder. Specifically, Black and co-workers (1988) identified alcoholism as a predictor of poor treatment response. In the McLean cohort (Tohen et al. 1990a), the presence of alcoholism in a manic patient predicted a shorter time in remission. Currently, we can only speculate about the relationship between relapse to mania and alcoholism. It is often unclear whether alcoholism is the cause or the result of relapse in manic patients. The presence of affective symptoms between episodes has been associated with higher risk of relapse, and these may also predispose patients to alcoholism. Alternately, alcohol abuse may represent a form of "self treatment" of dysphoria, insomnia, or other symptoms that may precede relapse. The possible interrelationship of mild affective symptoms, alcoholism, and relapse needs to be further evaluated. Finally, it is also possible that alcoholism negatively influences the course of bipolar disorder, both through its direct effects on mood and behavior, and by compromising compliance with psychiatric treatment.

A frequent problem in studies of relapse in MDI is that relapse rates are often reported analyzing the information cross-sectionally. This approach has been criticized in the literature (Keller et al. 1982). More recent studies (Keller et al. 1986; Tohen et al. 1990a) have used survival analysis methodology (Cox 1972; Kalbfleish and Prentice 1980), both to study relapse that has occurred and to estimate the probability of future relapses. Survival curves can also be a very useful descriptive tool. For example, Figure 8–1 illustrates the month-to-month probability of remaining in remission for a group of bipolar patients discharged (in remission) from McLean Hospital. The sample is divided by the presence or absence of a history of alcoholism (Tohen 1988). The figure shows that by 6 months post-discharge, the probability of remaining in remission was 67% (6/9 x 100) for patients with a history of alcoholism and 64% (42/66 x 100) for patients without such history. However, 3 years after the index hospitalization, 22% of MDI patients with a history of alcoholism were still in remission, compared to 35% of those without an alcoholism history.

Survival analysis curves can also be used to estimate the probability that a

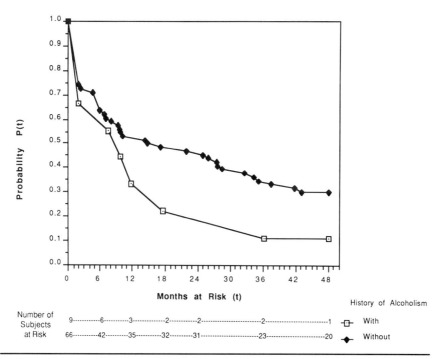

FIGURE 8–1. Cumulative probability of not relapsing into a manic or major depressive episode stratified by presence or absence of a history of alcoholism.

patient will remain in remission based on how long he or she has already been in remission. For example, in Figure 8–1, for manic patients with a history of alcoholism, we can calculate the probability of their remaining in remission for 4 years after being in remission for 1 year (30%/53% = 57%). Similarly, the probability of remaining in remission 4 years after already being in remission for 3 years is 30%/34% = 88%. In other words, for this particular subgroup of patients, the longer the patient has been in remission, the higher the probability that he or she will remain in remission. Clearly, survival curves can be helpful in the planning of mental health services for patients with MDI and other disorders.

Psychosocial Adjustment in Manic Patients

The psychosocial impairment caused by a manic episode can be extreme. Winokur and colleagues (1969) reported that close to 80% of subjects who suffered from recurrent mania lost their jobs. The literature on this subject has been inconsistent in defining the parameters of psychosocial outcome. Indeed, in most studies, outcome assessment consists of applying a combination of psychosocial and relapse/remission variables. Until recently, with the exception of the Iowa 500 study (Tsuang et al. 1979), psychosocial outcome per se has not been clearly operationalized. This 40-year retrospective study used structured diagnostic and outcome instruments and experienced minimal loss of patients to follow-up. Good outcome in residential and occupational adjustment was found in 69% and 67% of patients, respectively. In this regard, data from the McLean cohort (Tohen 1988) were quite similar. At the 4-year evaluation, 72% of patients were rated as good in terms of their occupational status, and 80% were rated as good with respect to their residential status.

In a study conducted at McLean, Dion and colleagues (1988) followed a cohort of 67 patients prospectively for 6 months after discharge and compared their functional outcome to their symptomatic outcome. After 6 months, most were rated symptom-free; however, one-third of the cohort was considered disabled, and only 21% were working at their previous level. Thus, although short-term treatment is effective in symptom amelioration, it does not necessary lead to rapid restoration of occupational functioning. These data also suggest that in manic patients discharged from an inpatient setting, follow-up treatment should focus on their rehabilitative needs so as to restore previous levels of functioning. The current trend toward shorter hospitalizations means that aftercare planning should address not only symptom amelioration but psychosocial rehabilitation as well.

Chronicity and Mortality in Mania

Chronicity

Clinicians are well aware that patients with mania are often in need of long-term treatment; however, the literature on chronicity in mania is confusing, primarily because of problems in definition. For example, a number of current nosological classifications do not even recognize the chronicity of mania. Indeed, the latest version of the World Health Organization's (WHO) International Classification of Diseases (ICD-9; 1978) does not include the term "chronicity" in describing the affective disorders. Also, in the latest edition of the *Diagnostic and Statistical Manual of Mental Disorders* (DSM-III-R; American Psychiatric Association 1987), "deterioration from previous level of functioning" is used as a criterion for diagnosis only in schizophrenia. In part, this is a continuation of Kraepelin's (1921) original separation of dementia praecox from manic-depressive illness, based largely on deteriorating course and poor outcome in the latter—despite clear indications that MDI is a chronic, and sometimes debilitating, illness.

The chronicity problem has been addressed in a number of studies. Fukuda and colleagues (1983) in Japan found that 6.2% of 1,066 patients were described as chronically ill. Zis and Goodwin (1979) concluded that 20–85% of manic patients had at least three relapses, and Coryell and Winokur (1982) estimated that 15–53% of manic patients will develop a chronic course. Inconsistent prevalence rates for chronicity appear to stem from varying definitions of chronicity and the variable length of follow-up in these studies. When chronicity is defined as chronic hospitalization for 5 years or more, the proportion of chronic cases may be as low as 0.8% (Wertham 1929). When chronicity is defined as inability to work and/or function socially, it can be as high as 54% (Shobe and Brion 1971).

In the McLean Hospital sample (Tohen 1988, 1991), the criteria for chronicity included one or more of the following: 1) the continuous presence of interepisodic symptoms; 2) psychosocial dysfunction; 3) multiple relapses and hospitalizations; or 4) continuous hospitalization because of severe symptoms and psychosocial dysfunction. Depending on how chronicity was defined, chronicity rates varied. At 4-year follow-up, 2 patients (2.7%) had been hospitalized for more than 1 year. After including those who had been living in a halfway house for more than 12 months, the number of chronic patients increased to 10 (14%). If chronicity was defined as the occurrence of multiple relapses, 21 patients (28%) had 4 or more during the 4-year follow-up period. If the definition of chronicity was the presence of prominent interepisodic symptoms, half of the patients would have qualified for chronicity. After 4 years, 20–30% sustained psychosocial disability, manifested by inability to work competitively or inability to live independently. Regardless of how chronicity was defined, up to 60% of the McLean sample required varying degrees of psychiatric treatment due either to continuous hospitalization, relapses and remissions, sustained psychosocial dysfunction, prominent symptoms between episodes, or a combination of these factors. Clearly, we are dealing with a population that needs varying types of long-term care.

Mortality

Suicide is a major contributor to mortality in patients with manic-depressive illness. The best approach to determine the proportion of deaths caused by suicide is to study mortality in a cohort comprised of deceased patients. In carrying out such studies, Taschev (1974) found that in 652 deceased bipolar patients, 27% had committed suicide, whereas Tsuang and colleagues (1979) found that 11% of patients with mania committed suicide. In the McLean cohort, 4% of subjects committed suicide (Tohen 1988, Tohen et al. 1990a).

Applying Outcome Data to Clinical Practice

A major problem in applying outcome data to clinical practice is the difficulty in generalizing from published studies that, for the most part, have been carried out in major academic centers, where the study population is likely to include a disproportionate number of the more difficult-to-treat patients, including those suffering from multiple recurrences of mania. As a result, most studies of course and outcome in patients with MDI have included individuals with multiple hospitalizations.

In addition, the presence and frequency of previous affective episodes is not always controlled for in outcome studies. This is important because the literature suggests that a pattern of previous affective (i.e., manic or depressive) episodes predicts future recurrences (Bratfos and Haug 1968; Keller et al. 1983; Tohen et al. 1990a). Thus, in the absence of data about prior episodes, it is difficult to determine if poor outcome is solely related to established chronicity as opposed to independent premorbid risk factors.

The study of "first-episode" patients is also preferable in research on both etiology and clinical course. With regard to the former, causal factors can be better differentiated from manifestations of the illness itself. In addition, cause and effect associations can be more easily evaluated (MacMahon and Pugh 1970) in first-episode patients. In this context, our group (Tohen et al. 1990b) conducted a 4-year follow-up study of 24 first-episode manic patients discharged from McLean Hospital in remission. Over a 4-year period, 11 patients remained in remission and 13 relapsed. Relapse was more likely to occur at the beginning of the follow-up period, with depression the more common manifestation. In comparison, the 1969 study done by Winokur and colleagues, which included multi-episode patients, reported a relapse rate of 50% within the first 6 months; whereas in the McLean sample of multi-episode patients (Tohen et al. 1990b), the relapse rate was 30% over the same time period.

In terms of clinical course, the "first-episode" McLean cohort (Tohen et al. 1990b) did fairly well at 4-year follow-up. Thirteen patients (54%) were asymptomatic and had either no or very mild psychosocial impairment. It is also possible that some of the 11 patients who had not relapsed by the fourth year will never have another major affective episode. This is important from a nosological point of view in that there may be a single-episode subtype of manic patients.

Again, the data support the notion that outcome in mania is heterogeneous, ranging from a chronic deteriorating course to a single episode with no psychosocial deterioration.

Summary

Mania is an illness with variable course. Some patients suffer from a single episode, followed by full recovery and no future hospitalization. Others follow a downhill chronic course with continuous or frequent hospitalization and functional deterioration. In serving the needs of these patients, it is desirable to identify meaningful patterns of illness and factors that affect onset, clinical course, response to treatment, and long-term prognosis. Carefully done, outcome studies are a vital part of this process.

References

American Psychiatric Association: Diagnostic and Statistic Manual of Mental Disorders, 3rd Edition, Revised. Washington, DC, American Psychiatric Association, 1987

Angst J: The course of affective disorders. Psychopathology 19(suppl):47–52, 1968

Baastrup PC, Poulsen JC, Schou M, et al: (1970). Prophylactic lithium: Double-blind discontinuation in manic-depressive and recurrent depressive disorders. Lancet 2:326–330, 1970

Black DW, Winokur G, Hubert J, et al: Predictors of immediate response in the treatment of mania: The importance of comorbidity. Biol Psychiatry 24:191–198, 1988

Bratfos O, Haug JO: The course of manic-depressive psychosis. Acta Psychiatr Scand 44:89–112, 1968

Carlson GA, Kotin J, Davenport YB, et al: Follow-up of 53 bipolar manic-depressive patients. Br J Psychiatry 124:134–139, 1974

Cassidy WL, Flanagan NB, Spellman M: Clinical observations in manic-depressive disease. JAMA 164:1535–1546, 1955

Chalmers TC, Smith H, Blackburn B, et al: A method for assessing the quality of a randomized control trial. Controlled Clin Trials 2:31–49, 1981

Clayton PJ: The epidemiology of bipolar affective disorder. Compr Psychiatry 22:32–43, 1981

Coppen A, Noguera R, Bailey J, et al: Prophylactic lithium in affective disorders. Lancet 2:275–279, 1971

Coryell W, Winokur G: Course and outcome, in Handbook of Affective Disorders. Edited by Paykel E. New York, Guilford, 1982, pp 93–106

Cox DR: Regression models and life tables. Journal of the Royal Statistical Society Series B 34:187–220, 1972

Cundall RL, Brooks PW, Murray LG: A controlled evaluation of lithium prophylaxis in affective disorders. Psychol Med 2:308–311, 1972

Davis JM: Overview: Maintenance therapy in Psychiatry II Affective Disorders. Am J Psychiatry 133:1–13, 1976

Dion GL, Tohen M, Anthony WA, et al: Symptoms and functioning of patients with bipolar disorder six months after hospitalization. Hosp Community Psychiatry 39:652–657, 1988

Dunner DL, Fleiss JL, Fieve RR: The course of development of mania in patients with recurrent depression. Am J Psychiatry 133:905–909, 1976

Fahndrich E, Wirtz EF: Verlaufspradikotoren affecktiver psychosen. Schweiz Arch Neurol Psychiatr 138:17–30, 1987

Falret JP: Memoire sur la Folie Circulaire, Forme de maladie mentale characterisee par la reproduction successive et reguliere de l'etat manique, de l'etat melancolique, et d'un intervalle lucide plus ou moins prolongue. Bulletin de l'Academie de Medecine 19:382–415, 1854

Fauman MA: Quality assurance monitoring in psychiatry. Am J Psychiatry 146:1121–1129, 1989

Fukuda K, Etoh T, Iwadat T, et al: The course and prognosis of manic-depressive psychosis: A quantitative analysis of episodes and intervals. Tohoku J Exp Med 139:299–307, 1983

Goodnick PJ, Fieve RR, Schegel A, et al: Predictors of interepisode symptoms and relapse in affective disorder patients treated with lithium carbonate. Am J Psychiatry 144:367–369, 1987

Goodwin FK, Jamison KR: The naturalistic course of manic-depressive illness, in Neurobiology of Mood Disorders. Edited by Post RM, Ballenger JC. Baltimore, Williams & Wilkins, 1984, pp 20–37

Hastings DW: Follow-up results in psychiatric illness. Am J Psychiatry 114:1057–1060, 1958

Himmeloch JM, Mulla D, Neil JF, et al: Incidence and significance of mixed affective state in a bipolar population. Arch Gen Psychiatry 33:1062–1066, 1976

Joint Commission on Accreditation of Hospitals: Monitoring and evaluation of the quality and appropriateness of care: a hospital example. QRB 12:326–330, 1986

Kalbfleisch JD, Prentice RL: The Statistical Analysis of Failure Time Data. New York, John Wiley, 1980

Keller MB, Shapiro RW, Lavori PW, et al: Recovery in major depressive disorder. Arch Gen Psychiatry 39:905–910, 1982

Keller MB, Lavori PW, Endicott J, et al: "Double depression": Two year follow-up. Am J Psychiatry 140:689–694, 1983

Keller MB, Lavori PW, Coryell N, et al: Differential outcome of pure manic, mixed/cycling and pure depressive episodes in patients with bipolar illness. JAMA 255:3138–3142, 1986

Kotin J, Goodwin F: Depression during mania: Clinical observations and theoretical implications. Br J Psychiatry 129:679–686, 1972

Kraepelin E: Lectures on Clinical Psychiatry. New York, W Wood & Co., 1904, pp 11–20

Kukopulos A, Reginaldi D, Laddomada P, et al: Course of the manic-depressive cycle and changes caused by treatments. Pharmakopsychiatrica 13:156–167, 1980

Lavori PW, Keller MB, Klerman GL: Relapse in affective disorders: A reanalysis of the literature using life table methods. J Psychiatr Res 18:13–25, 1984

MacMahon B, Pugh TF: Epidemiology Principles and Methods. Boston, Little, Brown, 1970, pp 17–27

Morgan HG: The incidence of depressive symptoms during recovery from hypomania. Br J Psychiatry 120:537–539, 1972

Nunn CMH: Mixed affective states and the natural history of manic-depressive psychosis. Br J Psychiatry 134:153–160, 1979

Post RM, Uhde TW, Ballenger JC: Prophylactic efficacy of carbamazepine in manic-depressive illness. Am J Psychiatry 140:1602–1604, 1983

Post RM, Rubinow DR, Uhde TW, et al: Dysphoric mania on clinical and biological correlates. Arch Gen Psychiatry 446:353–358, 1989

Prien RF, Caffey EM, Klett J: Prophylactic efficacy of lithium carbonate in manic-depressive illness. Report of the Veterans Administration and National Institute of Health Collaborative Study Group. Arch Gen Psychiatry 28:337–341, 1973

Regier DA, Myers JK, Kramer M, et al: The NIMH Epidemiologic Catchment Area (ECA) Program: Historical context, major objectives, and study population characteristics. Arch Gen Psychiatry 41:934–941, 1984

Regier DA, Boyd JH, Burke JD, et al: One-month prevalence of mental disorders in the United States. Arch Gen Psychiatry 45:977–986, 1988

Robins LN, Helzer JE, Weissman MM, et al: Lifetime prevalence of specific psychiatric disorders in the United States. Arch Gen Psychiatry 41:949–958, 1984

Rosenthal N, Rosenthal LN, Stallone F, et al: Psychosis as a predictor of response to lithium maintenance treatment in bipolar affective disorder. J Affective Disord 1:237–245, 1979

Rothman KJ: Modern Epidemiology. Boston, Little, Brown, 1986, pp 206–207

Sackett DL, Gent M: Controversy in counting and attributing events in clinical trials. N Engl J Med 301:14101412, 1979

Shobe FO, Brion P: Long term prognosis in manic-depressive illness. Arch Gen Psychiatry 24:334–337, 1971

Stallone F, Shelley E, Mendlewicz J: The use of lithium in affective disorders: III, A double-blind study of prophylaxis in bipolar illness. Am J Psychiatry 130:1006–1010, 1973

Taschev T: The course and prognosis of depression on the basis of 652 patients deceased, in Classification and Prediction of Outcome of Depression. Edited by Angst J. New York, FK Schattauer Verlag, 1974, pp 156–172

Tohen M: Outcome in bipolar disorder. Unpublished doctoral dissertation, Harvard University, Cambridge, MA, 1988

Tohen M: Arguments made for chronic mania as nosological entity. The Psychiatric Times 8:15–18, 1991

Tohen M, Waternaux CM, Tsuang MT: Outcome in mania: A four year prospective study utilizing survival analysis. Arch Gen Psychiatry 47:1106–1111, 1990a

Tohen M, Waternaux CM, Tsuang MT, et al: Four year follow-up of twenty-four first episode manic patients. J Affective Disord 19:79–86, 1990b

Tsuang MT, Woolson RF, Fleming JA: Long term outcome of major psychosis: I, Schizophrenia and affective disorders compared with psychiatrically symptom-free surgical conditions. Arch Gen Psychiatry 36:1295–1301, 1979

Tsuang MT, Tohen M, Murphy JM: Psychiatric Epidemiology in the New Harvard Guide to Psychiatry. Edited by Nicholi AM. Cambridge, MA, Harvard University Press, 1988, pp 761–779

Wertham FI: A group of benign chronic psychoses: Prolonged manic excitements. Am J

Psychiatry 9:17–78, 1929

Winokur G, Clayton PJ, Reich T: Manic-depressive Illness. St. Louis, MO, CV Mosby, 1969, pp 79–80, 96–106

World Health Organization: Mental Disorders: Glossary and Guide to Their Classification in Accordance With the Ninth Revision of the International Classification of Diseases, Chapter V. Geneva, World Health Organization, 1978

Zarin DA, Pass TM: Lithium and the single episode. Medical Care 25(suppl):76–84, 1987

Zis AP, Goodwin FK: Major affective disorder as a recurrent illness: A critical review. Arch Gen Psychiatry 36:835–839, 1979

❖ 9 ❖

The Effectiveness of Alcoholism Treatment: Evidence from Outcome Studies

James R. McKay, Ph.D.
Ronald T. Murphy, Ph.D.
Richard Longabaugh, Ed.D.

According to recent epidemiological studies, alcohol abuse or dependence is the most common psychiatric disorder among men and in the top five among women (Robins et al. 1984). In a sample of almost 20,000 adults, taken from five sites across the country, 13.5% met DSM-III criteria (American Psychiatric Association 1987) for alcohol abuse or dependence at some point in their lifetimes (Robins et al. 1988). For many years, people with alcohol disorders, despite their large numbers, were usually avoided by health care providers on the grounds that they were "hopeless." The picture, however, has certainly changed over the last 20 years. There has been a tremendous upsurge in interest in, and commitment to, treating alcohol abusers, as evidenced by the rapid growth in number of alcohol and drug abuse treatment units (U.S. Department of Health and Human Services 1981).

Many alcoholics are treated in inpatient or residential programs, which are typically 2–4 weeks in length and often based heavily on the Alcoholics Anonymous (AA) approach to recovery. Other treatment approaches have been developed, ranging from "brief interventions" to larger scale programs designed to improve the alcoholic's family, work, and leisure environments. Treatment providers are now faced with the problem of how to choose from a burgeoning list of treatment options. The purpose of this chapter is to provide an overview of the effectiveness of various treatments for alcohol disorders. Based on findings from controlled studies, we will attempt to draw conclusions about what sorts of treatments appear effective and which patients benefit most from the various approaches. We will also draw on the literature to suggest ways in which psychiatric hospitals can improve alcoholism treatment services.

We have restricted our review to controlled studies because they provide the best test of the effectiveness of treatment (Holder et al., in press). In controlled studies, one or more treatments are compared with each other and/or some sort of no-treatment control group. To ensure that the treatment and control groups are as equivalent as possible, patients are either randomly assigned or matched on relevant individual difference variables. Although many uncontrolled studies of treatments for alcoholism have also appeared in the literature, the outcomes are difficult to interpret because of many confounding factors and the lack of proper comparison groups (Holder et al., in press; Miller and Hester 1980).

The Evolution of Alcoholism Treatment Research

Early studies on the efficacy of alcoholism treatment were characterized by poor methodology and inconsistent results (Emrick 1975; Longabaugh 1988). By the late 1970s, however, the National Institute on Alcohol Abuse and Alcoholism (NIAAA) and other government granting agencies had begun to fund alcoholism treatment outcome studies, and the quality of the research started to improve. Unfortunately, the treatments that were evaluated did not appear to consistently bring about long-term changes in drinking behavior. Although most patients seemed to be somewhat better after treatment, in many studies up to two-thirds of the patients relapsed within 3 months (Hunt et al. 1971; Longabaugh 1988).

The limited efficacy of alcoholism treatment may have stemmed in part from the heterogeneity of alcoholics and alcohol problems (Pattison 1985). Recent research suggests that alcoholics can be divided into various subtypes, based on personality characteristics, family history, biological factors, and severity of alcohol abuse and related symptoms (Cloninger 1987; Schuckit 1987; Tarter and Edwards 1988; Zucker 1987). Moreover, there are other groups of alcoholics, such as dual-diagnosis patients, adolescents, and women, that differ in many obvious and important ways from the prototypical adult male alcohol abuser. In order to be effective, treatments for alcoholism may need to be adapted to the specific needs of different types of patients (Miller and Hester 1986a). Although the search has continued for *the* treatment for "alcoholism," the great variance among alcohol abusers has led most researchers and clinicians to conclude that a number of effective treatments are needed.

Much of the research in the alcoholism treatment field is thus now geared toward determining which kinds of patients benefit from what kinds of interventions, or "patient-treatment matching." Although many treatment facilities make efforts to match patients to appropriate treatments (Nirenberg and Maisto

1990), controlled studies of matching have only recently begun to appear in the literature. Excellent reviews of the theory behind patient-treatment matching and the problems commonly encountered with this approach can be found in the literature (Finney and Moos 1986; Longabaugh 1986; Miller 1989). The rationale behind patient-treatment matching research is to identify specific patient characteristics that interact with various treatment interventions to produce differential outcomes. This can be done in a variety of ways, including clinical judgment, patient preference, and statistical analyses. Patient-treatment matches are then evaluated in controlled studies by seeing whether patients matched to treatments have better outcomes than those who are not matched. Matches generated by well-articulated theories appear to be more productive than those identified through purely empirical strategies (Finney and Moos 1986).

An example of a study designed to investigate patient-treatment matching issues is the BETA project, conducted at Butler Hospital (Longabaugh et al., in press). In this outpatient study, alcohol-abusing patients were randomly assigned to one of three treatment conditions: 1) cognitive-behavioral therapy for the patient, 2) cognitive-behavioral therapy for the patient and conjoint therapy with a significant other, and 3) cognitive-behavioral and conjoint therapies plus occupational counseling. Each treatment condition was planned to last a maximum of 20 sessions, and patients were followed up for 18 months.

One of the matching hypotheses tested in the study was that patients will benefit from each condition to the degree they are having difficulties that are specifically treated by that condition. Thus, patients with occupational problems will benefit most from the third condition, patients with relationship problems will do best in the second condition, and so forth. A second hypothesis concerned patients' degree of investment in their various social environments. For example, patients with a high degree of investment in their interpersonal relationships were predicted to be more affected by the treatment conditions with conjoint therapy and the behavior of people they are close to during the follow-up. The results of the study will be discussed later in this chapter.

Commonly Used Treatment Approaches

In this section, we review controlled studies on the effectiveness of four of the more common alcoholism treatment approaches: residential or inpatient treatment, psychotherapy, self-help groups, and pharmacotherapy. Results of patient-treatment matching studies are discussed as well, along with implications for hospital-based treatment programs.

Residential Treatment

❧ Although it seems reasonable to assume that alcoholics treated in inpatient or residential programs would do better than those receiving less intense interventions, the evidence indicates that all patients do not. Two thorough reviews of controlled studies of the effectiveness of inpatient versus non-inpatient treatment, independently compiled (Longabaugh 1988; Miller and Hester 1986b), concluded that inpatient treatment was not superior to partial residential (day treatment or halfway house) or outpatient treatment. In more than a dozen studies, with follow-ups ranging from 3–24 months, patients treated in inpatient programs did not have better drinking outcomes. Length of stay in residential programs was also unrelated to drinking outcomes in eight controlled studies (Longabaugh 1988).

However, inpatient treatment does appear to be superior to less intensive treatments for certain types of patients. A number of studies have found that patients with either less social support or stability, a greater degree of alcohol dependence or problem severity, or a greater degree of psychiatric comorbidity seem to benefit more from inpatient treatment (McLellan et al. 1983; Miller and Hester 1986b; Nace 1990; Orford et al. 1976). In addition, alcoholic patients who are engaging in extremely self-destructive behavior or who are acutely suicidal or violent may require inpatient care (Miller 1989; Nace 1990).

A large study carried out by McLellan and colleagues (1983) provided impressive evidence of the importance of properly matching patients to treatments. A total of 372 male substance abuse patients were treated in 4 programs, 2 of which were 60-day inpatient therapeutic communities. Patients in each program were considered as either matched or mismatched to treatment, based on criteria the authors had devised in a previous study. Patients with at least moderate degrees of psychiatric impairment or family, work, or legal problems were seen as needing inpatient treatment. For drug-abusing patients, the criteria for inpatient treatment also included moderate to severe drug abuse and/or medical problems. At the 6-month follow-up, patients who had been properly matched to inpatient treatment had significantly better outcomes—as measured by lower alcohol and drug use severity, fewer family problems, and less psychiatric impairment—than those who had been mismatched.

It appears that residential treatment programs are not the first treatment of choice for most alcohol abusers, given their lack of overall effectiveness and high cost (Holder et al., in press). Residential programs should instead concentrate their efforts on attracting patients who need inpatient services, as well as designing programs to address the specific needs of more disturbed patients with fewer supports. Inpatient psychiatric facilities would seem particularly well-suited to treat alcoholic patients who are suicidal, severely depressed, or suffering from some other major psychiatric problem.

Psychotherapy

Holder and co-workers (in press) recently reviewed the literature on the effectiveness of individual and group psychotherapy with alcoholics. The authors examined well-controlled studies in which either supportive counseling, psychodynamic, cognitive, or group therapy interventions were employed. Psychotherapy led to better drinking outcomes than the comparison groups (e.g., no treatment, minimal treatment, placebo, or another treatment modality) in only 7 of 35 studies. All psychotherapy approaches fared equally badly, with the exception of cognitive therapy, which showed some indications of effectiveness.

Despite these disappointing findings, there is reason for cautious optimism. First, it is not clear that the carefully controlled research on the efficacy of psychotherapy as a treatment for alcoholism has been a proper test of the interventions studied. In most of these studies, alcoholics received a fairly brief course of therapy soon after detoxification or upon completion of an inpatient program. Psychotherapy may be more effective somewhat later in the recovery process, after the alcoholic has achieved sobriety. The timing of such interventions is largely unresearched, however, making it impossible to draw any conclusions.

Evidence from controlled studies also suggests that certain types of patients benefit more from particular kinds of psychotherapy. Patients with a low "conceptual level"—those with a preference for simpler rules, fewer abstract cognitive constructs, and greater dependence on authority—do better with more directive and structured treatments, whereas the opposite is true for those with high conceptual level (McLachlan 1972, 1974; Miller and Hester 1986a). Patients with low self-esteem appear to do particularly poorly in confrontational groups (Annis and Chan 1983). In a recent study of the effectiveness of group therapy, alcoholics who were high on measures of sociopathy and psychopathology did better in coping skills groups, whereas alcoholics low in sociopathy did better in interactional groups (Kadden et al. 1989).

Self-Help Groups

AA and other mutual self-help groups are generally well thought of by most treatment providers. Anecdotal reports given by clinicians and AA members about the effectiveness of AA suggest that those who stay in AA stay sober. However, there have been no properly designed, carefully controlled studies of the effectiveness of AA (McCrady and Irvine 1989; Miller and Hester 1986a). Given the popularity of AA, it has been virtually impossible to conduct a study in which patients would be randomly assigned to AA or some other treatment (or no treatment at all). We also do not know what aspects of the AA program are particularly efficacious and whether this efficacy varies across different types of patients or even from one AA group to another.

However, it is clear that some patients take to AA while others do not. Although the data are not particularly compelling, there is some evidence that patients with greater severity of drinking problems, affective rather than cognitive focus, and a concern about purpose and meaning in life are good candidates for AA, as well as those with better interpersonal skills and a high need for affiliation (Emrick 1987; McCrady and Irvine 1989).

The efficacy of AA has important implications for residential programs, as so many of them are based around the AA program. For example, the efficacy of AA-based versus other types of residential programs has not been properly tested. Studies of this sort have been difficult to do, however, partly because of the influence of supporters of AA who often believe that self-help programs will work for anyone who seriously tries them. Creative research efforts are needed to determine which patients will benefit most from AA, either in the context of inpatient treatment or as an outpatient approach to maintaining sobriety.

Pharmacotherapy

Although a wide variety of drugs have been tried as treatments for alcoholics, we confine this review to the two most widely used approaches, disulfiram (Antabuse) and psychotropic medications.

Disulfiram, the most widely used antidipsotropic medication in the United States, is used to deter alcoholics from drinking by producing an aversive reaction after alcohol is ingested. Despite its widespread use, controlled research indicates that disulfiram is effective only with a highly specific subset of patients, in certain settings, and under specific clinical conditions. In addition, the side effects of disulfiram and potential danger of disulfiram-ethanol reaction contraindicate its use in patients with a wide array of medical and psychiatric conditions. In addition, disulfiram should not be used by pregnant women (Fuller 1989).

Most controlled studies have demonstrated that the benefit obtained by disulfiram therapy is largely accounted for by a placebo effect rather than the drug itself. However, several studies concluded that a certain subset of patients are more likely to benefit from disulfiram than from placebo or no treatment. For example, in a large Veterans Administration (VA) multicenter study (Fuller et al. 1986), older and more socially stable men who relapsed during follow-up had fewer drinking days if they were in the treatment condition receiving 250 mg of disulfiram daily.

These results replicated an earlier study (Baekeland et al. 1971), in which middle-aged and/or more socially stable men were more likely to benefit from disulfiram. The following characteristics were also associated with good outcome with disulfiram in this study: 1) a longer history of heavy drinking; 2) a history of delirium tremens; 3) good motivation, as manifested by contact with AA and/or abstinence at intake; and 4) not being treated with antidepressant medication. According to Fuller (1989), "The middle-aged alcoholic who has relapsed, has some degree of social stability, and is not significantly depressed is the most suitable candidate for disulfiram therapy" (p. 119).

There is also strong evidence for the effectiveness of disulfiram in preventing relapse when used in a comprehensive behavior therapy treatment program. In several such programs, a contract was drawn up which specified that disulfiram ingestion was to be monitored by a significant other (Azrin et al. 1982; O'Farrell et al. 1985). Because compliance is a major obstacle to the effectiveness of disulfiram treatment, this sort of behavioral contracting may be an important component of the treatment.

A number of drugs have proved effective in lessening suffering during detoxification (for a review, see Miller et al. 1989). Here, we will review the effectiveness of psychotropic medication during the rehabilitation phase of treatment. The medications that have been used most frequently are lithium, antidepressants, and tranquilizers. At this point, results from controlled studies indicate that these drugs do not consistently produce decreases in drinking (Miller and Hester 1986a; Miller et al. 1989).

Approximately 20–30% of alcoholics are thought to have an underlying affective disorder or some other psychiatric problem that existed prior to the onset of alcohol abuse. This group has been labeled "secondary alcoholics" (Schuckit 1987). There is some evidence that alcoholics with an underlying psychiatric disorder can benefit from psychotropic medications. Some patients with affective disorders, for example, will drink less if lithium or antidepressants are added to their standard treatments. Unfortunately, the results of controlled studies have been inconsistent and have not provided compelling evidence that lithium and antidepressants lead to reduced drinking in alcoholics with affective disorders (Miller and Hester 1986a; Miller et al. 1989).

Alcoholics frequently report anxiety during recovery, and anxiety and other negative mood states have been implicated in relapse (Marlatt and Gordon 1985). This seems to suggest that alcoholics could benefit from tranquilizers and other antianxiety agents. However, the evidence from controlled studies strongly indicates that they do not (Holder et al., in press; Miller et al. 1989). This may be because many of these drugs are mood-altering and are frequently abused by alcoholics. Some alcoholics suffer from various panic and phobic disorders that surface once they stop drinking. Antianxiety or antidepressant

medication may prove helpful in diminishing panic and anxiety in these patients, which could in turn reduce drinking, but properly controlled studies have
not yet been carried out.

In conclusion, psychotropic medications appear to be helpful for some alcoholics, but the appropriate patient-treatment matches have not been worked out
well as yet. Because of the risk of toxicity, overdose, and abuse, treatment of
alcoholics with drugs such as lithium and antidepressants must be undertaken
with extreme caution. Given the risks in using medication, it would be enor-
mously helpful to know more about which patients will benefit from which
drugs. More controlled studies in this area are needed.

Alternative Treatment Approaches

Brief Interventions

Some alcoholics appear to benefit as much from a session or two of "advice"
concerning their abusive drinking and need for moderation as from lengthy in-
or outpatient treatment. In studies of this type of intervention, the "advice"
given has typically consisted of a thorough assessment of the scope of the
patient's alcohol abuse, followed by a single counseling session. Patients in some
studies have also been given a self-help manual to take home (Miller and Munoz
1982). Brief interventions of this sort have proven surprisingly effective. In more
than a dozen controlled studies conducted since 1977, brief intervention was at
least as effective as the interventions it was compared to in practically every
case.

How are we to understand these findings? Obviously, many alcoholics need
considerably more than an hour or two of advice to make changes in their
drinking. Minimal treatment may work for some patients because they were
simply ready to change (Prochaska and DiClemente 1986). These are the patients who would get better no matter what intervention was used. Others may
be impressed by the directness of a physician who "lays it on the line" about
their drinking. Alcoholics who still have much to lose, as well as people who are
at the problem drinking stage, may be more likely candidates for brief intervention. However, more research is needed to determine both the active ingredients
of brief intervention and who will benefit from it.

What treatment providers can learn from studies of brief interventions is that
it is important to be direct as well as supportive when talking with patients
about their alcohol problems. Any patient who is treated in a psychiatric facility
should be given a thorough drug and alcohol assessment and informed fully of
the results. For some patients, this will be enough to get them to make some
changes in their drinking.

Therapies Directed at the post-treatment Environment

Although the success rate for the interventions described previously can probably be improved through careful patient-treatment matching, relapse rates will
undoubtedly remain high. This is because difficulties and stressors in the recovering alcoholic's social and work environments play major roles in the recovery
process (Longabaugh 1988).

In two studies, 31–59% of the variance in drinking outcomes at 2 years after
treatment was attributable to post-treatment environmental factors (Cronkite
and Moos 1980; Finney et al. 1980). Although the interventions discussed in
this chapter can have an effect on the post-treatment environment (particularly
AA), they are primarily concerned with change within the alcoholic. Another
group of interventions, developed more recently, aim instead to improve the
quality of the alcoholic's social and work environments. They are focused largely
on interpersonal processes and typically have a behavioral or cognitive/behav-
ioral orientation. We will review here the effectiveness of such interventions,
including marital and family therapy and several so-called "broad spectrum"
approaches.

Marital and family therapies.   The state of the alcoholic's relationship with
family or significant others can be one of the more critical factors in the post-
treatment environment (Moos and Moos 1984). A wide range of conjoint therapies have been tried with alcoholics, including educational, interactional, and
behavioral marital therapies. Various forms of family therapy have been utilized
as well, although none have been tested with controlled studies. However, several forms of marital therapy have been carefully evaluated, and the results are
encouraging.

In their review of marital therapy, Holder and co-workers (in press) found
that of the 10 controlled studies in the literature, 9 found marital therapy to be
better than no treatment or a different treatment intervention. In these studies,
behavioral marital therapy (BMT) fared particularly well. For example, O'Farrell
and co-workers (1985) contrasted BMT and interactional marital therapy with a
no-treatment control group. Both treatment groups showed greater improvements on a variety of indices of marital adjustment compared to controls,
and the BMT groups also enjoyed a greater degree of sobriety over a short-term
follow-up. Two other studies conducted at Butler Hospital found a "crossover"
effect in which BMT groups began to look better than other groups, in terms of
drinking outcomes, after the first year of follow-up (McCrady et al. 1986; Stout
et al. 1990). This is an exciting finding, as the efficacy of treatment usually
declines rather than increases over time. These researchers also found that patients in conjoint therapy are less likely to drop out of treatment (Noel et al.
1987) and that therapy aimed at improving the marriage as a whole (e.g., BMT)

seems to work better than couples therapy that is focused strictly on alcohol related problems (McCrady 1986).

Despite these impressive outcomes, conjoint therapies are obviously not an option for all alcoholics. The patient must have some family members or significant others who are willing to participate in treatment. Another important variable to consider before recommending conjoint therapy is the patient's degree of social investment—in other words, how important relationships are to the patient. The study by Longabaugh and colleagues (in press) described previously generated several provocative findings, with implications for patient-treatment matching. Patients high in social investment did better in the conditions that included conjoint therapy compared to those in the condition that did not, but only if they received support for their sobriety from family and friends. Those who did not receive such support had the worst outcomes of all patients in the study. Patients low in social investment were also negatively affected by the social support fostered by the conjoint treatment. Thus, conjoint therapy was only beneficial for patients high in social investment and with family and friends who were supportive of sobriety. These findings highlight the complexity of appropriate patient-treatment matching. Not only do the characteristics of the person and treatment need to be considered, but also those of the person's post-treatment environment.

Broad spectrum approaches. These treatment interventions are designed to address other problems in the alcoholic's life that may be related to alcohol abuse. The interventions we will review here are social skills and stress-management training. We will also discuss the effectiveness of several comprehensive interventions, which attempt to improve the alcoholic's social and work situations as well as decrease drinking.

Social skills training (SST) interventions are designed to improve the patient's ability to interact with others. According to the model on which SST is based, patients drink in an attempt to cope with social situations that are particularly difficult for them. Although there is no "standard" SST intervention, most seek to improve communication and assertiveness skills through modeling, rehearsal, and cognitive restructuring. The treatment can be delivered on either an inpatient or outpatient basis. Controlled studies of SST have shown that it is effective in reducing the severity of post-treatment drinking (Chaney 1989; Holder et al., in press). In general, however, these studies have not utilized comparison groups that make it possible to draw conclusions about the most important components of SST.

In a recent study, male subjects who had completed a standard inpatient treatment program received either communication skills training or cognitive behavioral mood management training. Subjects in the communication skills condition drank significantly less alcohol on drinking days during follow-up

(Monti et al. 1990). The study also generated results with implications for patient-treatment matching. Cognitive-behavioral training was effective for patients who had lower anxiety or weaker urges to drink during treatment and for those patients with more education. Communication skills training benefited a broader range of patients, regardless of their education, anxiety, or urge to drink (Rohsenow et al. 1991).

A number of studies have considered the effectiveness of various forms of stress-management training, including exercise, relaxation, and meditation. The results have been mixed. In the controlled studies reviewed by Holder and colleagues (in press), patients treated with stress management therapies of one sort or another did better than controls in 6 out of 10 studies. The relative effectiveness of different types of stress management therapy has not been well researched, nor have patient-treatment matching issues. As can be imagined, it appears that patients high in anxiety are more likely to benefit from stress-management therapy (Rosenberg 1979), although more work is clearly needed before any conclusions can be drawn about who benefits most from which approach.

Comprehensive interventions show a great deal of initial promise. Smith (1985, 1986) reported on the effectiveness of a particular halfway house program, which featured contact with recovering alcoholic program staff, daily AA meetings, and a work program. Compared to matched subjects treated with hospital-based detoxification only, a substantially higher percentage of men and women in the halfway house enjoyed continuous abstinence during the 14–18 month follow-up.

The "Community Reinforcement Approach" (CRA), developed by Azrin and colleagues, consists of a number of behavioral interventions, including conjoint therapy, job-finding training, counseling focused on alcohol-free social and recreational activities, and monitored administration of disulfiram (Azrin 1976; Hunt and Azrin 1973). One of the unique features of CRA is the use of an alcohol-free social club, which recovering alcoholics are encouraged to attend. The overall goal of CRA is to make sobriety more rewarding than drinking.

When pitted against other interventions, CRA has done extremely well. In a study in which patients were randomly assigned to CRA or to a standard hospital treatment program, those getting CRA drank less, spent fewer days away from home, worked more days, and were institutionalized less over a 24-month follow-up (Azrin 1976). The same counselors administered both the hospital program and CRA, which makes the large differences in outcomes all the more striking. A second controlled study contrasted CRA, administration of disulfiram with a behavioral compliance program, and regular outpatient treatment (Azrin et al. 1982). Once again, those treated with CRA did substantially better on all outcome measures than those in the other treatment conditions. However, the authors observed that married patients did equally well in the CRA and disulfiram groups.

Conclusions

In this chapter, we have provided an overview of the effectiveness of various treatments for alcohol disorders by considering the results from controlled treatment outcome studies. This is not meant to be an exhaustive review of the literature. We have not covered all treatment approaches, nor have we included every relevant study. Readers who are interested in more information can consult excellent reviews by Hester and Miller (1989), Longabaugh (1988), and Miller and Hester (1986a). With these limitations in mind, we present the following conclusions.

First, it is now clear that treatments for alcohol abuse can lead to substantial reductions in drinking and drug use. In studies by Azrin (1976), McCrady (1986), and Stout et al. (1990), for example, patients were abstinent on an average of 80% or more of the days of follow-ups ranging from 18 to 24 months. Treatment has also been shown to bring about improvements in family functioning, marital satisfaction, and psychiatric impairments (McCrady et al. 1986; McLellan et al. 1983; O'Farrell et al. 1985).

Thus, the relevant question is no longer "Are treatments for alcoholism effective?" but rather "Which alcoholic patients benefit most from what treatments?" Controlled studies of patient-treatment matching are generating some of the most exciting and encouraging results in the field. However, because matching studies are a relatively recent phenomenon in alcoholism treatment, only a few findings have been replicated. And so we are currently left with a number of enticing leads but little confirmation or certainty. The good news is that studies of matching are becoming increasingly common, sophisticated, and rigorous. Furthermore, the development of a new generation of reliable and valid assessment instruments promises to expand the list of patient characteristics that can be matched on (Sobell et al. 1988).

Second, surprisingly little is known about the effectiveness of what are arguably the two most popular treatments for alcoholism: the 28-day inpatient program and AA. Although it is clear that some patients benefit from these interventions, a considerable amount of research is still needed before we can say with any certainty who will do so. What research does show is that patients with either psychiatric comorbidity, greater alcohol dependence, or little social support appear to benefit from more-intensive as opposed to less-intensive interventions. However, the majority of people treated in 28-day inpatient programs do not fit that profile. There may be other, as yet unidentified patient characteristics that predict greater success in more intensive programs. Inpatient programs could bolster support for their efficacy by conducting studies to determine the characteristics of patients who benefit from treatment and publishing the results.

Finally, a number of treatment approaches that are less commonly used appear to show great promise. These include behavioral marital therapy, social skills training, and the community reinforcement approach. Hospital-based treatment programs should consider implementing these treatments for appropriate patients if they have not already done so. Marital therapy and social skills training can be done in group as well as individual modalities, and manuals are available to teach the techniques to clinicians (cf. Chaney 1989; McCrady et al. 1986). These interventions can be done on an outpatient basis or begun while patients are hospitalized and continued following discharge.

Health care insurance providers are less and less willing to fund inpatient treatment. The studies we have reviewed here suggest that many alcoholics can derive substantial benefit from being treated with less costly interventions, including partial hospitalization, halfway houses, and various forms of outpatient therapy. Hospital-based programs that want to remain viable through the 1990s will need to place more emphasis on the development of less-intensive programs as part of their overall treatment package. As more is known about which patients need inpatient hospitalization, it will be easier for the full-service hospital-based treatment facility to direct patients into the proper treatment or sequence of treatments.

References

American Psychiatric Association: Diagnostic and Statistical Manual of Mental Disorders, 3rd Edition, Revised. Washington, DC, American Psychiatric Association, 1987

Annis HM, Chan D: The differential treatment model: Empirical evidence from a personality typology of adult offenders. Criminal Justice and Behavior 10:159–173, 1983

Azrin NH: Improvements in the community reinforcement approach to alcoholism. Behav Res Ther 14:339–348, 1976

Azrin NH, Sisson RW, Meyers R, et al: A social-systems approach to resocializing alcoholics in the community. J Stud Alcohol 43:1115–1123, 1982

Baekeland F, Lundwall L, Kissin B, et al: Correlates of outcome in disulfiram treatment. J Nerv Ment Dis 153:1–9, 1971

Chaney EF: Social skills training, in Handbook of Alcoholism Treatment Approaches. Edited by Hester RK, Miller WR. New York, Pergamon, 1989, pp 206–221

Cloninger CR: Neurogenetic adaptive mechanisms in alcoholism. Science 236:410–416, 1987

Cronkite RC, Moos RH: Determinants of the post-treatment functioning of alcoholic patients: A conceptual framework. J Consult Clin Psychol 48(3):305–316, 1980

Emrick CD: A review of psychologically oriented treatment of alcoholism: II. The relative effectiveness of treatment versus no treatment. J Stud Alcohol 36(1):88–103, 1975

Emrick CD: Alcoholics Anonymous: Affiliation processes and effectiveness as treatment. Alcoholism: Clinical and Experimental Research 11:416–423, 1987

Finney JW, Moos RH: Matching patients with treatment: Conceptual and methodological issues. J Stud Alcohol 47(2):122–134, 1986

Finney JW, Moos RH, Mewborn CR: Posttreatment experiences and treatment outcome of alcoholic patients six months and two years after hospitalization. J Consult Clin Psychol 48(1):17–29, 1980

Fuller RK: Antidipsotropic medications, in Handbook of Alcoholism Treatment Approaches. Edited by Hester RK, Miller WR. New York, Pergamon, 1989, pp 117–127

Fuller RK, Branchey L, Brightwell DR, et al: Disulfiram treatment of alcoholism: A Veterans Administration cooperative study. J Nerv Ment Dis 256:1449–1455, 1986

Hester RK, Miller WR (eds): Handbook of Alcoholism Treatment Approaches. New York, Pergamon, 1989

Holder HD, Longabaugh R, Miller WR, et al: The cost effectiveness of treatment for alcohol problems: A first approximation. J Stud Alcohol (in press)

Hunt GM, Azrin NH: A community reinforcement approach to alcoholism. Behav Res Ther 11:91–104, 1973

Hunt WA, Barnett L, Branch L: Relapse rates in addiction programs. J Clin Psychol 27:455–456, 1971

Kadden RM, Cooney NL, Getter H, et al: Matching alcoholics to coping skills or interactional therapies: Posttreatment results. J Consult Clin Psychol 57(6):698–704, 1989

Longabaugh R: The matching hypothesis: Theoretical and empirical status. Paper presented at the American Psychological Association Symposium on the Matching Hypothesis in Alcoholism Treatment, Washington, DC, August 1986

Longabaugh R: Longitudinal outcome studies, in Alcoholism: Origins and outcome. Edited by Rose RM, Barrett J. New York, Raven, 1988, pp 267–280

Longabaugh R, Beattie M, Noel N, et al: The effect of social investment on treatment outcome. J Stud Alcohol (in press)

Marlatt GA, Gordon JR (eds): Relapse Prevention. New York, Guilford, 1985

McCrady BS: The family in the change process, in Treating Addictive Behaviors. Edited by Miller WR, Heather N. New York, Plenum, 1986, pp 305–318

McCrady BS, Irvine S: Self-help groups. In Handbook of Alcoholism Treatment Approaches. Edited by Hester RK, Miller WR. New York, Pergamon, 1989, pp 153–169

McCrady BS, Noel NE, Abrams DB, et al: Comparative effectiveness of three types of spouse involvement in outpatient behavioral alcoholism treatment. J Stud Alcohol 47(6):459–467, 1986

McLachlan JF: Benefit from group therapy as a function of patient-therapist match on conceptual level. Psychotherapy: Theory, Research, and Practice 9:317–323, 1972

McLachlan JF: Therapy strategies, personality orientation and recovery from alcoholism. Canadian Psychiatric Association Journal 19:25–30, 1974

McLellan AT, Woody GE, Luborsky L, et al: Increased effectiveness of substance abuse treatment: A prospective study of patient-treatment "matching." J Nerv Ment Dis 171:597–605, 1983

Miller WR: Matching individual with interventions, in Handbook of Alcoholism Treatment Approaches. Edited by Hester RK, Miller WR. New York, Pergamon, 1989, pp 261–271

Miller WR, Hester RK: Treating the problem drinker: Modern approaches, in The Addictive Behaviors: Treatment of Alcoholism, Drug Abuse, Smoking, and Obesity. Edited by Miller WR. Oxford, Pergamon, 1980, pp 11–141

Miller WR, Hester RK: The effectiveness of alcoholism treatment: What research reveals, in Treating Addictive Behaviors: Process of Change. Edited by Miller WR, Heather N. New York, Plenum, 1986a, pp 121–174

Miller WR, Hester RK: Inpatient alcoholism treatment: Who benefits? Am Psychol 41(7):794–805, 1986b

Miller WR, Munoz RF: How to Control Your Drinking, Revised Edition. Albuquerque, NM, University of New Mexico Press, 1982

Miller SI, Frances RJ, Holmes DJ: Psychotropic medications. In Handbook of Alcoholism Treatment Approaches. Edited by Hester RK, Miller WR. New York, Pergamon, 1989, pp 231–241

Monti PM, Abrams DB, Binkoff JA, et al: Communication skills training, communication skills training with family, and cognitive behavioral mood management training for alcoholics. J Stud Alcohol 51:263–270, 1990

Moos RH, Moos BS: The process of recovery from alcoholism: III. Comparing functioning in families of alcoholics and matched control families. J Stud Alcohol 45:111–118, 1984

Nace EP: Inpatient treatment of alcoholism: A necessary part of the therapeutic armamentarium. The Psychiatric Hospital 21(1):9–31, 1990

Nirenberg TD, Maisto SA: The relationship between assessment and alcohol treatment. Int J Addict 25(11):1275–1285, 1990

Noel NE, McCrady BS, Stout RL, et al: Predictors of attrition from an outpatient alcoholism treatment program for couples. J Stud Alcohol 48:229–235, 1987

O'Farrell TJ, Cutter HS, Floyd FJ: Evaluating behavior marital therapy for male alcoholics: Effects on marital adjustment and communication from before to after treatment. Behavior Therapy 16:147–167, 1985

Orford J, Oppenheimer E, Edwards G: Abstinence or control: The outcome for excessive drinkers two years after consultation. Behav Res Ther 14:409–418, 1976

Pattison EM: The selection of treatment modalities for the alcoholic patient, in The Diagnosis and Treatment of Alcoholism. Edited by Mendelson JH, Mello NK. New York, McGraw-Hill, 1985, pp 189–294

Prochaska JO, DiClemente CC: Toward a comprehensive model of change, in Treating Addictive Behaviors: Process of Change. Edited by Miller WR, Heather N. New York, Plenum, 1986, pp 3–27

Robins LN, Helzer JE, Weissman M, et al: Lifetime prevalence of specific psychiatric disorders in three sites. Arch Gen Psychiatry 38:381–389, 1984

Robins LN, Helzer JE, Przybeck TR, et al: Alcohol disorders in the community: A report from the epidemiologic catchment area, in Alcoholism: Origins and Outcome. Edited by Rose RM, Barrett J. New York, Raven, 1988, pp 15–29

Rohsenow DJ, Monti PM, Binkoff JA, et al: Patient-treatment matching for alcoholic men in communication skills vs. cognitive-behavioral mood management training. Addict Behav 16:63–69, 1991

Rosenberg SD: Relaxation training and a differential assessment of alcoholism. Unpublished doctoral dissertation, California School of Professional Psychology, San Diego, 1979 (University Microfilms No. 80-04 362)

Schuckit MA: Biological vulnerability to alcoholism. J Consult Clin Psychol 55(3):301–309, 1987

Smith DI: Evaluation of a residential AA program for women. Alcohol Alcohol 20:315–327, 1985

Smith DI: Evaluation of a residential AA program. Int J Addict 21:33–49, 1986

Sobell LC, Sobell MB, Nirenberg TD: Behavioral assessment and treatment planning with alcohol and drug abusers: A review with an emphasis on clinical application. Clinical Psychology Review 8:19–54, 1988

Stout RL, McCrady BS, Longabaugh R, et al: Marital therapy helps maintain the effectiveness of alcohol treatment: Replication of an outcome crossover effect. Manuscript submitted for publication, 1990

Tarter RE, Edwards K: Psychological factors associated with the risk for alcoholism. Alcoholism: Clinical and Experimental Research 12(4):471–480, 1988

U.S. Department of Health and Human Services: Fourth special report to the U.S. Congress on alcohol and health (DHHS Publ No ADM-81-1080). Edited by Deluca JR. Washington, DC, U.S. Government Printing Office, 1981

Zucker RA: The four alcoholisms: A developmental account of the etiological process, in Nebraska Symposium on Motivation, Vol 34: Alcohol and Addictive Behaviors. Edited by Rivers PC. Lincoln, NE, University of Nebraska Press, 1987, pp 27–84

❖ 10 ❖ Outcome Studies in Patients with Eating Disorders

L. K. George Hsu, M.D.

Outcome studies in patients with eating disorders are conducted primarily to elucidate the course and prognosis of these disorders, although the findings may be useful for other purposes, such as the classification of the disorders. Therefore, apart from satisfying the intellectual curiosity of researchers, a knowledge of the course and prognosis of these sometimes chronic and fatal disorders may provide clinicians with a proper perspective on them and, at times, a proper focus in their treatment. Unfortunately, methodologically robust outcome studies for the eating disorders remain the exception rather than the rule. In an earlier review of outcome studies for anorexia nervosa published between 1954 and 1979, I have summarized the five most common methodological deficits: 1) incomplete clinical data and/or inadequate diagnostic criteria, 2) incomplete description of treatment, 3) poorly defined or inadequate outcome criteria, 4) short follow-up duration, and 5) incomplete follow-up data, including a high failure-to-follow rate. Other reviewers have come to similar conclusions (e.g., Steinhausen and Glanville 1983a; Swift 1982). Nevertheless, many of the outcome studies published in the last 10 years continue to suffer from similar methodological failings.

Needless to say, such failings prompt biased conclusions that, unfortunately, sometimes become widely and uncritically accepted. For instance, the conclusion that anorexia nervosa may, in time, become "transformed" into a mood disorder (Cantwell et al. 1977) is still widely quoted (e.g., Katz et al. 1984); and the finding that family therapy may affect a superior outcome (Rosman et al. 1977) is still held to have been proven (e.g., Minuchin 1984). In fact, neither of these findings has been subsequently confirmed (e.g., see Hsu 1988; Russell et al. 1987). Obviously, anorexia nervosa may still turn out to be a variant of a mood disorder, and family therapy may still prove to be the treatment of choice. The point I want to stress is that there is, at present, insufficient follow-up data to support such claims.

In this chapter, I will review the recent outcome studies for both anorexia

159

nervosa and bulimia nervosa, draw conclusions that bear upon certain issues of current interest, and suggest improvements for future studies.

Outcome of Anorexia Nervosa

The present review will focus on 17 studies that I could find published in English between 1980 and 1989. For a review of the earlier studies, the reader may turn to several articles (Hsu 1980; Schwartz and Thompson 1981; Steinhausen and Glanville 1983a; Swift 1982). I have excluded the excellent family versus individual therapy 1-year follow-up study of Russell and colleagues (1987), because the duration of follow-up is really too short to allow for meaningful comparison.

Because the outcome of anorexia nervosa is dependent on the duration of follow-up (Hsu 1988; Morgan and Russell 1975), I have separated the findings according to whether they are intermediate-term (minimum duration 4 years) or long-term (minimum duration at least 18 years). The short-term studies (minimum duration less than 4 years) are mentioned in comparison to the intermediate-term studies.

Intermediate Outcome

Four studies (Burns and Crisp 1984; Hall et al. 1984; Morgan et al. 1983; Tolstrup et al. 1985) fulfilled at least four of the five following criteria to qualify for a methodologically robust study: 1) well-defined diagnostic criteria, 2) follow-up duration of at least 4 years from onset of illness, 3) well-defined follow-up criteria, 4) low failure-to-trace rate, and 5) direct interview at follow-up in the majority of patients.

In Table 10–1, I have summarized the findings from the four studies using the Morgan and Russell general outcome categories, which all the four studies used (Morgan and Russell 1975):

- good outcome = body weight within ± 15% of normal and regular menstrual periods (normal libido in the male) in the last 6 months;
- intermediate = weight occasionally outside of ± 15% normal and/or amenorrhea or irregular periods (absent or decreased libido in the male) in the last 6 months; and
- poor = weight outside ± 15% normal in the last 6 months.

In addition, I have included a fifth study (Bassoe and Eskeland 1982), despite the fact that it has failed two of the five criteria: the failure to define normal weight and the use of questionnaires (an indirect method) for follow-up in the majority of patients. However, even allowing for some methodological differences among the studies and the fact that the Burns and Crisp study consists of only male patients, the data in these studies are quite uniform. At a minimum of 4 years after onset of illness, about 50% of patients have a good outcome in terms of body weight and menstrual status (or in the case of males, normal sexual functioning); about 25% are not fully recovered but have improved to a varying degree; and some 25% are unimproved and would still qualify for a diagnosis of anorexia nervosa. These figures compare well with the two earlier studies (Hsu et al. 1979; Morgan and Russell 1975), which used essentially the same methodology and design (Table 10–1).

The crude mortality at intermediate-term follow-up is usually less than 5% (Table 10–2). Here I have included two other studies. Steinhausen and Glanville (1983b) reported on 31 patients followed for 4 to 28 years after onset. Although 10 (32%) refused to participate in the follow-up, thus making the overall outcome pattern difficult to interpret, the authors are nevertheless able to ascertain that these patients are all alive. Patton (1988a) reported on a 4- to 15-year follow-up of 332 anorectic patients seen at the Royal Free Hospital in London and found a crude mortality rate of 3.3%, which represents a standardized mortality ratio (mortality rate compared to the expected mortality rate in the general population matched for sex and age and duration of study) of 6.01. This means that anorectic patients are six times more likely to die (from whatever causes) than women in the general population. Unfortunately, Patton did

TABLE 10–1. Weight and menstrual outcome (Morgan and Russell criteria) at intermediate-term follow-up for anorexia nervosa

Recent studies	Good (%)		Intermediate (%)		Poor (%)		Dead (%)		Unknown (%)	
1. Bassoe & Eskeland[a] 1982 (N = 77)	52	(68)	13	(17)	12	(16)	0		0	
2. Burns & Crisp 1984 (N = 27)	12	(44)	7	(26)	8	(30)	0		0	
3. Hall et al. 1984 (N = 50)	18	(36)	18	(36)	13	(26)	1	(2)	1	(2)
4. Morgan et al. 1983 (N = 78)	45	(58)	15	(19)	15	(19)	1	(1)	3	(4)
5. Tolstrup et al. 1985 (N = 151)	60	(40)	44	(29)	29	(19)	9	(6)	9	(6)
Mean %	49		25		22		2		2	
Previous studies										
1. Hsu et al. 1979 (N = 105)	47	(45)	32	(30)	21	(20)	2	(2)	3	(3)
2. Morgan & Russell 1975 (N = 41)	16	(39)	11	(27)	12	(29)	2	(5)	0	

[a] Taking only the 77 patients found for at least 4 years.

not report on the overall outcome pattern of his sample. In all these studies, the most common causes of death are suicide or complications of anorexia nervosa (Table 10–2).

For comparison, I have presented the findings of four short-term studies (with the minimum duration of follow-up being 2 years; Table 10–3), again using the Morgan and Russell criteria. By and large, the outcome pattern is more variable. Because these are studies of shorter duration, the crude mortality rate is lower than in the intermediate-term studies. Finally, I have summarized the findings of six studies that, in my opinion, have too large a failure-to-trace rate (Table 10–4). In addition, the range of follow-up duration in these studies is not uniform (from less than 2 years to more than 25 years), and the criteria used for reporting weight and menstrual outcome in some of them (e.g., Steinhausen and

TABLE 10–2. Intermediate-term mortality of anorexia nervosa

Recent studies	N/n Traced[b]	% Crude mortality (n)	Suicide
1. Bassoe & Eskeland[a] 1982	77/77	0	0
2. Burns & Crisp 1984	27/27	0	0
3. Hall et al. 1984	50/50	2 (1/50)	not determined
4. Morgan et al. 1983	78/75	1 (1/75)	1 (1/75)
5. Steinhausen & Glanville 1983b	31/31	0	0
6. Tolstrup et al. 1985	151/151	6 (9/151)	4 (6/151)
7. Patton 1988a	332/332	3 (11/332)	not reported
Previous studies 1. Hsu et al. 1979	105/102	2 (2/102)	0
2. Morgan & Russell 1975	41/41	5 (2/41)	3 (1/41)
3. Theander 1970	94/94	13 (12/94)	3 (3/94)

[a] Taking only the 77 followed for more than 4 years.
[b] Traced = Patients ascertained as not dead although they may not have participated in the follow-up.

TABLE 10–3. Short-term anorexia nervosa studies

	Good (%)		Intermediate (%)		Poor	(%)	Dead (%)		Unknown (%)	
1. Hawley 1985 (*N* = 21)	9	(43)	6	(29)	3	(14)	0		3	(14)[b]
2. Kohle & Mall 1983 (*N* = 36)	9	(25)	17	(47)	9	(25)	1	(3)	0	
3. Martin[a] 1985 (*N* = 22)	19	(86)	?		3	(14)	0		0	
4. Nussbaum et al.[a] 1985 (*N* = 70)	45	(64)	12	(17)	6	(9)	0	(?)	7	(10)

[a] Authors used different outcome classification.
[b] All known to be alive.

Glanville 1983a; Vandereycken and Pierloot 1983) were idiosyncratic, thus making data comparison difficult. Given these many methodological problems, the highly variable outcome pattern is expected.

Although data on weight and menstrual function are uniformly presented in many of these studies, the same cannot be said for data in the other outcome parameters. One major hurdle is the lack of agreed-upon systems for the reporting of such data. I will therefore simply summarize the findings, because a more detailed review is unlikely to be rewarding.

Eating pattern remains highly abnormal in many patients. Bulimia (undefined in terms of severity or frequency) is reported in 7% (Burns and Crisp 1984) to 40% (Hall et al. 1984) of patients, and vomiting (again undefined) in 11% (Burns and Crisp 1984) to 26% (Hall et al. 1984) of patients. Laxative abuse (undefined) was reported by only one study (Burns and Crisp 1984; 11% undefined). Preoccupation with weight or food was reported in about 60% of the patients (Burns and Crisp 1984; Hall et al. 1984). All the studies seem to indicate that eating patterns and eating attitudes may remain highly abnormal even among patients who have recovered in terms of weight and menses. Unfortunately, most of the data are nonstandardized, and the lack of solid basic data in this area is surprising. For instance, it is frustrating that there are no clear data to indicate how many patients would qualify for bulimia nervosa (with or without anorexia nervosa) at follow-up.

Mental status data also suffer from lack of uniform reporting. Three studies present outcome according to diagnostic categories (Hall et al. 1984; Tolstrup et al. 1985; Toner et al. 1986), but only the Toronto group (Toner et al. 1986) used a standardized interview for this purpose. Data focusing on symptoms (e.g., Burns and Crisp 1984) are unsatisfactory, because the severity and duration of the symptoms are undefined. Despite their high failure-to-trace rate, the finding

TABLE 10–4. Anorexia nervosa studies with large numbers of untraced patients

Study	Good (%)	Intermediate (%)	Poor (%)	Dead (%)	Unknown (%)
1. Becker et al.[a] 1981 (N = 38)	14 (37)	7 (18)	6 (16)	5 (13)	6 (16)
2. Santonastaso et al. 1987 (N = 55)	25 (45)	7 (13)	6 (11)	2 (4)	15 (27)
3. Steinhausen & Glanville 1983a (N = 31)	At least 6 (10)	?	At least 4 (13)	0	10 (32)
4. Toner et al.[a] 1986 (N = 149)	23 (15)	16 (11)	16 (11)	5 (3)	89 (60)
5. Touyz & Beumont 1984 (N = 49)	18 (37)	9 (18)	4 (8)	2 (4)	16 (33)
6. Vandereycken & Pierloot 1983 (N = 26)[b]	At least 15 (56)	?	?	?	About 50% overall

[a] Different outcome category used by authors.
[b] Taking only patients followed for at least 5 years.

of Toner and colleagues (1986) of a high prevalence (60% lifetime) of affective disorders (mainly major depression) and anxiety disorders (mainly obsessive-compulsive disorder) should alert future researchers to pay specific attention to this area. In particular, the Toronto group found that the restrictive anorectic patients have a higher 1-year incidence of major depression (35% versus 19%) and obsessive compulsive disorder (23% versus 10%), whereas the bulimic ano-rectic patients have a higher incidence of substance use disorders (43% versus 0%). This may indicate heterogeneity within the anorexia nervosa syndrome, as others have suggested (e.g., Halmi et al. 1986). Unfortunately, the authors did not indicate whether such disorders coexist with a concurrent eating disorder. Several studies have suggested that affective symptoms are more common among those that remain anorectic (e.g., Burns and Crisp 1984; Hall et al. 1984). All the studies agree that schizophrenia is probably not more common than ex-pected.

Psychosocial and psychosexual functioning are also not reported in a stan-dardized fashion. Most studies suggest that better psychosocial functioning (in-cluding sexual attitudes) occurs among those whose anorectic symptoms have improved. Several studies reported the percentage of patients married at follow-up (e.g., Burns and Crisp 1984, 30%; Hall et al. 1984, 40%) or of those that have borne children (e.g., Bassoe and Eskeland 1982, 29% of females), but without comparison groups such data are difficult to interpret. In the Danish study (Brinch et al. 1988), 50 of 140 women had borne children during the follow-up interval (mean, 12.5 years), whereas none of the 11 males had fathered a child. The patients were older at age of first delivery than the national average (26.1 years versus 24.1 years), and the number of children per woman patient was 0.6, compared to the national average of 1.7 for women aged 32. At the time of pregnancy, 36 of the 50 patients were considered to have recovered from their anorectic illness. Overall, the mothers had a better outcome than the nonmothers. In the offspring, perinatal complications were common, prematurity was twice the expected rate, and perinatal mortality six times the expected rate. Unfortunately, the authors did not report on such details as whether there was a correlation between prenatal complication or mortality and the mother's clinical status. Clearly, more data are needed in this area. Work and school performance are almost always satisfactory at follow-up, even among patients who are still anorectic.

Prognostic indicators varied among the series, and methodological differences (such as criteria for each prognostic item and statistical methods used) probably accounted for such discrepancies. Table 10–5 lists those factors predictive of poor outcome identified by at least three of the seven studies (four recent and three previous). Four factors have been found by four of the studies to predict a poor outcome: longer duration of illness, lower minimum weight, previous treatment that failed to bring about a lasting remission, and a premorbid disturbed relationship with the family. The first three factors suggest the presence of a severe, chronic, and treatment-resistant illness, and they therefore make intuitive sense (i.e., chronicity begets chronicity). The last factor (poor relationship with family) suggests either a family system interaction disturbance or else a disturbed personality in the patient. Unfortunately, the criteria for assessing quality of family relationships or premorbid personality are poorly defined; and because the assessment is retrospective, subjective bias cannot be reliably excluded.

In summary, the outcome at a minimum of 4 years after onset of illness in properly diagnosed anorectic patients is quite uniform in terms of weight and menstrual functioning. About 75% have improved to a varying degree, 5% have died, and the remainder have not improved. Therefore, any study reporting a significantly different outcome pattern should be examined in terms of its adherence to the methodological criteria described previously.

Beyond the weight, menstrual, and mortality data, few generalizations can be made. Available data suggest that those who have recovered from their emaciation and amenorrhea are less likely to suffer from affective or anxiety symptoms. Schizophrenic symptoms are not more frequent than expected. Psychosocial (except perhaps work or school performance) and psychosexual functioning are

TABLE 10–5. Prognostic indicators for poor outcome

	Theander 1970	Morgan and Russell 1975	Hsu et al. 1979	Morgan et al. 1983	Burns and Crisp 1984	Hall et al. 1984	Steinhausen and Glanville 1983b
Longer duration of illness		X	X	X	X		
Lower minimum weight	X	X	X		X		X
Later age of onset	X	X	X		Possible		
Vomiting			X			Possible	
Being married			X			X	
Personality/social difficulties		X	X	X	Possible		
Disturbed relationship with family		X	X	X	X		
Previous treatment		X	X	X	X		X

better in those who have recovered from their anorectic symptoms. Among the prognostic indicators, those that suggest the presence of a severe, chronic, and treatment-resistant illness are more likely to predict a worse outcome.

Long-Term Outcome of Anorexia Nervosa

If there was any optimism over the intermediate-term outcome of anorexia nervosa, it was shattered when Theander (1985) in Lund, Sweden, published his long-term follow-up of the 94 patients that he originally reported on in 1970 (see Table 10–6). The crude mortality rate, at a minimum of 24 years (mean of 33 years) after onset of illness, was 20% (19/94). Five patients (5%) had died of suicide, 12 (13%) of the complications of anorexia nervosa, and 2 (2%) of cancer. This grim outlook is ameliorated somewhat by the finding that more patients have recovered at the 24-year follow-up (71%) than at the 6-year follow-up (52%). Unfortunately, Theander did not report the standardized mortality ratio of his cohort. A third finding of significance in Theander's study is that about half of the patients that died (11/19, 12%) had succumbed within 8 years of onset of illness (i.e., early deaths), and the remainder (8/19, 9%) after 17 years (i.e., late deaths). Some investigators (i.e., Crisp 1980; Hsu 1990) have suggested that the lower rate of early deaths in the recent studies may be related to more effective treatment.

Russell at the Maudsley Hospital, London, has also recently completed a long-term follow-up (minimum of 18 years, mean of 20 years from time of admission to the hospital) of patients on whom he had reported earlier (Morgan and

TABLE 10–6.   20-year outcome of anorexia nervosa

			Crude mortality				
	0–12 years	(%)	12–24 years	(%)	Total	(%)	SMR
Theander 1985 (*N* = 94)	10	(11)	9	(10)	19	(20)	?
Ratnasuriya et al. 1989 (*N* = 41)	2	(5)	5	(12)	7	(17)	?
Hsu & Callender (unpublished) (*N* = 63)	3	(5)	5	(8)	8	(13)	471
Hsu & Crisp (unpublished) (*N* = 105)	2	(2)	2	(2)	4	(4)	136
Patton 1988a (*N* = 332)	?		?		11	(3)	601

Russell 1975). The results (Ratnasuriya et al. 1989) indicated that 30% (n = 12) have recovered according to weight and menstrual function, 33% (n = 13) had an intermediate outcome, 20% (n = 8) a poor outcome, and 17% (n = 7) had died. Of those that died, three (7%) were due to suicide, three (7%) due to complications of the illness, and one (2%) due to an unrelated cause (murder). Thus, a similarly high long-term mortality rate is seen in the Maudsley cohort. However, the overall good outcome pattern reported by the Swedish study is not confirmed by the Maudsley study. If anything, the Maudsley group had a worse outcome at 20-year follow-up than at 5-year follow-up. This discrepancy could probably be explained by the fact that the Maudsley patients are younger. At 20-year follow-up, their mean age is 40 years, whereas the Swedish cohort at 24-year follow-up has a mean age of 51 years (i.e., the illness in the Maudsley cohort may still not have run its full course). Of significance is the lower early mortality (2/41, 5%) in the Maudsley series, which, as previously mentioned, may be due to better treatment. However, the benefits of treatment do not seem to extend beyond 12 years, because the late mortality rate (5/41, 12%) is actually higher in Maudsley than in Lund. The high suicide rate is particularly disturbing.

I have conducted a preliminary long-term follow-up (minimum 17 years from onset) of the St. George's cohort (N = 105, all female) under Professor Crisp in St. George's Hospital, London, a cohort that I have previously reported on (Hsu et al. 1979). For comparison, I have also followed 63 female patients entered into the Aberdeen Case Register between 1965 and 1973. They represent patients that were treated in catchment area medical or psychiatric facilities and not referred to a specialist clinic, as is the case for many of the other published series. At the time of follow-up in 1989, 97 of the 105 St. George's patients were known to be alive; 4 (4/105, 4%) had died (2 from complications of anorexia nervosa, 1 from suicide, and 1 from cancer); and 4 were untraced, although not recorded as dead at either the National Health Central Registry or the Birth and

TABLE 10–7. Causes of death in long-term studies

	Anorexia nervosa (%)		Suicide (%)		Other (%)		Total (%)	
St. George's (N = 105)	2	(2%)	1	(1%)	1	(1%) Cancer	4	(4%)
Aberdeen (N = 63)	3	(5%)	4	(6%)	1	(2%) Cancer	8	(13%)
Sweden (N = 94)	12	(13%)	5	(5%)	2	(2%)	19	(20%)
Maudsley (N = 41)	3	(7%)	3	(7%)	1	(2%) Murder	7	(17%)

Death Registry. Of the 63 Aberdeen patients, 53 were alive, 8 (8/63, 13%) had died, and 2 were untraced (again not recorded as dead). The data are summarized in Table 10–7.

Because this is a preliminary study primarily conducted to determine the feasibility of a full-scale follow-up, the overall outcome pattern in the two cohorts was not studied. The relatively low early mortality of the Aberdeen series is consistent with the Maudsley finding; and the standardized mortality ratio of the Aberdeen cohort is similar to that of the Royal Free Hospital series (Patton 1988a), which in fact had a shorter follow-up interval. Again, these findings lend support to the contention that better treatment may reduce early mortality. For the St. George's cohort, the low overall mortality rate and standardized mortality ratio are unexpected. Because patient selection factors are unlikely to have worked in its favor (being a specialist center, St. George's Hospital tends to treat more chronic and treatment-resistant cases), its low mortality strengthens the case that competent and comprehensive treatment may reduce not only early mortality but also late mortality. Effective treatment may also have contributed to St. George's lower suicide rate (Table 10–7). Whereas in the other three series the suicide rate was 5–7%, the St. George's cohort had only one suicide (jumped from height). Again, it is possible that the illness might not have run its full course in either the Aberdeen (mean age 40.9 ± 7.5 years at follow-up) or St. George's (mean age 38.8 ± 6.7 years) patients in view of their relatively young age in comparison to Theander's patients in Lund.

Clearly, it is still too early to come to a definite conclusion about the long-term outcome for anorexia nervosa. However, from the 300 patients in the four series, it is clear that, in time, about 1 out of 7 patients (14%) may die from suicide or complications of the illness. It is gratifying to find that treatment seems to have at least prevented early deaths. However, the overall outcome pattern is still unclear and must await further study.

Outcome of Bulimia Nervosa

Because bulimia nervosa was not delineated from anorexia nervosa until the late 1970s, it is perhaps not surprising that outcome studies are fewer and of shorter follow-up duration than those for anorexia nervosa. For our present purpose, I will confine my review to cases with a normal weight.

Short-Term Outcome of Bulimia Nervosa

I have been able to find nine studies that have at least 1-year follow-up from time of evaluation (Table 10–8).

Apart from the studies by Fairburn and colleagues (Fairburn et al. 1986) and

TABLE 10–8. Short-term outcome of bulimia nervosa

Author	N/n followed	Index treatment[a]	Duration (months)	Follow-up method	Bulimia nervosa[b] nondiagnosable (%)	Diagnosable (%)	Outcome body weight	Further treatment
1. Abraham et al. 1983	51/43	OP, I	14–72	Interview	65 (?)	35 (?)	Normal	ND
2. Fairburn 1981	11/6	OP, I	12	ND[c]	83	17	Normal	None
3. Fairburn et al. 1986	24/22	OP, I	12	Interview	100	—	Normal	None
4. Hsu and Holder 1986	56/48	OP, I	12–35	Telephone	75	25	Normal	ND
5. Johnson et al. 1986	12/6	OP, I	12	ND	83	17	ND	ND
6. Lacey 1983	30/28	OP, I, G	Up to 24	ND	100	—	Normal	11%
7. Russell et al. 1987	23/23	IP, OP, I, F	12	Interview	At least 21	ND	Mostly normal	ND
8. Wilson et al. 1986	17/11	OP, G	12	Interview	73	27	Normal	36%
9. Yager et al. 1987	?/392	ND	20	Postal questionnaire	43 (?)	57 (?)	ND	ND

[a] OP = outpatient; IP = inpatient; I = individual; G = group; F = family.
[b] Percentages are based on patients successfully traced for follow-up.
[c] ND = not described.

Lacey (1983), which have remarkably good results, the other studies found that about 75% of patients who have been treated are not diagnosable for a bulimic disorder at follow-up, although some of these patients may still have occasional episodes. All the studies are treatment studies (i.e., patients underwent treatment at the respective centers) except for the one by Yager and colleagues (Yager et al. 1987), which recruited patients from the community at large. Perhaps it is for the lack of specific treatment that the patients in the Yager study fared worse, because all the available controlled, randomized studies indicate that some form of cognitive behavioral treatment is superior to nonspecific or supportive therapy (Fairburn et al. 1986; Freeman et al. 1985; Kirkley et al. 1985; Lacey 1983; Lee and Rush 1986; Mitchell et al. 1990; Ordman and Kirschenbaum 1985; Russell et al. 1987; Wilson et al. 1986). Similarly, most of the controlled medication trials suggest that antidepressants are superior to placebo in decreasing bulimic episodes (Agras et al. 1987; Barlow et al. 1988; Horne et al. 1988; Hughes et al. 1986; Kennedy et al. 1988; Mitchell et al. 1989; Pope et al. 1983, 1989; Walsh et al. 1988). Thus, it is clear from the available evidence that cognitive behavioral therapy and antidepressants are effective in the short term for bulimia nervosa.

Intermediate-Term Outcome Studies

Four studies have a follow-up duration of over 2 years (Table 10–9). Overall, 16–50% are still diagnosable as having bulimia nervosa at follow-up, whereas 9–37% are still having occasional episodes. Again, the three studies (Brotman et al. 1988; Hsu and Sobkiewicz 1989; Mitchell et al. 1989) that used specific treatment seemed to have a better outcome than the one that used nonspecific treatment (Swift et al. 1987). However, the duration of follow-up in these studies are still relatively brief (not longer than 5 years), and thus the long-term outcome of bulimia nervosa remains to be clarified. With regard to mental status, the data are incomplete. Swift and colleagues (1987) found major depression at follow-up to be uncommon. Brotman and colleagues (1988) did not report such data, and the findings of the two studies using predominantly telephone follow-up could not be evaluated. Prognostic indicators were not examined in these studies.

Current Issues of Interest

I will use the findings to answer two questions that I believe are of interest to clinicians and investigators: 1) Are the eating disorders variants of other disorders such as the affective disorders? and 2) Do the findings shed any light on the pathogenesis of the eating disorders? In answering the second question, I will

TABLE 10–9. Intermediate-term outcome of bulimia nervosa

Author	N/n followed	Index Treatment[a]	Duration (months)	Follow-up method	Bulimia nervosa[b] nondiagnosable (%)	Diagnosable (%)	Outcome body weight	Further treatment
1. Brotman et al. 1988	12/12c	OP, I, G, M	24–60	ND	58 in remission	17 (25 marked improvement)	ND	ND
2. Hsu & Sobkiewicz 1989	45/35	OP, I	48–60	Mostly telephone	47	16 (plus 16% symptomatic but nondiagnosable)	Normal 2% underweight	30%
3. Mitchell et al. 1989	100/91	OP, G	24–60	Telephone	66	25 (plus 9% symptomatic but nondiagnosable)	Normal 1% underweight 7% overweight	ND
4. Swift et al. 1987	38/30	IP, OP (?)	24–60	Interview	13	50 (plus 37% symptomatic but nondiagnosable)	Normal	100%

[a] OP = outpatient; IP = inpatient; I = individual; G = group; F = family.
[b] Percentages are based on patients successfully traced for follow-up.
[c] Taking only patients followed for at least 2 years.

also review two longitudinal (i.e., follow-up) studies of dieters who were not initially diagnosable as suffering from an eating disorder.

Eating Disorders and Other Psychiatric Disorders

The debate on whether the eating disorders are variants of affective disorders is not entirely academic, because it has implications, not only for research, but also for treatment. I should point out at the outset that follow-up data alone can never settle the question of whether an eating disorder is a variant of an affective disorder. At best, they may provide evidence that is more or less consistent with the hypothesis.

For our present purpose, the statement "An eating disorder is a variant of an affective disorder" is taken to mean "An eating disorder has a biological abnormality that is the same as the one that occurs in an affective disorder." This definition is similar to the one proposed by Pope and Hudson (1988). However, because no biological abnormality has yet been identified consistently for either an affective or eating disorder, the arguments are necessarily speculative. Arguments presented eloquently on either side of the debate have focused on evidence from phenomenology, course and outcome, family history, biological abnormalities, and treatment response of the disorders (e.g., Pope and Hudson 1988; Strober and Katz 1987). It is with the course and outcome data that I am primarily concerned here.

In contrast to the episodic nature of an affective disorder (e.g., Keller 1985), anorectic and bulimic disorders are generally more protracted and tend to run a longer course (e.g., Hsu 1988). Furthermore, available evidence (and this could change as better studies are conducted) indicates that, in the patients who qualify for both an eating and affective disorder, the disorders often develop concurrently, although in some patients they subsequently may diverge with respect to the pattern of resolution or recurrence (Strober and Katz 1987). At follow-up, those that are free from an anorectic (Hall et al. 1984) or bulimic illness (Swift et al. 1987) are less likely to demonstrate affective symptoms. The most common diagnosis at follow-up, apart from anorexia nervosa, seems to be bulimia nervosa, not major depression (Hsu 1988). These findings do not readily support the view that the eating disorders are in fact affective disorders disguised with a different manifestation. However, as previously mentioned, the findings also do not definitely refute the hypothesis that the two disorders are, in fact, one.

More recently, the idea first proposed more than 50 years ago (Palmer and Jones 1939; Rahman et al. 1939)—that anorexia nervosa may be related to an obsessive-compulsive disorder—has been revived (e.g., Rothenberg 1986). The possibility that the two disorders may share a common disturbance in the serotonin neurotransmitter system is intriguing (Morley and Blundell 1988). From the perspective of course and outcome, not much can be said due to the lack of data. Toner and colleagues (1986) found a high prevalence of obsessive-compulsive disorder among their patients at follow-up, more so for the restrictors (39% lifetime, 23% last year) than the bulimic patients (29% lifetime, 10% last year). Unfortunately, whether the obsessive-compulsive symptoms occur in the context of an unresolved eating disorder is unclear.

Obviously, the same question of classification and nosology can be raised with respect to the relationship between the eating disorders and any of the other psychiatric disorders (such as psychoactive substance use disorders) or between anorexia and bulimia nervosa and restrictive and bulimic anorexia nervosa. For the moment, the follow-up data are incomplete and thus not very helpful on the issue of classification of the eating disorders.

Pathogenesis of the Eating Disorders

The question of classification, important though it is, is not as interesting to me as the question of the role affective disturbances play in the pathogenesis of an eating disorder (Hsu 1989). Is it possible that normal adolescent dieting is more likely to develop into an eating disorder if the dieter is also depressed or anxious? Unfortunately, longitudinal data on the pathogenesis of the eating disorders is almost nonexistent. Do the outcome data shed any light on this important issue?

The available data support an "accretion" model of the pathogenesis of the eating disorders. First, most studies indicate that the "weight phobia" persists even in those who have recovered. According to self-reports, these patients claim that they have somehow lost the "willpower" to starve themselves despite the fact that they still feel too fat. Furthermore, the data suggest that restrictive anorexia nervosa gives way, in time, to bulimia nervosa, but the reverse is not true (i.e., bulimic patients rarely revert to restrictive anorexia nervosa; Hsu and Sobkiewicz 1989). From such outcome data, a tentative model of the pathogenesis of the eating disorders may therefore be constructed: weight phobia leads to restrictive dieting behavior that, in turn, leads to bulimic behavior in some patients. This model also seems to be consistent with the patients' subjective reports regarding the onset of their eating disorder.

Two British longitudinal studies specifically addressed some of these issues. In a survey of 720 patients aged 16–35 attending four London general practices, King (1989) used the Eating Attitudes Test (EAT-26, Garner et al. 1982) to identify 76 high EAT scorers (71 female, 5 male). On interview, he found that 21 of the female high scorers showed significant bulimic symptomatology, and 36 were dieters. He also interviewed a random sample of 40 low scorers and found none to show any eating disorder symptomatology. At 12- to 18-month postal follow-up, he found 25% (9/36) of the dieters to have developed ominous bulimic symptoms, and only 10% (4/36) to be no longer dieting. Thus, the findings suggest that dieting behavior is a significant risk factor for the development of bulimic symptomatology. Unfortunately, he did not identify the other risk factors that turn dieting into an eating disorder. In a survey of 1,010 teenage girls from eight London schools, Patton and colleagues (Patton 1988b; Patton et al. 1990), again using the EAT-26, found 9.3% of the girls to be high scorers. On interview of these high scorers, they found that 22 showed significant bulimic symptomatology, and 61 were dieters.

At 1-year follow-up interview, 13 (21%) of the dieters had developed significant bulimic symptoms, whereas only 3 of the 98 (3%) nondieters did the same. The authors concluded that the relative risk for dieters developing an eating disorder is 7.9 times greater than that for nondieters. Among the risk factors studied, only a high score on the General Health Questionnaire (Goldberg and Hiller 1979), a measure of mainly affective symptomatology, predicted the development of an eating disorder in the dieters. There is therefore some support for the model that affective symptoms in a teenage dieter may turn the dieting behavior into a bulimic disorder. Neither of the studies found any cases of restrictive anorexia nervosa to have developed during the follow-up period; thus, the risk factors for the development of this disorder are unknown.

Clearly, much more data are needed in this vital area. Traditionally, most experts (e.g., Bruch 1970; Crisp 1980) have held the view that normal adolescent dieting is a transient phenomenon not related to the onset of anorexia nervosa. If dieting should prove to be a primary risk factor for the pathogenesis of an eating disorder, and if affective symptoms could turn "normal" dieting behavior into an eating disorder, then more specific preventive and treatment measures may be developed and implemented.

Conclusion

I hope you, the reader, have become convinced of the importance of the five criteria that I have listed previously in this chapter. If you have not, there are useful articles listed in Table 10–4. Even in these conscientiously conducted studies, the difficulty in summarizing the outcome data, let alone interpreting them, presents the case convincingly that some uniformity in the methodology of conducting and reporting outcome studies is needed. In particular, a high refusal (i.e., refuse to be followed) or untraced rate (over 15%) makes the finding difficult to interpret. I believe that we cannot assume that the outcome in this refusal (or untraced) group is similar to the successfully followed (or traced) group simply because the two are similar in terms of their baseline variables

(Toner et al. 1986). This is true for two reasons: the prognostic indicators are few and relatively weak, and the patients that refuse follow-up are likely to have done so because of a worse outcome (Hsu et al. 1979).

Future studies may benefit from attention to three other issues: 1) the use of standardized interviews and questionnaires, 2) the adoption of a more uniform way of reporting the findings, and 3) the study of the outcome of subclinical cases.

The importance of using standardized interviews and questionnaires is obvious, and some recent studies are using such measures (e.g., Swift et al. 1987; Toner et al. 1986). I hope this trend will continue so that outcome data, particularly those on mental status and psychosocial functioning, may become easier to interpret and more comparable among studies.

In terms of reporting outcome findings, more studies are using the Morgan and Russell outcome category (Morgan and Russell 1975) or the category developed by Garfinkel and colleagues (Garfinkel et al. 1977) to summarize the data on weight and menstrual function. However, I believe that weight and menstrual outcome should also be reported separately (i.e., in addition to the outcome categories). A global outcome score combining outcome rating in all areas is unhelpful if reported alone. It is also better to present outcome data in each area separately and in terms of standardized measures. Furthermore, it is important to report on the diagnostic status (whether full or partial syndrome of the patients at outcome) and to present the data separately for those who are still anorectic or bulimic and those who are not. This may allow other investigators to tease out the relationship between eating disorder symptoms and affective or anxiety symptoms. The significance, for the purpose of classification of a major depressive episode occurring with a concurrent unresolved anorectic illness and one occurring in a long-recovered anorectic patient, may be debatable, but at least the data should be clearly presented.

Finally, mortality should be reported in terms of the crude mortality rate, the standardized mortality ratio, and the causes of death. Mortality data presented in this way will allow us to assess the relative risk for increased mortality in the eating disorders. To exclude those deaths deemed not to be related directly to the eating disorder, as some have done (e.g., Theander 1985; Touyz and Beumont 1984) confuses rather than clarifies the data.

In summary, there has been some progress in our understanding of the intermediate outcome of the eating disorders, and a beginning has been made in our efforts to clarify the long-term outcome of anorexia nervosa. Unfortunately, it seems that there are still too many studies that produce data that are uninterpretable, including some studies that attempt to address the question of treatment efficacy without a proper design (e.g., Becker et al. 1981; Kohle and Mall 1983). Furthermore, the outcome of subclinical cases (or partial syndromes) has so far been neglected. A knowledge of the outcome of a carefully defined cohort (i.e., using clearly defined criteria to indicate why the subjects are subclinical instead of being "full syndromes" or "non-cases") may allow us to determine the relationship between full and partial syndrome and how best to classify the eating disorders. It may also help us to know what the risk factors are in the pathogenesis of the eating disorders.

References

Abraham S, Myra M, Llewellyn-Jones D: A study of outcome. International Journal of Eating Disorders 2:175–180, 1983

Agras WS, Dorian B, Kirkley BG, et al: Imipramine in the treatment of bulimia: A double-blind controlled study. International Journal of Eating Disorders 6:29–38, 1987

Barlow J, Blouin J, Blouin A, et al: Treatment of bulimia with desipramine: A double-blind crossover study. Can J Psychiatry 33:129–133, 1988

Bassoe HH, Eskeland I: A prospective study of 133 patients with anorexia nervosa: Treatment and outcome. Acta Psychiatr Scand 65:127–133, 1982

Becker H, Korner P, Stoffler A: Psychodynamics and therapeutic aspects of anorexia nervosa: A study of family dynamics and prognosis. Psychother Psychosom 36:816, 1981

Brinch M, Isager T, Tolstrup K: Anorexia nervosa and motherhood: Reproductional pattern and mothering behavior of 50 women. Acta Psychiatr Scand 77:90–104, 1988

Brotman AW, Herzog DB, Hamburg P: Long-term course in 14 bulimic patients treated with psychotherapy. J Clin Psychiatry 49(4):157–160, 1988

Bruch H: Psychotherapy in primary anorexia nervosa. J Nerv Ment Dis 150:51–67, 1970

Burns T, Crisp AH: Outcome of anorexia nervosa in males. Br J Psychiatry 145:319–325, 1984

Cantwell DP, Sturzenberger S, Burroughs J, et al: Anorexia nervosa: An affective disorder? Arch Gen Psychiatry 34:1087–1093, 1977

Crisp AH: Anorexia Nervosa: Let Me Be. London, Plenum, 1980, pp 4, 28, 84, 125

Fairburn CG: A cognitive behavioral approach to the management of bulimia. Psychol Med 11:707–711, 1981

Fairburn CG, Kirk J, O'Connor M, et al: A comparison of two psychological treatments for bulimia nervosa. Behav Res Ther 24:629–643, 1986

Freeman C, Sinclair F, Turnbull J, et al: Psychotherapy for bulimia: A controlled study. J Psychiatr Res 19:473–478, 1985

Garfinkel PE, Moldolfsky H, Garner DM: The outcome of anorexia nervosa, significance of clinical features, body image, and behavior modification, in Anorexia Nervosa. Edited by Vigersky AK. New York, Raven, 1977, pp 315–329

Garner DM, Olmsted MP, Bohr Y, et al: The eating attitudes test: Psychometric features and clinical correlates. Psychol Med 12:871–878, 1982

Goldberg DP, Hiller VF: A scaled version of the general health questionnaire. Psychol Med 9:139–145, 1979

Hall A, Slim E, Hawker F, et al: Anorexia nervosa: Long-term outcome in 50 female patients. Br J Psychiatry 145:407–413, 1984

Halmi KA, Eckert E, LaDu TJ, et al: Anorexia nervosa: Treatment efficacy of cyproheptadine and amitriptyline. Arch Gen Psychiatry 43:177–181, 1986

Hawley RM: The outcome of anorexia nervosa in younger subjects. Br J Psychiatry 146:657–660, 1985

Horne RL, Ferguson JM, Pope HG, et al: Treatment of bulimia with bupropion: A multicenter controlled trial. J Clin Psychiatry 49:262–266, 1988

Hsu LKG: Outcome of anorexia nervosa: A review of the literature (1954–1978). Arch Gen Psychiatry 37:1041–1046, 1980

Hsu LKG: The outcome of anorexia nervosa: A reappraisal. Psychol Med 18:807–812, 1988

Hsu LKG: The gender gap in the eating disorders: Why are the eating disorders more common in women? Clinical Psychology Review 9:393–407, 1989

Hsu LKG: The experiential aspects of bulimia nervosa: Implications for cognitive behavioral therapy. Behav Modif 14:50–65, 1990

Hsu LKG, Callender JS: Twenty year mortality in the Aberdeen Case Register cohort of anorexia nervosa patients. Unpublished manuscript, 1989

Hsu LKG, Crisp AH: Twenty year mortality in the St. George's cohort of anorexia nervosa patients. Unpublished manuscript, 1989

Hsu LKG, Holder D: Bulimia nervosa: treatment and short-term outcome. Psychol Med 16:65–70, 1986

Hsu LKG, Sobkiewicz TA: Bulimia nervosa: Four to six year outcome. Psychol Med 19:1035–1038, 1989

Hsu LKG, Crisp AH, Harding B: Outcome of anorexia nervosa. Lancet 1:62–65, 1979

Hughes PL, Wells LA, Cunningham CJ, et al: Treatment of bulimia with desipramine: A double-blind, placebo-controlled study. Arch Gen Psychiatry 43:182–186, 1986

Johnson WG, Schlundt DG, Jarrell MP: Exposure with response prevention, training in energy balance and problem solving therapy for bulimia nervosa. International Journal of Eating Disorders 5:35–45, 1986

Katz JL, Kuperberg A, Pollack CP, et al: Is there a relationship between eating disorder and affective disorder? New evidence from sleep recordings. Am J Psychiatry 14:753–759, 1984

Keller MB: Chronic and recurrent affective disorders: Incidence, course, and influencing factors, in Chronic Treatments in Neuropsychiatry. Edited by Kemali D, Racagni G. New York, Raven, 1985, pp 111–120

Kennedy SH, Piran N, Warsh JJ, et al: A trial of isocarboxazid in the treatment of bulimia nervosa. J Clin Psychopharmacol 8:391–396, 1988

King M: Eating disorders in a general practice population. Prevalence, characteristics and follow-up at 12 to 18 months. Psychol Med Monogr Suppl 14:3–34, 1989

Kirkley BB, Schneider JA, Agras W, et al: Comparison of two group treatments for bulimia. J Consult Clin Psychol 53:43–48, 1985

Kohle K, Mall H: Follow-up study of 36 anorexia nervosa patients treated on an integrated internistic-psychosomatic ward. International Journal of Eating Disorders 2(4):215–219, 1983

Lacey JH: Bulimia nervosa, binge eating and psychogenetic vomiting: A controlled treatment study and long-term outcome. British Medical Journal 286:1609–1613, 1983

Lee N, Rush PAJ: Cognitive-behavioral group therapy for bulimia. International Journal of Eating Disorders 5:599–613, 1986

Martin FE: The treatment and outcome of anorexia nervosa in adolescents: A prospective study and five year follow-up. J Psychiatr Res 19(2/3):509–514, 1985

Minuchin S: An interview with Salvador Minuchin. Family Therapy Networker 8:31–32, 1984

Mitchell JE, Pyle RL, Hatsukami D, et al: A 2 to 5 year follow-up study of patients treated for bulimia. International Journal of Eating Disorders 8:157–165, 1989

Mitchell JE, Pyle RL, Eckert ED, et al: A comparison study of antidepressants and structured intensive group psychotherapy in the treatment of bulimia nervosa. Arch Gen Psychiatry 47(2):149–160, 1990

Morgan HG, Russell GFM: Value of family background and clinical features as predictors of long-term outcome in anorexia nervosa: Four year follow-up study of 41 patients. Psychol Med 5:355–371, 1975

Morgan HG, Purgold J, Welbourne J: Management and outcome in anorexia nervosa: A standardized prognostic study. Br J Psychiatry 143:282–287, 1983

Morley JE, Blundell JE: The neurobiological basis of eating disorders: Some formulations. Biol Psychiatry 23:53–78, 1988

Nussbaum M, Shenker IR, Baird D, et al: Follow-up investigation in patients with anorexia nervosa. J Pediatr 106:835–840, 1985

Ordman AM, Kirschenbaum DS: Cognitive-behavioral therapy for bulimia: An initial outcome study. J Consult Clin Psychol 53:305–313, 1985

Palmer RL, Jones MS: Anorexia nervosa as a manifestation of compulsion neurosis. Archives of Neurological Psychiatry 41:856–861, 1939

Patton GC: Mortality in eating disorders. Psychol Med 18:947–952, 1988a

Patton GC: The spectrum of eating disorders. Psychosomatic Research 32(6):579–584, 1988b

Patton GC, Johnson-Sabine E, Wood K, et al: Abnormal eating attitudes in London schoolgirls—a prospective epidemiological study: Outcome at twelve month follow-up. Psychol Med 20:383–394, 1990

Pope HG, Jr., Hudson JI: Is bulimia nervosa a heterogeneous disorder? Lessons from the history of medicine. International Journal of Eating Disorders 7:155–166, 1988

Pope HG, Jr., Hudson JI, Jonas JM, et al: Bulimia treated with imipramine: A placebo-controlled, double-blind study. Am J Psychiatry 140:554–558, 1983

Pope HG, Keck PE, McElroy SL, et al: A placebo-controlled study of trazodone in bulimia nervosa. J Clin Psychopharmacol 9(4):254–259, 1989

Rahman L, Richardson HB, Ripley HS: Anorexia nervosa with psychiatric observations. Psychosom Med 1:335–365, 1939

Ratnasuriya RH, Eisler I, Szmukler GI, et al: Outcome and prognostic factors after 20 years of anorexia nervosa, in Psychobiology of Human Eating Disorders. Edited by Schneider LH, Cooper SJ, Halmi KA. Ann N Y Acad Sci 575:567–568, 1989

Rosman BL, Minuchin S, Baker L, et al: A family approach to anorexia nervosa: Study, treatment, and outcome, in Anorexia Nervosa. Edited by Vigersky RA. New York, Raven, 1977, pp 341–348

Rothenberg A: Eating disorder as a modern obsessive-compulsive syndrome. Psychiatry 49:45–53, 1986

Russell GFM, Szmukler GI, Dare C, et al: An evaluation of family therapy in anorexia nervosa and bulimia nervosa. Arch Gen Psychiatry 44:1047–1056, 1987

Santonastaso P, Favaretto G, Canton G: Anorexia nervosa in Italy: Clinical features and outcome in a long-term follow-up study. Psychopathology 20:8–17, 1987

Schwartz DM, Thompson MG: Do anorectics get well? Current research and future needs. Am J Psychiatry 44:319–323, 1981

Steinhausen HC, Glanville K: A long-term follow-up of adolescent anorexia nervosa. Acta Psychiatr Scand 68:1–10, 1983a

Steinhausen HC, Glanville K: Retrospective and prospective follow-up studies in anorexia nervosa. International Journal of Eating Disorders 2(4):221–235, 1983b

Strober M, Katz JL: Do eating disorders and affective disorders share a common etiology? International Journal of Eating Disorders 6:171–180, 1987

Swift WJ: The long-term outcome of early onset anorexia nervosa: A critical review. Journal of the American Academy of Child Psychiatry 21:38–46, 1982

Swift WJ, Ritholz M, Kalin NH, et al: A follow-up study of thirty hospitalized bulimics. Psychosom Med 49:45–55, 1987

Theander S: Anorexia nervosa: A psychiatric investigation of 94 female patients. Acta Psychiatr Scand Suppl 214:1–194, 1970

Theander S: Outcome and prognosis in anorexia nervosa and bulimia: Some results of previous investigations, compared with those of a Swedish long-term study. J Psychiatr Res 19:493–508, 1985

Tolstrup K, Brinch M, Isager T, et al: Long-term outcome of 151 cases of anorexia nervosa: The Copenhagen anorexia nervosa follow-up study. Acta Psychiatr Scand 71:380–387, 1985

Toner BB, Garfinkel PE, Garner DM: Long-term follow-up of anorexia nervosa. Psychosom Med 48:520–529, 1986

Touyz SW, Beumont PJV: Anorexia nervosa: A follow-up investigation. Med J Aust 141:219–222, 1984

Vandereycken W, Pierloot R: Long-term outcome research in anorexia nervosa: The problem of patient selection and follow-up duration. International Journal of Eating Disorders 2(4/5):237–242, 1983

Walsh BT, Gladis M, Roose SP, et al: Phenelzine vs placebo in 50 patients with bulimia. Arch Gen Psychiatry 45(5):471–478, 1988

Wilson AJ, Rossiter E, Kleifeld EL, et al: Cognitive-behavioral treatment of bulimia nervosa: A controlled evaluation. Behav Res Ther 24:277–288, 1986

Yager J, Landsverk J, Edelstein CK: A 20-month follow-up study of 628 women with eating disorders. I: Course and severity. Am J Psychiatry 144:1172–1177, 1987

❖ 11 ❖ Outcome Studies of Borderline Personality Disorder

Mary C. Zanarini, Ed.D.
Deborah L. Chauncey, A.B.
Tana A. Grady, M.D.
John G. Gunderson, M.D.

Borderline personality disorder (BPD) is a common psychiatric disorder; a recent review estimated that 11% of outpatients and 19% of inpatients meet current criteria for BPD (Widiger and Frances 1989). It is also a disorder that has generated a tremendous amount of research interest. A recent MEDLINE computer search indicated that more than 100 empirical studies of borderline psychopathology have been published in the past decade. Taken together, these studies have suggested that BPD is a valid disorder that 1) has a distinctive phenomenology, 2) "breeds true" in first-degree relatives, and 3) may be more closely associated with a childhood history of abuse than of neglect (Gunderson and Zanarini 1989; Zanarini et al. 1990).

However, little is known about the types of treatment that are most effective for these particularly-difficult-to-treat patients. Only prospective studies of the long-term course of BPD will permit a naturalistic assessment of the factors most closely associated with patients' improvement and recovery. Unfortunately, no such studies have yet been conducted. However, eight short-term prospective studies and four long-term follow-back studies have been conducted. We will review the results of these studies in the following sections.

Short-Term Outcome of BPD

Grinker and associates (1968) followed up 41 of 51 broadly defined "borderline syndrome" patients at a mean of 2.5 years after hospitalization (see Table 11–1 for details of this and subsequent short-term studies). They found that 66% of the patients described themselves as worse off, the same, or only marginally improved since their hospitalization. Approximately one-third of the patients

TABLE 11–1. Short-term follow-up studies of borderline personality disorder (BPD)

Study	BPD criteria/N	Control group(s)	Trace rate (%)[a]
Grinker et al. 1968	unspecified criteria ($N = 41$)	none	80
Werble 1970	unspecified criteria ($N = 28$)	none	55
Gunderson et al. 1975	loose criteria ($N = 24$)	29 schizophrenic patients	100
Carpenter and Gunderson 1977	loose criteria ($N = 14$)	20 schizophrenic patients	58
Pope et al. 1983	DSM-III criteria (via retrospective chart review) ($N = 27$)	27 schizophrenic patients 35 schizoaffective patients 18 bipolar patients	82
Akiskal et al. 1985	Gunderson-Singer and DSM-III criteria ($N = 100$)	57 schizophrenic patients 50 patients with personality disorder 50 bipolar patients 40 unipolar patients	100
Barasch et al. 1985	DIB and DSM-III (via interview) ($N = 10$)	20 patients with other personality disorders	38
Perry and Cooper 1985	DSM-III and BPS (via interview) ($N = 30$)	10 APD patients 15 bipolar II patients	57
Tucker et al. 1987	"severe personality disorder" by DSM-III (via clinical interview) ($N = 40$)	none	65
Modestin and Villiger 1989	DSM-III BPD (via clinical interview) ($N = 18$)	17 patients with other personality disorders	69

[a] Rate of BPD patients.

required rehospitalization during the follow-up period. The majority of the patients were occupationally stable, but worked in low-level jobs and were not upwardly mobile. The patient's social functioning was comparatively more impaired. Only 17% had an "active" social life, and the modal group of patients had social lives described as "limited leisure-time activities involving transient contact with people" (p. 133). In addition, nearly one-half of the patients had troubled or minimal relationships with their families.

Werble (1970) published a 6- to 7-year follow-up of 28 of the same patients. She found that most patients lived in the community; about half had been rehospitalized, but their hospitalizations tended to be brief. There had been little improvement in the patients' overall functioning over this period, and their social functioning had deteriorated slightly. However, there was no evidence that they were becoming schizophrenic. The majority of patients continued to work but were socially isolated, with few contacts with either family or friends. Werble wrote, "The stability in the life styles of the group is confirmed by the steady picture of employment that they present. [But] with very few exceptions, adaptations are made within very narrow constricted limits . . . whatever stable equilibria they achieve is very costly. There are very few human object relations in their lives" (p. 7).

Gunderson and colleagues (1975) studied the 2-year course of a group of 24 patients given a borderline diagnosis on the basis of brief psychotic experiences, diagnostic uncertainty, and the absence of nuclear schizophrenic symptoms. The BPD patients were matched by age, sex, race, and socioeconomic status with 29 schizophrenic patients. Gunderson and colleagues found that, on average, these patients had been employed part- to full-time for about one-half to two-thirds of the year prior to follow-up. They had social contacts about once every 2 weeks, and had been hospitalized for less than 3 months during the previous year. Their signs and symptoms were described as "moderate some of the time." In every area, the borderline patients remained as functionally impaired as the schizophrenic control group. These borderline patients did not develop symptoms resembling schizophrenia, but they remained "a confusing and often changing diagnostic group."

Carpenter and Gunderson (1977) followed up 14 of the original 24 patients at 5 years. The functioning of the borderline group was still indistinguishable from that of the schizophrenic group, except that the borderline patients maintained the quality of their social contacts, whereas those of the schizophrenic patients deteriorated. Relatively few patients had required hospitalization. Although several were "loners," most met regularly with friends. Almost all patients were employed continuously, although some were underemployed and some worked ineffectively. Overall, the functioning of these patients had not significantly changed since their 2-year follow-up.

Pope and associates (1983) were the first to use DSM-III criteria (American Psychiatric Association 1980) in a study of the short-term course of BPD. This was a "follow-back" study that diagnosed patients via retrospective chart review. The investigators followed 27 of 33 patients with DSM-III BPD for 4 to 7 years after their index hospitalization. No borderline patients developed schizophrenia during the follow-up period, and the borderline diagnosis was found to be fairly stable over time. Eighteen of the 27 patients (66.7%) had a probable or definite diagnosis of BPD at follow-up. However, the stability of the diagnosis did not ensure its distinctness—85% of the original cohort met DSM-III criteria for another "dramatic" cluster personality disorder, and 67% met DSM-III criteria for a substance use disorder.

As a whole, the group of patients with BPD had a significantly worse outcome than control groups with bipolar or schizoaffective disorders. They were similar to a schizophrenic control group on most outcome indices, except that the BPD patients had significantly better occupational functioning than the schizophrenics.

Pope and colleagues were also the first to study comorbid diagnoses of borderline patients and their effect on outcome. Thirteen of the patients they followed had "pure" BPD, whereas 14 had BPD plus a concurrent major affective disorder (MAD). At follow-up, the BPD patients with MAD were functioning significantly better than the "pure" BPD group on two measures of functioning: social functioning and freedom from symptoms. The researchers attributed the better functioning of the BPD-with-MAD group to the fact that these patients were more likely to have had a positive response to medication.

Akiskal and co-workers (1985) followed 100 borderline outpatients who met DSM-III criteria on the basis of a clinical interview over a period of 6 months to 3 years. They found that during the follow-up period, 52% of the borderline patients they studied developed affective disorders. Twenty-nine patients developed an episode of major depression, 4 developed manic episodes, 11 developed hypomanic episodes, and 8 developed mixed affective disorders. Many (45%) of these patients had a diagnosis of concurrent affective disorder at the beginning of the study—primarily dysthymic, cyclothymic, or bipolar II disorders. But even in the group that had no initial diagnosis of affective disorder, 11 (20%) had an episode of major depression, and 4 (7%) committed suicide. Akiskal and associates concluded that "borderline disorders are located predominantly on the border of affective rather than schizophrenic psychoses" (p. 45), and hypothesized that what we call borderline personality might represent an atypical, subaffective form of bipolar disorder.

Perry and Cooper (1985) compared a group of 30 borderline patients (out of an original cohort of 53) with a group of patients diagnosed as having DSM-III antisocial personality disorder (APD, the best-validated "dramatic cluster" personality disorder) and a group of patients with bipolar II disorder 1 to 3 years after their initial assessment. They used a semistructured diagnostic interview to assess the presence of BPD. In addition, they were the first researchers to give their subjects a definite BPD diagnosis only if they met both DSM-III and additional criteria: a sufficient score on the Borderline Personality Scale (BPS; Perry 1985), a reliable rating scale that assesses borderline psychopathology and includes areas not covered in the DSM-III criteria.

With regard to global functioning, Perry and Cooper (1985) found that the mean Global Assessment Scale (GAS; Endicott et al. 1976) score for their BPD group was 52.6, which is considered to be in the "fair" range. They also found no differences among their three groups at 2- to 3-year follow-up. However, border-line pathology, assessed as a continuous variable, was predictive of both lower GAS scores and greater variability in functioning.

Perry and Cooper (1985) did find several differences between BPD and APD patients during the follow-up period. They found that psychiatric health care use was significantly predicted by borderline psychopathology after controlling for sex. They also found that in borderline patients without antisocial pathology, there was a significant association between a borderline diagnosis and symptoms of anxiety and depression during the follow-up period. An APD diagnosis was not associated with affective symptoms, and the presence of antisocial symptoms in a borderline patient reversed the relationship between borderline and affec-tive symptoms. In addition, a BPD diagnosis was less strongly associated with drug and alcohol abuse and with antisocial symptoms during the follow-up period than was an APD diagnosis.

Barasch and colleagues (1985) conducted a 3-year follow-up of 10 patients with DSM-III diagnosed BPD and a reference group of 20 patients with other DSM-III personality-disorder diagnoses. They used a semistructured clinical in-terview to assess the presence of DSM-III Axis II disorders and found that the two groups were similar with respect to their "fair" level of functioning and the slight degree of their improvement over the follow-up period. (The BPD group has a mean GAS score of 51.4 at baseline and 59.2 at follow-up—a nonsignifi-cant difference.) Forty percent of each group developed a major depressive epi-sode during the follow-up period. Thus, neither the degree of their impairment nor their level of affective symptomatology distinguished the two groups.

In addition, Barasch and colleagues (1985) assessed the degree of stability of the borderline diagnosis over the follow-up period. Sixty percent of the BPD group met DSM-III criteria for BPD at follow-up, and 30% met four (rather than five) DSM-III criteria. Of the 20 nonborderline subjects, only three met DSM-III BPD criteria at follow-up. The authors concluded that BPD was a stable diagnosis over time and that it was neither a variant of a major depression nor a nonspecific label for "severe" personality disorders.

Modestin and Villiger (1989) also compared patients with BPD to patients with other personality disorders. They conducted a 4-1/2-year follow-up study of 18 DSM-III diagnosed borderline patients and 17 personality-disordered patients with heterogeneous nonborderline ICD-9 (World Health Organization 1978) diagnoses. They found that BPD patients were quite impaired, with about 70% only working part-time or receiving a disability pension. However, they func-tioned at about the same vocational and social level as the other personality-disordered patients, with the exception that significantly fewer were married. Modestin and Villiger also found that BPD patients were more often rehospitalized, but their hospitalizations were of shorter duration. However, both groups exhibited the same high level of depressive and anxiety symptoms.

Tucker and colleagues (1987) did a prospective study of 40 patients with "borderline disorders"—not DSM-III BPD—who were hospitalized on a specialized long-term treatment unit. They found that patients at follow-up 2 years post-discharge exhibited less suicidal ideation and behavior, were more likely to be in continuous psychotherapy, and had more close friendships and positive relationships than at baseline. Those patients hospitalized for more than 12 months were less likely to be rehospitalized and more likely to be in continuous psychotherapy during the first year following discharge, but these differences disappeared after the first year. The mean GAS score for this sample was 29.7 at admission, 41.6 at discharge, 50.3 1 year after discharge, and 56.5 2 years after discharge, indicating that these patients moved from the incapacitated to the fair range of functioning.

The generalizability of the results of these studies has been limited by a number of methodological problems. These problems have included small sample sizes, absence of control groups, lack of explicit criteria for BPD, use of unstructured assessment techniques for making diagnoses, nonblind assessment of outcome status, limited assessment of outcome functioning, and very little focus on prediction of outcome.

Despite these limitations, three major findings concerning the short-term course of BPD have emerged from these studies. First, borderline patients continued to have substantial difficulty functioning 6 months to 7 years after their initial assessment, particularly in the areas of social functioning and needing continuing psychiatric care. Second, their level of functioning was very similar to that of patients with both schizophrenia and other forms of personality disorder. Third, BPD patients did not go on to develop schizophrenia but retained the "stable instability" characteristic of a borderline diagnosis.

Long-Term Outcome of BPD

Plakun and associates (1985) conducted a follow-back study of 237 patients who had been hospitalized between 1950 and 1976 at Austen Riggs, a private psychiatric hospital in western Massachusetts (see Table 11–2 for details of this and subsequent long-term studies). They had originally mailed out a 50-item questionnaire to the 878 patients who had been hospitalized for at least 2 months, and they received a 27% response rate. Among these patients, who were diagnosed through chart review according to DSM-III criteria, were the following patient groups: 61 borderline patients, 19 schizophrenic patients, 24 patients with major affective disorder, 13 schizotypal patients, and 19 patients with schizoid personality disorder.

These groups were compared on their baseline and follow-up functioning using their mean GAS scores. All borderline groups except those with a comorbid schizotypal personality disorder achieved a higher baseline GAS score than the schizophrenic controls but equivalent to the affective controls. However, the functioning of borderline patients with and without a concurrent affective disorder was basically the same.

At a mean follow-up period of 15 years, the borderline patients achieved a mean GAS of 67, a score in the good range of functioning. Both the 54 "aggregated" borderlines (all but those with a concomitant major affective disorder) and the borderline patients with a comorbid schizotypal disorder achieved a higher mean GAS than the schizophrenic patients, the latter group moving from being the lowest functioning borderline subgroup to the highest. In addition, borderline patients without a comorbid affective disorder were functioning significantly better than those with a comorbid affective disorder.

McGlashan (1986a) followed up all inpatients treated at Chestnut Lodge between 1950 and 1975 who met the following criteria: 1) index admission of at least 90 days, 2) age between 16 and 55, and 3) absence of an organic brain

TABLE 11–2. Long-term follow-up studies of borderline personality disorder (BPD)

Study	BPD criteria/N	Control group(s)	Trace rate (%)[a]
Plakun et al. 1985	Retrospective DSM-III diagnosis (N = 63)	19 schizophrenic patients 24 patients with major affective disorder 13 patients with schizotypal PD 19 patients with schizoid PD	27
McGlashan 1986a	Retrospective DSM-III and DIB diagnosis (N = 81 "pure" BPD)	163 schizophrenic patients 44 patients with unipolar depression	72
Paris et al. 1987	Retrospective DIB diagnosis (N = 100)	None	32
Stone et al. 1987	Retrospective DSM-III and "psychostructural" diagnosis (N = 251)	89 schizophrenic patients 55 schizoaffective patients	84

[a] Rate for first two studies is for all patients, whereas rate for last two studies is for borderline patients.

syndrome. Follow-up information was obtained on 446 patients, resulting in a trace rate of 72%. Follow-up information was collected by the use of a semi-structured clinical interview with the patient or an informant, with most of the follow-up interviews being conducted by phone. Most comparisons focused on 81 patients meeting current criteria for BPD only, 163 who met current criteria for schizophrenia, and 44 who met current criteria for major depression, with diagnoses being derived through retrospective chart review.

McGlashan found that his borderline patients achieved an overall Health Sickness Rating Scale (HSRS; Luborsky 1962) score of 64 a mean of 15 years after their index admission (range 2–32 years). This mean rating represents a good level of functioning and was equal to that of depressed controls but significantly higher than that of schizophrenic patients. However, closer examination reveals that 5% of this borderline cohort were functioning in the incapacitated range, 16% in the marginal range, 26% in the moderate range, 37% in the good range, and 16% in the recovered range. Thus, about half of the borderline patients (53%) were functioning in the good-recovered range and about half (47%) were functioning in the moderate-incapacitated range. In addition, 3% of the traced borderline patients had committed suicide.

In terms of instrumental functioning, borderline patients worked about half the time at reasonably complex jobs. They also met with friends about once every other week. About half were married or living with a sexual partner, and about half avoided intimate relationships entirely. In terms of further treatment, the average borderline patient was rehospitalized one or two more times, spending about 8% of the follow-up period as an inpatient. They used psychosocial treatments during about one-third of the follow-up period (35%) and psychotropic medications about one-fourth of the time (22%). Almost half (46%) were in some form of psychiatric treatment at the time of their follow-up interview. These figures were very similar to those achieved by the depressed controls. However, the borderline patients functioned significantly better than schizophrenic patients in the instrumental realm and used significantly less psychiatric treatment than these psychotic controls.

McGlashan found that overall functioning was significantly related to both length of follow-up period and comorbid disorders. In terms of length of follow-up, he found that patients who were followed 10–19 years had significantly better overall functioning than those followed 9 years or less and about the same as those followed 20 years or more. He also found that overall functioning for these patients followed the pattern of an inverted U, with functioning improving through their 20s and 30s, peaking in their 40s, and declining in their 50s.

In terms of comorbid disorders, McGlashan found that "pure" borderline patients functioned better than borderline patients with a comorbid depression, who in turn functioned better than borderline patients with a comorbid schizophrenic disorder, who in turn functioned better than "pure" schizophrenic patients. He also found that "pure" borderline patients and those with a comorbid schizotypal disorder (McGlashan 1986b) or comorbid antisocial traits (Heinssen et al. 1989) achieved about the same overall outcome.

Paris and colleagues (1987) reviewed the charts of all patients hospitalized for psychiatric reasons at the Jewish General Hospital in Montreal between 1958 and 1978. Three hundred twenty-two patients met retrospective Diagnostic Interview for Borderlines (DIB) criteria (Gunderson et al. 1981) for BPD, and 100 of these patients (31.5%) were reinterviewed a mean of 15 years after their index admission. The researchers found that all aspects of their borderline psychopathology as measured by a live DIB interview had decreased significantly. They also found that only 25% of these patients still met DIB criteria for BPD.

In terms of overall functioning, these borderline patients achieved a mean HSRS score of 63, a score indicating a good global outcome. They also achieved a mean work score of 3.8, indicating frequent job changes without unemployment. Their social participation score was 3.2—close to a level described as limited leisure time with transient social contact. In terms of further treatment, they had a mean of 1.3 rehospitalizations and a mean of 1.9 years of further treatment. Overall, there was great variability in the amount of treatment received, but most of the patients' treatment histories were chaotic and intermittent. Of the 165 patients who could be located, 14 (8.5%) had committed suicide.

Stone and co-workers (1987) followed up 464 (84%) of the 550 patients hospitalized at the New York State Psychiatric Institute between 1963 and 1976 meeting the following inclusion criteria: 1) stay of at least 3 months, 2) age under 40, and 3) IQ of 90 or higher. Most of this group of patients were selected for their potential to benefit from intensive psychotherapy. However, a substantial minority were admitted because of their family's VIP status. Stone made retrospective DSM-III diagnoses after reviewing each patient's chart and then attempted to personally contact each patient, most of whom he had known during their index hospitalization. He was able to trace 251 (84%) of the 299 patients meeting DSM-III criteria for BPD and/or Kernberg's structural criteria for borderline personality organization (Kernberg 1977) and interviewed relatives or other informants when patients were unavailable. Stone found that the average GAS score of this group of patients a mean of 16 years after their index admission was 67. This score, which indicates a good level of functioning, was significantly higher than that achieved by schizophrenic controls. Almost half of the borderline patients received a GAS score in the recovered range (42%), 30% received a GAS score in the good range, 17% in the fair range, and 11% in the marginal-incapacitated range. This distribution was also significantly different from that attained by the schizophrenic patients in the study; less than 3% of these patients receiving GAS scores in the recovered range.

In terms of more specific spheres of follow-up functioning, 56% of the borderline patients had worked at least three-quarters of the time, 17% had worked about half the time, and 17% worked less than half the time or not at all. More than half of the borderlines (55%) worked at complex jobs, 43% worked at relatively uncomplicated jobs, and 2% worked at very simple jobs. Less than half (47%) had ever married, and less than a quarter (22%) had children. However, only 25% had ever been rehospitalized, and these hospitalizations tended to be brief. In addition, borderline patients functioned better in each of these spheres than schizophrenic patients. Despite these generally optimistic findings, it is important to note that 7.6% of the overall group of borderline patients and 8.9% of the DSM-III borderlines committed suicide, both rates being similar to those found for schizophrenic patients (9.0%) and substantially lower than those found for schizoaffective (23.6%) patients.

Despite the consistency of the findings in these four studies, the generalizability of their results is limited by a number of methodological problems. These problems have included use of highly variable chart material as the basis for diagnoses, assessment of post-hospital functioning at only one point in time, absence of detailed information concerning follow-up functioning, use of mailed questionnaires or telephone interviews as the only or primary source of information, use of upper-middle-class inpatient samples from tertiary facilities, lack of independence of baseline and follow-up data, absence of controls or failure to use near-neighbor Axis II controls, the wide range of follow-up periods in each study, and the presence of different age cohorts.

Despite these limitations, three major findings have emerged from these studies. First, the functioning of borderline patients over time is highly variable, with some functioning very well, many continuing to have substantial difficulty in a number of areas of their lives, and 3–10% of these patients committing suicide. Second, borderline patients seem to function better vocationally than they do interpersonally. Third, borderline patients function better overall than schizophrenics and about the same as affectively-disordered patients.

Prediction of Outcome

Although a number of factors have been examined for their predictive power, comorbidity with other disorders has been the most frequently assessed. Comorbidity with four other disorders—major affective disorder, antisocial personality disorder, schizotypal personality disorder, and substance abuse—has been repeatedly examined with conflicting conclusions. As we have noted, Pope and colleagues (1983) found that their borderline patients with a history of MAD were functioning better 4 to 7 years after their initial assessment than border-lines without a history of MAD. Paris and associates (1987) found no relation-ship between a history of affective disorder and outcome in their borderline cohort, whereas both Plakun and co-workers (1985) and McGlashan (1986a) found that those borderlines with a history of affective disorder were functioning worse than those without such a history. Only Stone (1989) has replicated the Pope findings that a history of affective disorder is related to a better outcome. However, Stone found that this overall result was due to the poorer outcomes attained by male borderlines without a history of affective disorder, patients who often met DSM-III criteria for antisocial personality disorder and serious sub-stance abuse. Stone found these latter disorders to be associated with a poor outcome in BPD. As a result of these more refined analyses, he has suggested that it is not the presence of an affective disorder that bodes well for borderline patients but rather the absence of a history of antisocial personality disorder and serious alcohol and/or drug abuse.

McGlashan has recently found that borderline patients (usually male) with antisocial features do as well in the long term as borderline patients without such traits (Heinssen et al. 1989). This difference between his results and Stone's findings is probably because Stone was studying patients who actually met DSM-III criteria for APD. These patients were not admitted to Chestnut Lodge; thus, McGlashan and his colleagues were studying patients without a full-blown antisocial disorder. Plakun and colleagues (1985) found that comor-bidity with schizotypal personality disorder boded well for borderline patients, whereas McGlashan (1986b) and Stone (1989) found that it had no overall effect; both pure and mixed cohorts achieving the same level of outcome. This difference may be due to the much lower trace rate found in the Plakun study (1985) compared with those of McGlashan and Stone, the better functioning schizotypal borderlines being more likely to respond than those who were doing poorly.

A number of other factors have been associated with a better outcome. Both McGlashan (1985) and Stone (1989) found that a high IQ is a good prognostic factor. Stone (1989) also found that artistic talent and physical attractiveness (if female) are associated with a better outcome. Plakun (1988) has found that the absence of parental divorce or of narcissistic entitlement and the presence of self-destructive acts during the index admission are all related to a better overall outcome.

A number of other factors have also been associated with a poor outcome. McGlashan (1985) found that both affective instability and greater length of previous hospitalizations boded poorly for patients, whereas Paris and colleagues (1987, 1988) found that the presence of dysphoria, a family history of mental illness, a younger age when first seen, and the presence of maternal psychopathology boded poorly. Stone (1989) found that a childhood history of parental brutality boded poorly as well.

Suicide among borderline patients has been found to be positively correlated with three factors: 1) the number of previous attempts, 2) a higher educational level (Paris et al. 1989), and 3) the density of borderline psychopathology as measured by the number of DSM-III criteria met (Stone 1989).

These findings are marked by their inconsistency, which may be due to the limited information concerning predictor variables that could be culled from retrospective chart review. It may also be that the failure to study predictor variables that emerge during the follow-up period (e.g., attainment of a stable intimate relationship) has led to difficulties in identifying the strongest predictor variables.

Conclusions

The studies reviewed above suggest that BPD is a very serious disorder with a heterogeneous outcome. Future studies of the long-term course and outcome of BPD should be prospective in nature. They should also involve large enough samples of borderline patients to assess the effect of various factors, such as comorbidity, sex, and socioeconomic background, on outcome. Perhaps more importantly, these studies will need to focus on what Zanarini and colleagues (1989) have referred to as pathways to health—factors such as sustained psychotherapy that, alone or in concert, may help borderline patients to begin the long climb to health.

References

Akiskal HS, Chen SE, Davis GC, et al: Borderline: an adjective in search of a noun. J Clin Psychiatry 46:41–48, 1985

American Psychiatric Association: Diagnostic and Statistical Manual of Mental Disorders, 3rd Edition. Washington, DC, American Psychiatric Association, 1980

Barasch A, Frances A, Hurt S, et al: The stability and distinctness of borderline personality disorder. Am J Psychiatry 142:1484–1486, 1985

Carpenter WT, Gunderson JG: Five year follow-up comparison of borderline and schizophrenic patients. Compr Psychiatry 18:567–571, 1977

Endicott J, Spitzer RL, Fleiss JL, et al: The Global Assessment Scale: A procedure for measuring overall severity of psychiatric disturbance. Arch Gen Psychiatry 33:766–771, 1976

Grinker RR, Werble B, Drye RC: The Borderline Syndrome: A Behavioral Study of Ego-Functions. New York, Basic Books, 1968, pp 126–140

Gunderson JG, Zanarini MC: Pathogenesis of borderline personality, in Review of Psychiatry, Vol 8. Edited by Tasman A, Hales RE, Frances AJ. Washington, DC, American

Psychiatric Press, 1989, pp 25–48

Gunderson JG, Carpenter WT, Strauss JS: Borderline and schizophrenic patients: a comparative study. Am J Psychiatry 132:1257–1264, 1975

Gunderson JG, Kolb JE, Austin V: The diagnostic interview for borderline patients. Am J Psychiatry 138:896–903, 1981

Heinssen RK, McGlashan TH, Fenton WS: Antisocial traits in borderline personality. Paper presented at the annual meeting of the American Psychiatric Association, San Francisco, CA, May 1989

Kernberg OF: The structural diagnosis of borderline personality organization, in Borderline Personality Disorders. Edited by Hartocollis P. New York, International Universities Press, 1977, pp 87–121

Luborsky L: Clinician's judgements of mental health: a proposed scale. Arch Gen Psychiatry 7:407–417, 1962

McGlashan TH: The prediction of outcome in borderline personality disorder: Part V of the Chestnut Lodge follow-up study, in The Borderline: Current Empirical Research. Edited by McGlashan TH. Washington, DC, American Psychiatric Press, 1985, pp 61–98

McGlashan TH: The Chestnut Lodge follow-up study: III. long-term outcome of borderline personalities. Arch Gen Psychiatry 43:20–30, 1986a

McGlashan TH: Schizotypal personality disorder: Chestnut Lodge follow-up study: VI. long-term follow-up perspectives. Arch Gen Psychiatry 43:329–334, 1986b

Modestin J, Villiger C: Follow-up study on borderline versus nonborderline disorders. Compr Psychiatry 30:236–244, 1989

Paris J, Brown R, Nowlis D: Long-term follow-up of borderline patients in a general hospital. Compr Psychiatry 28:530–535, 1987

Paris J, Nowlis D, Brown R: Developmental factors in the outcome of borderline personality disorder. Compr Psychiatry 29:147–150, 1988

Paris J, Nowlis D, Brown R: Predictors of suicide in borderline personality disorder. Can J Psychiatry 34:8–9, 1989

Perry JC: Depression in borderline personality disorder: lifetime prevalence at interview and longitudinal course of symptoms. Am J Psychiatry 142:15–21, 1985

Perry J, Cooper S: Psychodynamic symptoms and outcome in borderline and antisocial personality disorders and bipolar II affective disorder, in The Borderline: Current Empirical Research. Washington, DC, American Psychiatric Press, 1985, pp 19–41

Plakun EM, Burkhardt PE, Muller JP: 14-year follow-up of borderline and schizotypal personality disorders. Compr Psychiatry 26:448–455, 1985

Plakun EM: Outcome correlates of borderline patients. Paper presented at the annual meeting of the American Psychiatric Association, Montreal, Canada, May 1988

Pope HG, Jonas JM, Hudson JI, et al: The validity of DSM-III borderline personality disorder: a phenomenologic, family history, treatment response, and long-term follow-up study. Arch Gen Psychiatry 40:23–30, 1983

Stone MH, Stone DK, Hurt SW: Natural history of borderline patients treated by intensive hospitalization. Psychiatr Clin North Am 10:185–205, 1987

Stone MH: The course of borderline personality disorder, in Review of Psychiatry, Vol 8. Edited by Tasman A, Hales RE, Frances AJ. Washington, DC, American Psychiatric

Press, 1989, pp 103–125

Tucker L, Bauer SF, Wagner S, et al: Long-term hospital treatment of borderline patients: a descriptive outcome study. Am J Psychiatry 144:1443–1448, 1987

Werble B: Second follow-up study of borderline patients. Arch Gen Psychiatry 23:1–7, 1970

Widiger TA, Frances AJ: Epidemiology, diagnosis, and comorbidity of borderline personality disorder, in Review of Psychiatry, Vol 8. Edited by Tasman A, Hales RE, Frances AJ. Washington, DC, American Psychiatric Press, 1989, pp 8–24

World Health Organization: Mental Disorders: Glossary and Guide to Their Classification in Accordance with the Ninth Revision of the International Classification of Diseases. Geneva, World Health Organization, 1978

Zanarini MC, Gunderson JG, Chauncey DL, et al: A two- to six-year controlled follow-up of borderline personality disorder outpatients. Paper presented at the annual meeting of the American Psychiatric Association, San Francisco, CA, May 1989

Zanarini MC, Gunderson JG, Frankenburg FR, et al: Discriminating borderline personality disorder from other axis II disorders. Am J Psychiatry 147:161–167, 1990

❖ 12 ❖   Empirical Perspectives on Narcissism

Eric M. Plakun, M.D.

Since the publication in 1914 of Freud's paper "On Narcissism," psychoanalysts have recognized a narcissistic line of development that can become a prominent and organizing feature of a personality. In recent decades, there has been substantial controversy within psychoanalysis about how best to understand, conceptualize, and treat narcissistic patients. Otto Kernberg (1975, 1980) has been the most articulate spokesman for the ego psychological, object relations point of view concerning narcissism, whereas the late Heinz Kohut (1971, 1977) broke with traditional analytic concepts in his espousal of the self psychology point of view concerning narcissism. However, there is substantial evidence that both Kernberg and Kohut have been influenced by earlier psychoanalytic precursors such as W.R.D. Fairbairn (Sacksteder 1990). In part, it was the heated debate about narcissism in the decade preceding publication of DSM-III (American Psychiatric Association 1980) that led to the inclusion of narcissistic personality disorder (NPD) in DSM-III. It was, however, included in the absence of meaningful empirical data about the disorder—a problem recognized by authors of psychoanalytic papers on narcissism, who have often called for empirical data (Akhtar and Thomson 1982; Bursten 1982; Goldstein 1985; Nurnberg 1984). Indeed, Siever and Klar state in the 1986 *Annual Review of Psychiatry,* "There are to our knowledge no empirical studies of the criteria for narcissistic personality disorder. Its inclusion in DSM-III was based on the consensus of clinicians regarding its existence. . . . While narcissistic personality disorder is widely discussed in the psychodynamic literature, there are no data supporting the coherence, validity or reliability of the diagnostic group" (pp. 299, 301).

In some respects, the paucity of empirical research on NPD is no surprise, because the diagnosis has been of primary interest to psychoanalysts who often eschew empirical methodology for epistemological reasons. Even within psychoanalysis, there has been disagreement between those representing the ego psychologic, object relations point of view and self psychologists about how best to diagnose and conceptualize the disorder. Self psychologists reject the conflict/defense model and view NPD as a developmental arrest due to impaired parental mirroring/idealization. They prefer to make the diagnosis only through the emergence of specific selfobject transferences in the course of psychoanalysis. DSM-III and DSM-III-R (American Psychiatric Association 1987) have offered criterion sets for the NPD diagnosis that have become widely utilized and accepted, an essential step if empirical study is to occur.

Further, many narcissistic patients function highly, either not presenting for treatment at all or presenting primarily as outpatients. Those NPD patients who do require inpatient treatment often manifest significant comorbidity with an Axis I diagnosis such as a major affective disorder (MAD); substance abuse/dependence; or another Axis II disorder, such as borderline personality disorder, with impulsivity and self-destructiveness precipitating hospitalization. However, we are learning that the treatment of such syndromes as substance dependence and the affective disorders requires attention to comorbid diagnoses (including the personality disorders). Greater awareness about the longitudinal course and outcome of disorders such as NPD is thus desirable, even for those who practice primarily in short-term, nonanalytic inpatient settings.

Although the establishment of uniform criterion sets for NPD has been helpful, NPD patients are not frequently present in large numbers when samples of personality disorder patients are studied. Pfohl and his colleagues (1986) at the University of Iowa studied the internal consistency of DSM-III criteria in 131 personality disorder patients but found that only 5 met criteria for NPD. They were unable to calculate an overall kappa statistic for interrater agreement about the presence of the diagnosis because of its low frequency in their sample.

Borderline personality disorder (BPD), another new diagnosis in DSM-III, is closely related to NPD and has attracted the lion's share of research interest. Four landmark long-term retrospective follow-up studies have been published on BPD that, despite the methodologic weaknesses inherent in retrospective research designs, have contributed much information on BPD. Two of these studies came from member hospitals of the National Association of Private Psychiatric Hospitals (NAPPH): McGlashan's study of patients at Chestnut Lodge (1983, 1986) and our study at the Austen Riggs Center (Plakun et al. 1985, 1987). Other studies (Paris et al. 1987; Stone et al. 1987) have also presented longitudinal course and outcome data on BPD compared to other diagnostic groups, which have contributed to the establishment of the diagnostic validity of BPD as defined in DSM-III. The study we have conducted at the Austen Riggs Center has been the only research with a large enough sample of NPD patients to offer longitudinal course and outcome data on this diagnostic group, although McGlashan and Heinssen (1989) and Stone (1989) have published studies of BPD patients who also demonstrated narcissistic traits.

McGlashan and Heinssen (1989) found little difference at long-term follow-up between non-comorbid BPD patients and BPD patients with narcissistic traits. But at baseline, BPD patients with narcissistic traits demonstrated a non-significant trend toward more and longer previous hospitalizations. They also tended to be older at illness onset and at index hospitalization than non-comorbid BPD patients. At follow-up, there was a tendency falling short of significance for BPD patients with narcissistic traits to be functioning more poorly socially and vocationally, to have more problems with alcohol, to have been more likely to attempt suicide during the follow-up interval, and to have poorer global functioning than the non-comorbid BPD patients. Stone (1989) studied BPD patients from the P.I. 500 (Stone et al. 1987) who also had narcissistic traits falling short of or fulfilling criteria for NPD, reporting that long-term outcome of these narcissistic BPD patients was similar overall to long-term outcome of pure BPD patients. Stone found that more narcissistic BPD patients were men than was the case for other BPD patients, who were more often women. Narcissistic BPD patients also appeared to be at greater risk for successful suicide. The information these studies provide about the influence of narcissistic traits on BPD is valuable and welcome, but it does not provide data about non-comorbid NPD.

Ronningstam and Gunderson (1989) have developed a semistructured interview for narcissism (the Diagnostic Interview for Narcissism, or DIN), which assesses five dimensions of narcissism (grandiosity, interpersonal relations, reactiveness, affects and mood states, and social and moral adaptation) that are closely related to the DSM-III and DSM-III-R NPD criteria.

The DIN has been reported by Ronningstam and Gunderson to discriminate narcissistic from nonnarcissistic clinician-rated patients. The complete development of the DIN will allow reliable clinical diagnoses of NPD comparable to those provided by the diagnostic interview for borderlines (DIB) (Gunderson et al. 1981).

Richman and Flaherty (1990) studied gender differences in narcissistic styles, and their data suggest that some of the DSM-III and DSM-III-R criteria for NPD may be more representative of male than of female manifestations of narcissism. A scale developed by the researchers operationalizing DSM-III-R criteria failed to demonstrate a link between the criteria and low self-esteem or dysphoric mood in women medical students, but did demonstrate such a link in men. "Envy," as defined in the DSM-III-R NPD criteria, appeared to be a valid indicator in both sexes, but "interpersonal exploitativeness," "entitlement," and "lack of empathy" appeared more representative of male manifestations of narcissism.

Analysis of data from the Austen Riggs Center follow-up study has allowed us to assess four different empirical issues concerning NPD in an effort to explore the validity of this new diagnosis. The first issue addressed was how well

DSM-III criteria for NPD and BPD discriminated between these two closely related diagnoses (Plakun 1987). The validity of a new diagnostic entity can hardly be trusted if its defining criteria do not reliably distinguish it from a near neighbor diagnosis. The second issue studied was whether the premorbid psychiatric history, demographic characteristics, longitudinal course, and outcome of NPD patients could be distinguished from that of other well established diagnostic groups (in this case, schizophrenia and the major affective disorders), allowing assessment of the validity of the NPD diagnosis as a discrete entity (Plakun 1989). The third issue addressed was to what extent NPD differed from BPD in terms of demographic characteristics, psychiatric history, longitudinal course, and outcome (Plakun 1989). It is not enough to establish that NPD differs from schizophrenia and/or MAD. There must also be evidence that its history, course, and outcome appear distinct from a near neighbor diagnosis such as BPD. Finally, correlates of good and poor outcome in NPD were assessed, allowing comparison to outcome correlates for BPD (Plakun 1990, 1991). Before I summarize the findings of this research, a review of patient selection and methodology is appropriate.

Patients and Methods

All subjects were originally inpatients at the Austen Riggs Center, a long-term, fully open psychiatric hospital emphasizing intensive psychoanalytic psychotherapy at which the mean stay approaches 1-1/2 years.

Patients at the Center have generally failed to benefit from prior short-term hospitalization and/or outpatient treatment with or without medication, leading to referral for longer-term inpatient treatment. Despite generally being treatment failures, patients are selected for ability to work in a completely open setting and therefore are relatively high functioning. The most frequent diagnosis is BPD, with or without superimposed MAD, but substantial numbers of patients also meet criteria for schizophrenic spectrum disorders or other severe personality disorders including NPD. There is no privilege system, no restriction of patients' freedom, and there are no closed units. There is 24-hour nursing coverage and a doctor on call, a voluntary activity program, and a self-governing patient community with staff consultants. During the index hospitalization, patients receive 4–5 hours of individual psychotherapy each week from an experienced board eligible or certified psychiatrist or doctoral level clinical psychologist. Patients are referred from throughout the United States and from other countries.

In 1979, an effort was made to contact by mail the 878 patients treated for at least 2 months between 1950 and 1976 to compare their current functioning to that preceding admission. A 2-month stay was determined to be the minimum period permitting collection of data adequate enough to make retrospective DSM-III diagnoses. Of the former patients, 252 could not be located; 262 failed to respond to requests for participation; 33 refused participation; and 94 had died, primarily in the oldest group of patients treated between 1950 and 1960.

Of the domain of 878 former patients, 237 (or 27% of the total group but 45% of living former patients who could be located) responded to an invitation and completed detailed mailed follow-up questionnaires. This response rate compares favorably with the 25–30% for mailed questionnaires preferred by Warner and colleagues (1983) in their study of follow-up methods. The researchers noted that the lower response rate with mailed questionnaires, compared to in-person or telephone interviews, is compensated for by the minimization of responses intended to please the interviewer.

The sample consisted of 89 (38%) males and 148 (62%) females, with a mean age of 24.5 years (SD ± 7.7) at admission. The mean length of stay during the index hospitalization was 16.6 months (SD ± 10.6). The mean interval between admission and follow-up was 13.6 years (SD ± 6.6). The respondent sample proved representative of the entire population on the basis of respondent versus nonrespondent comparisons of admission variables, suggesting no significant difference between groups.

Each subject's hospital record contained preadmission and admission summaries, a detailed case history, nursing notes, and activities reports. Only variables for which blind raters could achieve adequate interrater agreement were utilized as baseline and follow-up measures. Retrospective DSM-III diagnoses based on portions of the case record were made by two raters blind to patient identity and clinical diagnosis for the 237 respondents. Interrater reliability was assessed on 25 patients leading to kappa coefficients of 0.81 ($Z = 2.79$, $P < .01$, 2-tailed) and 0.69 ($Z = 2.02$, $P < .05$, 2-tailed) for Axis I and Axis II disorders, respectively.

These compared favorably with the kappas of the DSM-III field trials, in which Axis I and Axis II kappas were 0.68 and 0.56, respectively. The kappa for BPD alone, among the jointly rated group of charts, was 0.78 ($Z = 0.81$, $P < .05$). For NPD, kappa was 1.0 ($Z = 1.47$, $P = .07$), indicating complete rater agreement on the presence or absence of NPD in all cases in the sample of 25 charts. The kappa of 1.0, falling just short of significance, reflects the infrequency of the NPD diagnosis in the sample; that is, most of the "agreement" in the kappa is about the absence of NPD. Certainly, kappa would not likely prove to be 1.0 for NPD among all 237 charts, but agreement of this degree in the reliability sample suggests adequate interrater agreement. DSM-III does not report kappas for individual Axis II diagnoses, so no comparison can be made. The two raters were in agreement about the presence or absence of individual NPD criteria between 75% (preoccupation with fantasies of success) and 90% (response to criticism) of the time, and about BPD criteria between 70% (unstable and intense relationships) and 95% (intolerance of being alone) of the time. Based on adequate demonstration of interrater agreement, the remaining patients were assigned DSM-III diagnoses but were also rated for the presence or absence of each Axis II criterion by one of the two raters. In recognition of the problem posed by the mixed monothetic and polythetic diagnostic system of DSM-III, which confounds study of individual criteria, NPD was diagnosed with a polythetic model requiring the presence of at least five of the eight total DSM-III NPD criteria, A through D and E1 through E4. Thus, although it was DSM-III criteria that were rated for NPD, the diagnosis was made using the polythetic system adopted in DSM-III-R. The BPD diagnosis also required at least five of the eight DSM-III BPD criteria.

Forty-four patients met criteria for BPD while free of MAD and NPD. Nineteen patients met criteria for NPD while free of MAD and BPD. Eight patients met criteria for both BPD and NPD while free of MAD, and they were excluded from subsequent comparisons. For the first study, examining the capacity of NPD and BPD criteria to distinguish between the two diagnoses, it was desirable to include BPD and NPD patients who nearly met criteria for the other diagnosis by meeting four of its criteria. Thus, all 44 BPD and 19 NPD patients were included. However, for the remainder of the comparisons, the use of as "pure" a group of BPD and NPD subjects as possible was desirable. Further, it is probably true that long-term NPD inpatients are more likely to display borderline traits than outpatients, a factor also favoring elimination of patients meeting four criteria from the reciprocal diagnosis from the BPD and NPD groups. Two NPD patients were thus eliminated, leaving a group of 17 NPD patients, among whom 3 met 5 NPD criteria, 2 met 7, and 12 met 6. Of these 17 NPD patients, 5 met 3 BPD criteria, 11 met 2, and 1 met 1. The most common BPD criterion found in 11 of the 17 NPD patients was "a pattern of unstable and intense relationships," probably reflecting the similarity of this criterion to the NPD criterion for overidealized and devalued relationships. Because 14 of the 17 NPD patients met 6 or more of the 8 NPD criteria, they were a strongly narcissistic group despite the presence of some borderline traits.

Eleven patients were eliminated from the original BPD group because they met more than three NPD criteria. Of the resulting group of 33 BPD patients, 2 met 3 NPD criteria, 8 met 2, and the remainder met 1 or none. Thus, more than two-thirds of the "pure" BPD patients were free or nearly free of NPD traits.

The Discrimination of NPD and BPD
Using DSM-III Criteria

As noted previously, all 44 BPD patients and 19 NPD patients were used in this study so that we could be conservative in assessing the ability of the criteria for each diagnosis to discriminate between them. Phi correlation coefficients with χ^2 were calculated for each of the 8 BPD and 8 NPD DSM-III criteria for the presence of the BPD diagnosis. Tables reporting the correlations are available in the original study (Plakun 1987). NPD criteria appeared substantially better at discriminating between the two diagnoses than BPD criteria. The highest correlation overall was that of the DSM-III NPD criterion for "grandiosity," which was found in 95% of NPD patients and only 16% of BPD patients, yielding a phi coefficient of correlation of 0.74 (P = .0001), suggesting this is the most prototypic NPD criterion for distinguishing the two diagnoses. "Exhibitionism" also was quite discriminating, appearing in 89% of NPD patients and only 16% of BPD patients, with a correlation coefficient of 0.70 (P = .0001). "Interpersonal exploitativeness" appeared in 84% of NPD patients and 24% of BPD patients, yielding a phi coefficient of correlation of 0.58 (P = .0001).

"Entitlement" was not very sensitive but appeared a highly specific criterion for distinguishing these two diagnoses, because it appeared in 47% of the NPD patients but only 2% of the BPD patients (phi = 0.52, P = .0001).

Although "cool indifference or overreaction" appeared in 95% of the NPD patients, it was also present in 48% of the BPD patients, producing a low but significant correlation (phi = 0.46, P = 0001). The only NPD criterion not to achieve significance was that for "overidealized and devalued relationships," which occurred in 32% of NPD patients and 18% of BPD patients (phi = 0.16, P = 0.2).

Among the BPD criteria, the most prototypic in discriminating between these two diagnoses appeared to be "impulsivity", which was present in 91% of BPD patients but also 42% of NPD patients (phi = 0.44, P = .0001). "Affective instability," "self damaging acts," "inappropriate intense anger," "intolerance of being alone," "chronic feelings of emptiness or boredom," and "identity disturbance" all yielded correlations in the 0.28 to 0.32 range and were significant at the P = .02 or better level. Both "intolerance of being alone" and "chronic feelings of emptiness or boredom" were low in sensitivity (present in 30% and 34% of BPD patients respectively), but highly specific (present in 0% and 5% of NPD patients respectively). The least discriminating criterion was that of "unstable and intense relationships," present in 89% of the BPD patients but also 63% of NPD patients, yielding a phi correlation coefficient of 0.21 (P = .08) and probably reflecting the similarity of this DSM-III BPD criterion to the "overidealized and devalued relationships" criterion of NPD.

Studies based on correlations alone can be deceptive because of intercorrelations between criteria, which were reported in the original study. To control for intercorrelation effects, maximum and minimum R^2 improvement stepwise regressions were performed rank ordering the ability of each BPD or NPD criterion to predict the presence of BPD. The complete sequence of the 16-variable regression is available in the original paper, but it is worth noting that again NPD criteria seemed superior to BPD criteria in discriminating between the two diagnoses. In the performance of the stepwise regressions, the predictive power gained by adding variables fell off sharply after the first five. Therefore, an additional maximum R^2 improvement stepwise regression extracting the best five variable model for distinguishing BPD from NPD was performed. This model accounts for 81% of the total variance in discriminating between the two diagnoses (df = 62, P <.001). Thus, in this sample of NPD and BPD patients, it was highly likely that a patient manifested NPD rather than BPD if he or she manifested "entitlement," "grandiosity," "preoccupation with fantasies of success," and "exhibitionism," but did not manifest "inappropriate, intense anger" from among the BPD criteria.

In summary, these data suggest that DSM-III criteria for NPD and BPD can reliably distinguish between the two diagnoses in a conservatively defined patient sample. It should be kept in mind that these data shed no light on the ability of these criteria to distinguish NPD or BPD from any other diagnosis. These findings also support the notion that grandiosity is the single most prototypic feature of NPD.

The Validity of Narcissistic Personality Disorder

In this study, 17 "pure" NPD patients were compared to 19 schizophrenics and 26 patients with a unipolar or bipolar MAD in terms of demographic and family history variables, preadmission psychiatric history variables, index hospitalization measures, and follow-up measures (Plakun 1989). This study follows the precedent set with BPD of exploring the validity of a new diagnosis by comparison to well-known and established psychiatric diagnoses. Tables reporting the detailed comparisons are available elsewhere (Plakun 1989). For our current purpose, an overall summary is in order.

No significant differences were found among the three diagnostic groups in terms of demographic features. But there was a tendency for NPD patients, like schizophrenics, to be equally divided between the two sexes, whereas more MAD patients were women. A family history of psychiatric illness tended to be relatively more common in schizophrenic and MAD patients than in NPD patients, but again, these differences fell short of significance.

Six groups of reliably rated preadmission measures were compared for the three diagnoses, including measures of social, vocational, and global functioning; previous outpatient and inpatient treatment; and symptoms. Overall, NPD tended to differ from schizophrenia, MAD, or both on 19 of the 25 preadmission measures employed. On 7 of the 19 differing measures, NPD tended to differ from schizophrenia more than from MAD. Five of these achieved statistical significance, with NPD patients (like MAD patients) more likely to be married, less likely to have been hospitalized in the year prior to the index admission, older at onset of their illness, and having a higher admission Global Assessment Scale score (Spitzer et al. 1973) than schizophrenic patients. On 4 of the 19 measures that differed, NPD patients tended to be distinct from those with MAD, but none of these measures achieved statistical significance. NPD appeared to differ from both MAD and schizophrenia on 8 of the 19 measures.

Seven measures of the index hospitalization were studied, including the frequency of treatment crises, highest maximum Full Scale IQ achieved, and mean length of stay. On four of the seven measures, the three diagnoses could not be distinguished, even on a trend level. On three measures, though, NPD again tended to differ more from schizophrenia than from MAD, including shorter length of stay, lower likelihood of discharge by transfer to another hospital, and greater likelihood of being discharged with the therapeutic goal rated as achieved by the therapist than was the case in schizophrenia.

At mean 14-year follow-up, the three diagnostic groups were again assessed in terms of social, vocational, and global functioning; follow-up interval outpatient and inpatient treatment; and symptoms. Of the total of 19 follow-up measures used to compare the 3 groups, NPD tended to differ from schizophrenia or MAD or both diagnoses on 15. On 6 of the 15 differing measures, NPD tended to be more distinct from schizophrenia than from MAD, including 2 measures of hospital treatment that achieved statistical significance.

Specifically, schizophrenic patients were rehospitalized a mean of 2.6 times in the follow-up interval, compared to 0.4 times for NPD patients and 0.8 times for MAD patients (analysis of variance with Duncan's Multiple Range Test, $F = 4.87$, df = 2, $P = .01$). Schizophrenic patients were significantly more likely to have been rehospitalized in the year before follow-up than either the MAD or NPD patients (analysis of variance with Duncan's Multiple Range Test, $F = 4.51$, df = 2, $P = .01$). Patients with NPD tended to differ more from those with MAD than from those with schizophrenia on four measures of social and vocational functioning and outpatient treatment. NPD patients resembled schizophrenic patients much more than they resembled MAD patients in the low percentage of patients (65% for NPD and 68% for schizophrenia) reporting satisfactory intimate relations at long-term follow-up, compared to 92% of MAD patients, a difference that approached statistical significance (χ^2 = 5.85, df = 2, P = .06). NPD tended to differ from both MAD and schizophrenia on 5 of the 15 measures.

As was the case for the preadmission measures, the preponderance of the data tends to suggest that NPD is a distinct entity, with some of the differences achieving statistical significance. However, the differences were less clear at follow-up than at admission. It should be noted that the general tendency of NPD to differ more from schizophrenia than from MAD, more clearly on preadmission than on follow-up measures, does not necessarily demonstrate a fundamental similarity between NPD and MAD but only the lack of a measurable difference on the variables tested.

Certainly more than one retrospective study is required to establish the validity of a new diagnostic entity, but overall trends in the data lend credence to the hypothesis that NPD is a valid diagnostic entity.

The Course and Outcome of NPD and BPD

Such psychoanalytic contributors as Kernberg (1975, 1980), Adler (1981, 1986), Rinsley (1985), and others have consistently included a view of NPD and BPD as near-neighbor diagnoses. This is reflected in the inclusion of NPD and BPD in the same personality disorder cluster in DSM-III and DSM-III-R. Comparison of BPD and NPD in terms of demographic characteristics, preadmission psychiatric history, measures of the index treatment, and longitudinal course and outcome advance study of the validity of NPD. Although, as noted previously, McGlashan and Heinssen (1989) and Stone (1989) have compared non-comorbid BPD patients to those with narcissistic traits, it is only in our sample of 17 "pure" NPD patients that a comparison between the two diagnoses in a more homogeneous form has been conducted (Plakun 1989). The 17 "pure" NPD patients described herein were compared to 33 "pure" BPD patients in terms of the same measures utilized in the preceding comparisons of NPD to schizophrenia and MAD. In the current comparisons, the lack of statistically significant differences should not be surprising, because the two diagnoses are so closely related.

A detailed report of the results of comparison of the two diagnoses is available elsewhere (Plakun 1989). Although the two diagnoses showed more similarities than differences, there were some notable findings. Although the difference was not statistically significant, NPD was equally common in both sexes, whereas in this sample 70% of BPD patients were women. A clear preponderance of women inpatients meeting criteria for BPD has also been reported by others (McGlashan 1986; Paris et al. 1987; Stone et al. 1987). Only one in five NPD patients compared to nearly two in five BPD patients had a family history of psychiatric illness. At admission, the cohorts of NPD and BPD patients were both in their mid-20s (25.9 and 25.4 years, respectively), but the average NPD patient first had contact with a mental health provider approximately 3 years earlier, as opposed to nearly 5 years earlier for BPD. BPD patients were more likely to have engaged in preadmission suicide attempts or nonsuicidal self-destructive behavior and more frequently had histories of alcohol or drug abuse. Perhaps surprisingly, NPD patients showed more social isolation on the Strauss-Carpenter Social Scale at admission (NPD = 2.5 and BPD = 3.2 on a 0 to 4 scale, analysis of variance with Duncan's Multiple Range Test, F = 3.69, df = 1, P = .06).

In terms of preadmission global functioning, the NPD patients also tended to be at a disadvantage compared to those with BPD as indicated by a lower mean total Strauss-Carpenter score at admission (8.8 compared to 9.6 on a 0 to 12 scale) and a greater percentage of seriously dysfunctional patients defined as those with an admission Global Assessment Scale score below 30 (18% of the NPD patients compared to only 3% of BPD patients, χ^2 = 3.3, P = .07). Such differences as those that emerged in the comparison of index hospitalization treatment experience were marginal, suggestive only of a slightly greater tendency toward impulsive behavior in BPD patients during treatment.

At mean 14-year follow-up, patients with NPD continued to show a trend toward greater impairment than those with BPD in terms of social and global functioning and rehospitalization history. Particularly noteworthy is the previously noted low percentage of NPD patients reporting satisfaction with intimate relations. Only 65% of NPD patients reported satisfaction with intimate relations, compared with 91% of BPD patients. During the follow-up interval, NPD patients had more rehospitalization (a mean total of 1.8 months compared to 0.6 months for BPD patients). NPD patients were twice as likely as BPD patients (24% compared to 12%) to have received no further psychotherapy in the follow-up interval, but NPD patients who returned to psychotherapy after discharge from the index hospitalization tended to remain in it longer (4.6 versus 3.7 years). Again, the differences are not significant, but 12% of the NPD patients compared to 6% of the BPD patients had been engaged in suicide attempts or gestures in the follow-up interval.

In terms of global functioning at follow-up, NPD patients had a lower mean Global Assessment Scale score at follow-up (64.7 compared to 66.6) and a smaller percentage of patients achieving one benchmark of good follow-up functioning: a Global Assessment Scale score of 60 or higher (65% of NPD patients compared to 76% of BPD patients).

Although the differences tend to be at a trend level, there is a suggestion that NPD patients are at a disadvantage socially and globally compared to BPD patients. These findings are reminiscent of those noted by McGlashan and Heinnsen (1989) and Stone (1989) in their studies of the effect of NPD traits on BPD course and outcome.

It has been reported by both McGlashan (1986) and Plakun (1989) that BPD outcome, as a function of length of follow-up, distributes in an inverted U pattern, with good and poor outcomes found in the first and third decades of follow-up, but with poor outcomes rare and good outcomes common in the second decade of follow-up. Such an inverted U distribution of outcomes as a function of length of follow-up interval was not found with NPD in this study, with good and poor outcomes present throughout.

In summary, the evidence described herein does not definitively distinguish BPD patients from those with NPD, but the differences found tend to suggest a difference in terms of sex distribution and family history. There is evidence NPD patients may be more impaired than BPD patients, especially with respect to social and global functioning. We must keep in mind that the NPD patients studied here had a severe enough form of the disorder to come to inpatient treatment at a hospital specializing in work with treatment-resistant patients.

It could not be assumed from these data that NPD outpatients would be at the same disadvantage as BPD outpatients. Taken in sum, the data suggest that at least a subset of NPD patients appear to have a disorder that is more disabling than BPD. Further, differences in sex distribution, family history, preadmission and follow-up social and global functioning, and global functioning as a function of length of follow-up interval suggest that one can discriminate between BPD and NPD, despite strong similarities.

Outcome Correlates of NPD and BPD

Outcome of the NPD and BPD patients described in this chapter was quite heterogeneous. All four of the long-term follow-up studies of BPD have attempted to assess factors responsible for outcome heterogeneity. The data presented by Stone and colleagues (1987) suggest that such factors as higher IQ, talent, and attractiveness, and the absence of substance abuse or of prominent antisocial traits were all associated with better outcome. Paris and colleagues (1987) found that dysphoria was correlated with negative global outcome and that a history of early conflict between the patient and his or her mother was associated with poor outcome in borderline patients (1988). Axis I comorbidity with a major affective disorder (McGlashan 1983, 1986; Plakun et al. 1985), Axis II comorbidity with schizotypal personality disorder (Plakun et al. 1987), or narcissistic traits falling short of or fulfilling criteria for NPD (McGlashan and Heinssen 1989; Stone 1989) have all been reported to influence outcome. But substantial outcome heterogeneity remains, even when efforts are made to study relatively "pure," non-comorbid, homogeneous groups of BPD patients.

Both McGlashan's (1985) study and ours at the Austen Riggs Center (Plakun 1991) have used the most ambitious approaches to the study of outcome heterogeneity in BPD, employing correlations with multiple independent dimensions of outcome and (in the case of McGlashan's study) also utilizing multiple regression and discriminant function analysis to assess outcome prediction. The strongest predictors of outcome in BPD to emerge in McGlashan's study included higher IQ, the absence of affective instability, the presence of distractibility, and a shorter length of hospitalization prior to the index admission. Of particular note is the fact that McGlashan's work found (and ours confirmed) that the principles of outcome prediction gleaned from studies of outcome in schizophrenia do not appear to hold true in the case of BPD. In schizophrenia, like tends to predict like (e.g., good social, vocational, or global functioning at baseline predicts good social, vocational, or global functioning at follow-up). In both studies, like predicted like only for hospitalization; BPD patients with a history of more hospitalization at baseline were more likely to have been rehospitalized during the follow-up interval. Further, demographic background variables and such symptoms as personality traits had substantial predictive value, which is not the case in outcome prediction in schizophrenia.

Plakun's (1991) study of outcome prediction in BPD used correlation coefficients to study more than 50 reliably rated predictors for seven dimensions of outcome in BPD patients, including measures of follow-up interval rehospitalization, assessments of vocational and social functioning and symptoms based on the year before follow-up (Strauss-Carpenter items), global functioning as measured by the Global Assessment Scale score at follow-up, a measure of the degree of satisfaction with intimate relationships, and the achievement of marriage or a stable relationship at follow-up. The most important predictors, selected because their correlations were significant at the $P = .01$ level or better and on multiple dimensions of outcome, demonstrated correlation of good outcome in BPD patients with the absence of a family history of parental divorce (associated with good vocational, global, symptom, and social outcome); shorter duration of prior hospitalizations at the time of index admission (associated with less rehospitalization in the follow-up interval); the absence of the narcissistic trait of "entitlement" (associated with good vocational, social, and global outcome); and the presence of self-destructive acts during the index hospitalization (associated with better intimate functioning and greater likelihood of achievement of marriage or a stable relationship at follow-up).

These findings confirmed McGlashan's (1985) demonstration of the significance of hospitalization as a predictor in BPD patients, but they also offer information about previously unreported predictors. The fact that a history of parental divorce is associated with poor outcome is reminiscent of the finding of Paris and colleagues (1988) that developmental conflict with the mother is associated with poor outcome in BPD. The finding that the presence of narcissistic "entitlement" in patients with BPD is associated with poor outcome is consistent with findings (McGlashan and Heinssen 1989; Stone 1989) that narcissistic traits are associated with poor outcome in BPD patients. The fact that the presence of self-destructive acts during the index hospitalization was associated with better outcome in BPD patients is an interesting and provocative one, which should not be interpreted to imply that self-destructive behavior is a good sign in itself. More likely, self-destructive behavior, which can be contained within the hospital setting and successfully worked through in psychotherapy, may serve as a marker that the treatment has become a meaningful therapeutic engagement. This point of view was espoused by Winnicott (1965), who noted that, in the course of intensive psychotherapy, acting out—which remains containable within the holding environment of the psychotherapy—may be a hopeful sign of useful therapeutic engagement.

Outcome prediction in NPD has been studied for the group of 17 relatively "pure," non-comorbid NPD patients described previously (Plakun 1990), allowing comparison to outcome predictors in BPD. In this study, the correlation coefficients of more than 50 reliably rated predictor variables were studied against the same seven dimensions of outcome assessed in BPD. Because correlation coefficients themselves are vulnerable to intercorrelation effects between predictor variables or between outcome dimensions, predictor versus predictor and outcome dimension versus outcome dimension intercorrelations were performed as well. The outcome dimension versus outcome dimension correlations demonstrated that the seven dimensions of outcome were relatively independent, except that global outcome tended to be related to some of the other individual dimensions. Analysis of predictor versus predictor intercorrelations were considered in assessing significant predictor versus outcome dimension intercorrelations.

None of the specific correlates of outcome in BPD were also found to correlate with outcome in NPD, but the general pattern persisted, with like tending not to predict like, and demographic background variables and such symptoms as personality disorder criteria appearing to have predictive value. Taking not only statistical significance but also significance over multiple dimensions as a standard, the most robust predictor of outcome for NPD was socioeconomic status at the time of the index admission. This sample of patients ranged from middle class to the highest socioeconomic class as measured by the Hollingshead-Redlich Scale. Lower (i.e., middle class) socioeconomic status was associated with good global, symptom, and social outcome. Shorter index hospitalization was also associated with good symptom and global outcome, but this was probably because of the intercorrelation of this variable with socioeconomic status. Wealthier patients may have stayed in the hospital longer because they could afford to.

The absence of schizotypal "suspiciousness or paranoid ideation" correlated with less rehospitalization and good vocational outcome, whereas the absence of schizotypal "ideas of reference" was associated with good global functioning. These correlations suggest paranoid traits are ominous in NPD. Being eldest in the sibship or an only child was associated with achievement of good intimate and vocational functioning at follow-up, perhaps suggesting that greater focus of parental interest or attention may mitigate some of the impairments that unfold later in patients predisposed to NPD temperamentally or dynamically.

Conclusion

As is apparent from the foregoing, there are few empirical studies of reliably diagnosed NPD patients. Most of the data presented here come from one relatively small group of NPD patients treated in an unusual inpatient setting. Therefore, caution in the interpretation of results is warranted. Nevertheless, the data presented from this study and others tend to support the coherence, validity, and reliability of the NPD diagnosis as defined in DSM-III and DSM-III-R, constituting an important first step in moving NPD from an exclusively psychoanalytic concept into the realm of empirical psychiatry. Taken in sum, the data presented suggest that NPD is a valid diagnostic entity that is found in a roughly equal distribution in both sexes; NPD is defined by diagnostic criteria that reliably discriminate it from BPD; NPD tends to differ in longitudinal course and outcome from schizophrenia more than from the major affective disorders; and, although resembling its near neighbor diagnosis of BPD in terms of longitudinal course and outcome, NPD shows evidence that it may be associated with poorer social and global functioning at baseline and follow-up. Finally, NPD patients from the highest socioeconomic classes tended not to do as well as those from the middle class, possibly because of a greater reliance on nonparent caretakers. Paranoid traits appeared to be particularly prognostically ominous, but being eldest in the sibship or an only child appeared to be prognostically favorable in NPD patients.

References

Adler G: The borderline-narcissistic personality disorder continuum. Am J Psychiatry 138:46–50, 1981

Adler G: Psychotherapy of the narcissistic personality disorder patient: Two contrasting approaches. Am J Psychiatry 143:430–436, 1986

Akhtar S, Thomson JA, Jr.: Overview: Narcissistic personality disorder. Am J Psychiatry 139:12–20, 1982

American Psychiatric Association: Diagnostic and Statistical Manual of Mental Disorders, 3rd Edition. Washington, DC, American Psychiatric Association, 1980

American Psychiatric Association: Diagnostic and Statistical Manual of Mental Disorders, 3rd Edition, Revised. Washington, DC, American Psychiatric Association, 1987

Bursten B: Narcissistic personalities in DSM-III. Compr Psychiatry 23:409–420, 1982

Freud S: On narcissism: An introduction (1914), in the Standard Edition of the Complete Psychological Works of Sigmund Freud, Vol 14. Translated and edited by Strachey J. London, Hogarth Press, 1957, pp 67–104

Goldstein WN: DSM-III and the narcissistic personality. Am J Psychother 39:4–16, 1985

Gunderson JG, Kolb JE, Austin V: The diagnostic interview for borderlines (DIB). Am J Psychiatry 138:896–903, 1981

Hollingshead AB, Redlich FC: Social Class and Mental Illness. New York, John Wiley, 1958

Kernberg O: Borderline Conditions and Pathological Narcissism. New York, Jason Aronson, 1975

Kernberg O: Internal World and External Reality. New York, Jason Aronson, 1980

Kohut H: The Analysis of the Self. New York, International Universities Press, 1971

Kohut H: The Restoration of the Self. New York, International Universities Press, 1977

McGlashan TH: The borderline syndrome: I. Testing three diagnostic systems. II. Is it a variant of schizophrenia or affective disorder? Arch Gen Psychiatry 40:1311–1323, 1983

McGlashan TH: The prediction of outcome in borderline personality disorder: Part V of the Chestnut Lodge follow-up study, in The Borderline: Current Empirical Research. Edited by McGlashan TH. Washington, DC, American Psychiatric Press, 1985, pp 63–98

McGlashan TH: The Chestnut Lodge follow-up study: III: Long-term outcome of borderline personalities. Arch Gen Psychiatry 43:20–30, 1986

McGlashan TH, Heinssen RK: Narcissistic, antisocial and non-comorbid subgroups of borderline personality disorder. Psychiatr Clin North Am 12:653–670, 1989

Nurnberg HG: Survey of psychotherapeutic approaches to narcissistic personality disorder. Hillside J Clin Psychiatry 6:204–220, 1984

Paris J, Brown R, Nowlis D: Long-term follow-up of borderline patients in a general hospital. Compr Psychiatry 28:530–535, 1987

Paris J, Nowlis D, Brown R: Developmental factors in the outcome of borderline personality disorder. Compr Psychiatry 29:147–150, 1988

Pfohl B, Coryell W, Zimmerman M, et al: DSM-III personality disorders: Diagnostic overlap and internal consistency of individual DSM-III criteria. Compr Psychiatry 27:21–34, 1986

Plakun EM: Distinguishing narcissistic and borderline personality disorders using DSM-III criteria. Compr Psychiatry 28:437–443, 1987

Plakun EM: Narcissistic personality disorder: A validity study and comparison to borderline personality disorder. Psychiatr Clin North Am 12:603–620, 1989

Plakun EM: An empirical overview of narcissistic personality disorder, in New Perspectives on Narcissism. Edited by Plakun EM. Washington, DC, American Psychiatric Press, 1990, pp 103–149

Plakun EM: Outcome prediction in borderline personality disorder. Journal of Personality Disorders 5:93–102, 1991

Plakun EM, Burkhardt PE, Muller JP: 14-year follow-up of borderline and schizotypal personality disorders. Compr Psychiatry 26:448–455, 1985

Plakun EM, Muller JP, Burkhardt PE: The significance of borderline and schizotypal overlap. Hillside J Clin Psychiatry 9:47–55, 1987

Richman JA, Flaherty JA: Gender differences in narcissistic styles. In New Perspectives on Narcissism. Edited by Plakun EM. Washington, DC, American Psychiatric Press, 1990, pp 73–100

Rinsley DB: Notes on the pathogenesis and nosology of borderline and narcissistic personality disorders. J Am Acad Psychoanal 13:317–328, 1985

Ronningstam E, Gunderson JG: Descriptive studies in narcissistic personality disorder. Psychiatr Clin North Am 12:585–601, 1989

Sacksteder J: Psychoanalytic conceptualizations of narcissism from Freud to Kernberg and Kohut, in New Perspectives on Narcissism. Edited by Plakun EM. Washington, DC, American Psychiatric Press, 1990, pp 3–69

Siever LJ, Klar H: A review of DSM-III criteria for the personality disorders, in American Psychiatric Association Annual Review, Vol 5. Edited by Frances AJ, Hales RE. Washington, DC, American Psychiatric Press, 1986, pp 299–301

Spitzer RL, Gibson M, Endicott J: Global Assessment Scale. New York, New York State Department of Mental Hygiene, 1973

Stone MH: Long-term follow-up of narcissistic/borderline patients. Psychiatr Clin North Am 12:621–641, 1989

Stone MH, Hurt SW, Stone DK: The PI 500: Long-term follow-up of borderline inpatients meeting DSM-III criteria. I. Global outcome. Journal of Personality Disorders 1:291–298, 1987

Warner JL, Berman JJ, Weyant JM, et al.: Assessing mental health program effectiveness: A comparison of three client follow-up methods. Evaluation Review 7:635–658, 1983

Winnicott DW: The Maturational Process and the Facilitating Environment. New York, International Universities Press, 1965, pp 203–216

❖ 13 ❖   Outcome Measurement: Tapping the Patient's Perspective

Susan V. Eisen, Ph.D.
Mollie C. Grob, M.S.W.
Diana L. Dill, Ed.D.

Introduction

For those interested in implementing systematic evaluation of psychiatric hospital treatment programs, a decision must be made as to what assessment procedures should be used. A number of excellent reviews of outcome measures are available, including a comprehensive critical review of mental health treatment outcome measures (Ciarlo et al. 1986); reviews of social adjustment measures (Kane et al. 1985; Wallace 1986; Weissman 1975; Weissman et al. 1981); a review of psychotherapy change measures (Waskow and Parloff 1975); and a sampler of measures relevant to mental health center evaluators (Hargreaves et al. 1977).

However, before choosing a measure, evaluators will need to decide what their goals are in conducting the evaluation, including what effects of treatment are to be measured and whose perspective is to be emphasized. There exist multiple perspectives on patient care within an inpatient setting—those of administrators, treaters, patients, and their collaterals—and these perspectives do not necessarily overlap. Hospital administrators may emphasize evaluation issues pertaining to their responsibility to coordinate service delivery and maintain organizational functioning. Treaters may emphasize evaluation issues concerning accuracy of diagnosis and efficacy of therapeutic interventions. Patients themselves may not agree with those who treat them about targets for therapeutic intervention, process of treatment, and acceptable standards for concluding treatment. Evaluators will need to decide which of these perspectives will inform their choice of measurement strategy.

In this chapter, we argue that emphasizing the patient's perspective has unique advantages to evaluators. For instance, patients as consumers of mental health services have become increasingly interested in providers who are respon-sive to their requests. The patient's perspective can be emphasized by 1) designing outcome measures around treatment goals defined by patients, 2) re-cruiting patients as evaluators of their progress (self-reports), and 3) assessing patient satisfaction with various aspects of treatment (the consumer model). The value of tapping the patient's perspective, as well as limitations of attending exclusively to the patient's perspective, are addressed in this chapter.

Most of the popular current outcome measures (for example, the Symptom Checklist 90 [SCL-90; Derogatis 1977], the Minnesota Multiphasic Personality Inventory [MMPI; Hathaway and McKinley 1956], and the Social Adjustment Scale—Self-Report [SAS; Weissman and Bothwell 1976]) have not been de-signed around treatment goals as defined by patients, but instead typically have emphasized psychiatric symptoms or difficulties in adaptation as they are defined by treaters. Patients do not necessarily present their problems in these terms. The variety of patient goals for treatment—for example, "to regain hope, to raise my physical energy, and become functional," "to stop feeling frightened all the time," or "to go back to work"—presents a measurement challenge to evaluators.

Phrasing evaluation measures in terms of patients' goals when initiating treat-ment would seem to be more relevant to patients. An additional advantage of incorporating the patient's perspective in goal-setting and treatment-planning is addressed by Shrauger and Osberg (1981): "Enlisting clients directly in making the decision regarding how they are to be treated may both increase the chance that treatment will meet their needs and produce greater feelings of responsibil-ity for any behavior change achieved" (p. 323; cf. Bowers 1975; Kopel and Arkowitz 1975). In support of this view, Eisen and Grob (1982a) found that psychiatric patients in a hospital-based rehabilitation program showed signifi-cant improvement (by their own reports and by independent reports made by patients' rehabilitation counselors) in goal areas they had identified at the start of treatment, but no change in goal areas they had not identified. In a related area, Eisenthal and colleagues (Eisenthal and Lazare 1976, 1977; Eisenthal et al. 1979) demonstrated that psychiatric patients initiated treatment with precon-ceived expectations about the forms of treatment that would help them (al-though these ideas were infrequently noted by intake workers) and that treatment adherence and satisfaction were greater in patients who received the forms of treatment they preferred.

Examples of measures that assess improvement in problems as they are identi-fied by the patient include the problem-focused nomenclature developed by Longabaugh and colleagues (Longabaugh et al. 1983), Target Complaints (Bat-tle et al. 1966), BASIS-17 (Eisen et al. 1986), and BASIS-32 (Eisen et al. 1989b, which we discuss in more detail later in this chapter). Other examples would be individualized treatment plans developed by patients in collaboration with their treaters, such as Goal-Attainment Scaling (Kiresuk and Sherman 1968).

Although few measures are designed around treatment goals as defined by patients, many of the most popular outcome measures have recruited patients to evaluate their progress, by using the self-report format—for example, the SCL-90 and the MMPI. A critical review of this measurement strategy follows in the next section, and the development of a self-report measure based on patient-identified goals is described. In addition, evaluators are increasingly tapping the perspective of the patient-as-consumer in terms of their satisfaction with various aspects of treatment. The advantages and limitations of satisfaction measures, as well as their complex relationship with treatment outcome measures, will be discussed in the final section of this chapter.

Self-Reports in Outcome Evaluation

Value and Limitations

Shrauger and Osberg (1981) suggested two major sources of skepticism that have negatively influenced attitudes toward the validity of self-reports. The first stems from the psychoanalytic concept of the unconscious, which assumes ". . . that people are usually unaware of some of their most important feelings and are, therefore, often not capable of appraising themselves competently. The effect of this view has been to make professionals question the validity of self-report data and focus more on their symbolic rather than on their obvious content" (p. 323).

The second source of skepticism noted by Shrauger and Osberg stems from response biases. Perhaps the most common bias is "social desirability," the tendency to present oneself in a favorable light, which in a clinical situation could mean denying problems or symptoms (Crowne and Marlowe 1964; Levitt and Reid 1981). Other biases include the "acquiescent response set" in which the respondent says "yes" to whatever is stated on the questionnaire, or "nay-saying," in which the respondent says "no" to everything. In the former case, exaggeration of problems may be reported, perhaps for secondary gain such as eligibility for disability payments. In the latter case, denial may occur, perhaps out of fear of negative consequences.

However, individuals who are assessing themselves are not the only ones who are subject to bias. Each type of informant brings his or her own bias to the assessment situation. In assessments done by significant others, Hogarty and Katz (1971) reported that mothers rated their adolescent children as significantly less pathological than did siblings; differences between ratings made by mothers versus fathers have also been reported (Crook et al. 1980). Hargreaves and colleagues (1977) suggested that therapists may be biased by their involvement and investment in the patient's treatment. Even "objective" interviewers or trained researchers may be biased for or against a particular type of treatment or toward a particular hypothesis (Ellsworth 1977). Possible racial/cultural and gender biases of independent raters have also been reported (Broverman et al. 1970; Weissman and Bothwell 1976). Another problem noted with reports by independent evaluators/interviewers, as well as with clinicians, is the tendency to see more impairment at intake because of close attention to problems possibly precipitating admission, and less impairment at the conclusion of treatment, at which point improvement is expected (Ciarlo et al. 1986).

Rather than discounting self-reports because of response biases, steps can be taken to minimize their effects. Guarantees of confidentiality and anonymity, separation of program evaluators from the clinical treatment staff, and thorough explanation to patients regarding goals and procedures of the evaluation process can all serve this purpose.

There are many advantages to self-report measures, chief among them that individuals know more about themselves than any external evaluator could learn and that people have the capacity to use their self-knowledge to draw inferences about their future behavior (Shrauger and Osberg 1981). In the case of intrapsychic symptoms or behaviors that are not directly observable by others, the patient may be the only one who has the knowledge to report. For patients who live alone, family members may have little information about the patient's symptoms or behavior (Willer and Biggin 1976). Even close family members who live with or near the patient may be shielded from knowledge about alcohol or drug abuse, for example, or even from depression or delusional thoughts. Another reason for using the self-report format is that it communicates respect to patients regarding their views as consumers of mental health services. Also, it is generally the easiest form of measure to administer and the least costly (Erickson 1975; Weissman and Bothwell 1976).

Reliability and Validity

The question of whether self-reported assessments are valid and reliable must be raised. In their review article, Shrauger and Osberg (1981) concluded that self-assessments appear to be at least as good, if not better predictors of reactions to therapeutic interventions than were other assessment measures. However, in most of the studies they reviewed, the subjects were outpatients; only one included psychiatric inpatients. With regard to prediction of post-hospital adjustment, results of six additional studies reviewed (all involving inpatients) were inconclusive. No clear advantage was found for any one particular assessment method. By contrast, Sappington and Michaux (1975) found that self-report measures completed at admission were better predictors of relapse (hospital readmission within 1 year) than were assessments based on professional evaluation.

Taken together, these results raise a question as to the appropriateness of generalizing findings from "normals" or outpatients to inpatients, and the ability of inpatients to make reliable and valid self-assessments. Are inpatients just too impaired to assess themselves in a meaningful way? A number of discussions of patient self-reports suggest that they cannot be used with the most impaired segment of the population who are unable to respond appropriately to the questions posed, particularly at the intake point (Ellsworth et al. 1968; Weissman 1975). However, the number of patients in this category is questionable. Greist and colleagues (1973) found that even actively psychotic inpatients were able to interact appropriately with a computerized interview to identify target problems.

Because self-reports have been used in a wide range of situations and populations and much has been written about their reliability and validity, we will limit this discussion primarily to their use in psychiatric inpatient populations, thus excluding the plethora of research done on outpatients, non-psychiatric medical patients, college students, and other non-inpatient populations (e.g., Castrogiovanni et al. 1989; Chesney et al. 1981; Conte et al. 1988; Klein et al. 1989; Lee and DeFrank 1988; Weissman et al. 1978; Winokur et al. 1982; Zimmerman and Coryell 1987, 1988).

A number of early studies (prior to 1970) suggested that inpatients may not be reliable sources of data about their mental health. Park and colleagues (1965) reported low but statistically significant correlations between self-report and psychiatrist ratings at admission of anxious neurotic patients. Ellsworth and associates (1968) obtained similar results among hospitalized schizophrenics, although agreement improved later. Similarly, May and Tuma (1964) found low correlations between schizophrenics' self-reported psychotic symptomatology as assessed by the MMPI and evaluations by nurses and therapists.

However, many events have taken place during the last 20 years that may justify changes in our approaches to patient assessment and evaluation of treatment. Among the more prominent are the rise of the community mental health movement and the decline of the large state hospital systems; increasing emphasis on patients' rights and treatment in less restricted settings; and advances in control of the symptoms that may limit a patient's ability to respond appropriately to assessment attempts.

Following is a review of the more recent literature (post-1970) dealing with reliability and validity of self-reports in psychiatric inpatient populations. Most of the work in this area has been done with respect to assessment of depression, alcohol abuse, other symptomatology, and social/community functioning.

Depression.   Assessment of depression has received more attention in the literature than any other area. Twelve studies involving inpatients are discussed in this section.

The Inventory to Diagnose Depression (IDD) developed by Zimmerman and colleagues (1986) and tested in a sample of psychiatric inpatients was found to have very high reliability (test-retest and split-half) and internal consistency (Cronbach's alpha was .92). In addition, scale scores were highly correlated ($r = .80$ or higher) with the Hamilton Rating Scale, the Beck Depression Inventory (BDI), and the Carroll Rating Scale. Correlations of the IDD with scales measuring the more psychological aspects of depression (Dysfunctional Attitude Scale, Hopelessness Scale, and Attributional Style Questionnaire) were also significant, although not as high (r ranging from .38 to .60). The IDD was also quite successful in diagnosing major depressive disorders, both according to DSM-III criteria (American Psychiatric Association 1980) and to the Schedule for Affective Disorders and Schizophrenia (SADS).

In a study designed to assess the value of depression rating scales for diagnosing major depression in cocaine abusers, Weiss and colleagues (1989) report that the BDI ". . . offered the best combination of sensitivity and specificity in screening for major depression" (p. 340). The SCL-90 and the Hamilton Rating Scale for Depression showed similar results but were not quite as good as the BDI. At the admission time point, all of the scales were highly sensitive but not very specific, whereas 4 weeks after admission (close to the discharge point), the pattern was reversed such that specificity was high and sensitivity low. The authors cautiously advise that these brief screening measures not be used as a substitute for comprehensive psychiatric evaluation.

Prusoff and colleagues (1972) reported moderate correlations (r ranging from .11 to .61) between clinical interview and self-report assessments in a combined sample of outpatients and inpatients, during acute depressive episodes. At a follow-up point 10 months later, when most patients were recovered, correlations were substantially higher (r ranging from .60 to .74). Separate results for inpatients were not reported, although the authors report that discrepancies were greater among the psychotically depressed patients. The authors offer the opinion that the clinician is the "better" rater, and that for psychotic or other severely ill patients, self-reports appear to be of limited value during the acute episode but are valuable in rating recovery.

Contrary to results reported by Prusoff and colleagues, Schaefer and his associates (1985) found correlations ranging from .45 to .79 between three different self-report depression measures obtained within 2 days of admission to a psychiatric hospital, and clinical ratings of depression based on DSM-III criteria as well as a 5-point global depression rating. In their study, higher validity coefficients were obtained for general psychiatric patients than for a group of chemically dependent patients. The Zung Depression scale emerged as the best of the self-report measures as a predictor of clinical ratings.

In a comparison of inpatients, outpatients, and normals on three self-report depression measures (BDI, Form E of the Depression Adjective Check List, and the Generalized Contentment Scale), reliability and concurrent validity did not differ between groups (Byerly and Carlson 1982). Highest reliability coefficients were obtained for the BDI (.86 for inpatients). Concurrent validity assessed by Pearson correlations among the three scales was also high (.73 for inpatients). Lowest correlations were obtained for nonpatients (ranging from .42 to .58). In addition, depression ratings successfully discriminated patients from nonpatients and diagnosed depressive patients from those not diagnosed as depressed.

As a component of depression, Fawcett and colleagues (1983) developed a measure of anhedonia that they tested on a sample of inpatients, outpatients, and nonpatients. The scale showed evidence of good reliability and successfully discriminated patients who met diagnostic criteria for major depressive disorder from nondepressive control subjects. In addition, among the depressive patients, anhedonia scores correlated significantly with other measures of depression.

In contrast to some of the promising results reported herein and the widespread use of self-report measures, in another review from a psychometric perspective, Boyle (1985) cited several previous reviews that are highly critical of the BDI, Zung, and several other self-report depression rating scales (i.e., Becker 1974; Carroll et al. 1973; Goodstein 1975; Kearns et al. 1982). Criticism focused on questionable reliability and validity, especially the adequacy of depression scales in discriminating depression from other emotional states.

Alcohol abuse.   Six studies provide data regarding reliability and validity of self-reported alcohol abuse among patients treated in an inpatient setting. In one study (McCrady et al. 1978), the researchers reported a correlation of .52 between patients' and spouses' reports of actual quantity and frequency of drinking during the month before hospitalization. On a measure of the consequences of drinking during the same time period, the correlation was .65. On more global measures of drinking, patient/spouse agreement was higher. When disagreements occurred, spouses underestimated drinking as frequently as did patients. From a study of hospitalized alcoholics (Hesselbrock et al. 1983), another research team concluded that ". . . information obtained from alcoholics is highly reliable and valid . . ." (p. 605).

Comparing alcoholics' self-reports of drinking with those of collateral informants 6 months after hospital discharge, Maisto and colleagues (1979) reported comparable results, with Pearson correlations ranging from .46 to .82 for different aspects of drinking behavior (all $P < .001$). A study of test-retest reliability of drinking patterns 7 to 8 years earlier found good reliability with r ranging from .52 to .88 (all $P < .0001$) between sessions occurring 2 to 3 weeks apart (Sobell et al. 1988).

Sobell and Sobell (1978) compared inpatient alcoholics' reports of drinking-related arrests, convictions, and hospitalizations with official records, and found

75% agreement—slightly but not significantly lower than the agreement rate for outpatients in the same study.

All of the studies reported in this section included patients who entered treatment for alcohol abuse. However, once an individual enters treatment for a problem, he or she may be less subject to denial or to a social desirability response bias than someone not in treatment for the problem. Thus, unreliability or lack of validity may be attenuated in these patients who have, in essence, already admitted that they have a problem.

Eisen and colleagues (1989a) used a variety of self-report measures of substance abuse in a sample of inpatients admitted to a hospital for other psychiatric problems. Even under these circumstances, correlations among three self-report measures of alcohol and drug abuse (quantity/frequency, MAST scores, and self-reported difficulty with alcohol or drugs) were highly significant (all $P < .001$), with r ranging from .45 to .69. Concordance of self-reported substance use with corresponding DSM-III-R diagnoses was lower (especially among women), which raises a question of whether in some cases substance abuse diagnoses were being missed in favor of other psychiatric disorders.

Other symptomatology. A recent paper discussed a self-report measure developed for assessment of thought disorder (McCarty et al. 1989). Preliminary results from 100 inpatients and normal subjects suggest high reliability (.81 to .94), good differentiation between patients and nonpatients, and no group differences in socially desirable or random responses. However, Harvey and Neale (1989) offered strong criticism of this approach, specifically with schizophrenic patients whose reports they do not consider to be reliable.

A number of studies used measures that encompass several different dimensions of symptomatology. In one study (Grob et al. 1978), researchers reported two outcome factors (functioning/improvement and helpfulness/satisfaction) that emerged from a 6-month follow-up study of psychiatric inpatients. These two factors appeared for both patients and family members. Correlations between patients and relatives were moderately high with respect to corresponding factors ($r = .58$ for functioning/improvement and $r = .51$ for helpfulness/satisfaction). Correlations between the two factors were much lower ($r = .23$ for patients and $r = .29$ for relatives).

In one of the first studies using the SCL-90 (Derogatis et al. 1973) in an inpatient population, Dinning and Evans (1977) found high convergent validity with the BDI and the MMPI. On the other hand, discriminant validity was fairly low, primarily because of the high intercorrelations among the SCL-90 subscales.

In a study of partial hospital patients (84% of whom had been previously hospitalized), patients' self-reported SCL-90 scores were significantly related to those of both independent evaluators and patients' therapists (Turner et al.

1983).

Social/community functioning.   Patient scores on the Denver Community Mental Health Questionnaire (DCMHQ), which measures community adjustment at follow-up, were highly correlated with corresponding assessments made by therapists ($r = .93$) and independent evaluators ($r = .76$; Turner et al. 1983). The same study also showed high correlations between patients' self-reported adjustment on the DCMHQ with those on a self-report version of the Personal Adjustment and Role Skills (PARS) questionnaire ($r = .65$). These correlations contrast with those reported by Ciarlo and Reihman (1977) for correspondence between clinician and self-report ratings on the DCMHQ, most of which were lower than .40. Correlations between clients and collaterals ranged from .52 to .87 in one study (Ciarlo and Reihman 1977) and from .28 to .78 in another (cited in Ciarlo et al. 1986, p. 192).

The Social Adjustment Scale (self-report form; Weissman and Bothwell 1976), although developed for outpatient groups, has been widely used among diverse samples including schizophrenic patients, depressive patients, alcoholic patients, and nonpatients. The reliability and validity data for the scale pertain to outpatient and other community samples, including a study indicating significant correspondence between the self-report version of the scale and the original interview format (r ranged from .40 to .76 and $r = .72$ for overall adjustment) and similar correspondence between patient self-rating in the acute phase of illness and those of a close relative (r ranged from .43 to .62 and $r = .62$ for overall adjustment). Mellsop and colleagues (1987) used a form of the SAS (SAS-M; Cooper et al. 1982) in a sample of inpatients and found that for patients diagnosed with depression, social adjustment at admission was more highly correlated with follow-up measures of psychiatric state rated by research team members ($r = .36$) than was the DSM-III Axis V rating ($r = -.11$). For those patients diagnosed with schizophrenia, the Axis V rating was more predictive ($r = .37$) than was the social adjustment score ($r = .21$); and for those with a personality disorder, the two measures were equally predictive ($r = .36$ for social adjustment, $r = .32$ for Axis V). Thus, schizophrenic patients' self-reports were not predictive of their follow-up status, whereas self-reports of depressive patients and of patients with personality disorders were.

The Self-Assessment Guide—a 55-item measure covering physical health, general affect, interpersonal skills, personal relations, use of leisure time, control of aggression, and employment—has shown adequate test-retest and split-half reliability, high correlation with another community adjustment scale, discrimination between hospitalized and nonrehospitalized groups, and sensitivity to change (Willer and Biggin 1976).

To sum up the results of the reliability and validity studies of self-report measures in the areas we have reviewed, we want to highlight the following.

With respect to depression, although a number of studies report high interrater reliability as well as concurrent and discriminant validity at both admission and follow-up points, some researchers caution against using self-reports until after the acute symptoms have subsided. They also warn about differential reliability and validity for particular diagnostic groups. For assessment of alcohol abuse, results are quite good; significant correlations between patients' self-reports and those of collateral informants, as well as with official records of drinking-related arrests, convictions, and hospitalizations, have been reported both pre- and post-treatment. For other symptomatology and social/community functioning, thorough assessments of reliability and validity among inpatients are infrequent, and results are complex, though promising.

Review of Available Measures for Generic Inpatient Evaluation

We reviewed measures cited in the literature that utilize a self-report format, cover a broad spectrum of psychopathology and social/community functioning, and have been used in psychiatric inpatient populations. Because of the need for assessment of diverse groups of patients who present for treatment at general psychiatric hospitals, we have not included specialized measures that assess only one dimension (e.g., depression, anxiety, self-esteem, substance abuse); measures that apply to a limited population (e.g., children, the elderly); or measures that have not been used or are not considered appropriate for inpatient samples.

It should also be noted that a number of widely used assessment techniques are based on information obtained from patients or clients in interviews varying in degree of structure (e.g., Psychiatric Status Schedule; Spitzer et al. 1970). However, we have not considered these true self-reports because they cannot be completed by the patient without the presence of an interviewer. This is an important practical consideration for any facility interested in conducting systematic, ongoing evaluation of treatment outcome that includes follow-up.

Existing scales that met our criteria can be grouped into three broad categories: 1) those that assess symptoms, states, or traits only; 2) those that assess social/community adjustment or functioning only; and 3) those that assess both symptoms and functioning. Measures assessing symptoms, states, or traits but not aspects of social or community adjustment, and those assessing adjustment but not symptoms, are mentioned because they have been widely used and may be appropriate for particular evaluation projects. However, in our view, assessment of both symptoms and functioning are vital to evaluation of the course and outcome of psychiatric illness and the effectiveness of hospital treatment programs.

The most commonly used self-report symptom scales (all reviewed in detail by Ciarlo et al. 1986) are 1) SCL-90-R, a 90-item symptom distress checklist

(Derogatis 1977); 2) MMPI, a 566-item true-false questionnaire (Hathaway and McKinley 1956); 3) Dupuy's General Well-Being Scale, a 33-item measure (discussed in Ciarlo et al. 1986, pp. 208–241); and 4) POMS, a 65-item scale (McNair et al. 1971). Although these self-report measures vary in length, and consequently in detail and specificity, they all measure the most common dimensions of symptomatology and psychopathology: depression, anxiety, somatization, and hostility. In addition, some include other features, such as psychotic symptoms, cognitive impairment, and aspects of personality functioning. They do not include items relating to social or community adjustment.

The most popular self-report measures of social/community functioning include 1) Social Adjustment Scale—Self-Report (SAS), a 42-item questionnaire (Weissman and Bothwell 1976); 2) Community Adaptation Schedule (Burnes and Roen 1967), a 217-item questionnaire; 3) the Personality and Social Network Adjustment Scale, containing 17 items rated on a 5-point scale (Clark 1968); 4) Self-Assessment Guide, a 55-item questionnaire (Willer and Biggin 1976); and 5) Progress Evaluation Scales, containing just seven items (Ihilevich et al. 1981). Each of these assesses occupational functioning, family relationships, and social life. In addition, some assess school functioning; household responsibilities; substance abuse; trouble with the law; recreation; and general "happiness," affect, or mood. None of them includes specific psychiatric symptoms.

The most popular All-Purpose Scales include 1) Denver Community Mental Health Questionnaire (DCMHQ), a 79-item multidimensional measure (Ciarlo and Reihman 1977); 2) Katz Adjustment Scales Form S (KAS), a 138-item self-report that has not been used or analyzed as extensively as the relative informant version of the scale (Katz and Lyerly 1963); 3) Major Problem Rating System, a 280-item computerized self-report comprising 44 categories of functioning, in which outcome is assessed only in areas identified as problems by clients (Stevenson et al. 1989); and 4) Target Complaints, an individualized measure of problem severity and improvement (Battle et al. 1966). Each of these "all-purpose" measures includes aspects of social and community functioning as well as specific symptomatology.

The Ideal Self-Report Measure

Ciarlo and colleagues (1986) outlined five major criteria that must be considered in the attempt to find the "ideal" self-report measure for evaluation of mental health treatment outcome:

1. Applicability to the appropriate target groups, independent of type of treatment.

2. Simple, teachable methodology and procedures, including use of measures with objective referents and multiple respondents.

3. Psychometric strength, including reliability, validity, sensitivity to change, freedom from respondent bias, and nonreactivity to situational factors.

4. Low cost.

5. Utility, including understandability to a wide audience, easy feedback, uncomplicated interpretation, usefulness to clinical services, and compatibility with clinical theories and practices.

When we consider these criteria for evaluation of the outcome of inpatient hospital treatment, specific elaborations emerge, especially with regard to methodology and procedures. A measure that will be used with newly admitted patients must be simply worded so that even the most severely impaired will be able to understand it. If a post-discharge follow-up is planned, the measure must also allow for a mail-in form that is brief and nonthreatening enough to maximize the response rate. The follow-up should also allow for a telephone interview that would not be a major imposition on the former patient. In terms of content area, for an inpatient population inclusion of specific symptoms as well as community functioning is important.

Of the available "combination" (symptoms and functioning) scales, none appears ideal. The length of measures such as the Katz Adjustment Scale and the Major Problem Rating System (MPRS) may be prohibitively time-consuming for a mail or telephone follow-up. Individualized techniques including target complaints and the MPRS do not allow for group comparisons, because assessments are not based on the same problems. (See Mintz and Kiesler 1982 for a complete discussion of individualized approaches to outcome evaluation.) On the other hand, individualized measures more closely reflect the patient's perspective than do standardized measures, because they ask the patient to identify the problems that are meaningful to him or her rather than to the clinician.

In our own efforts to initiate an outcome evaluation component for an inpatient population at McLean Hospital, we developed a measure that took into consideration the criteria reviewed. A major goal was to incorporate an individualized measurement approach into a standardized methodology. The development of this instrument is discussed in the next section.

BASIS-32

BASIS-32 was derived empirically from the open-ended reports of 354 newly admitted psychiatric inpatients about the problems that brought them to the hospital, as elicited by the Target Complaint Procedure (Battle et al. 1966). The patients were admitted to a variety of generic and specialized units and represented a broad spectrum of psychiatric disorders. Eight hundred ninety-seven individual problems, stated in the patients' own words, were obtained from the 354 patients. Twenty clinicians then sorted each of these 897 problems into 49 major categories based on their concept of which problems belonged together. A cluster analysis was performed to reduce the number of categories to be used as items in a structured interview or questionnaire.

The original form of BASIS contained 17 items (Eisen et al. 1986). It was later expanded to 32 items in order to 1) include symptoms previously assessed with a separate symptom scale, 2) obtain greater specificity in symptom and problem identification, 3) increase reliability, and 4) allow for scoring into subscales. BASIS-32 can be administered as a structured interview, given as a self-report, sent as a mailed follow-up, or done in a telephone interview.

When BASIS-32 is administered at the admission point, patients are asked to report the degree of difficulty they have been experiencing in each area during the week before admission to the hospital. Degree of difficulty is reported on a 5-point scale, from 0—no difficulty to 4—extreme difficulty. For every area in which some degree of difficulty is reported, patients are asked how long they have been experiencing difficulty in this area. Responses are coded on a 6-point chronicity scale, from 0—not a problem to 5—more than 5 years.

Versions of BASIS-32 have been developed for assessing patients at different time points during hospitalization or at discharge, and at a follow-up point after discharge. The time frame for these versions is 1 week. Parallel forms to be completed by family members and clinicians are also available.

BASIS-32 was first given to 387 psychiatric patients within 1 week of admission to McLean Hospital. By means of factor analysis using a varimax rotation, five factors were derived. This was followed by item analyses to arrive at scales with the highest possible internal consistency. The five subscales and their compositions appear in Table 13–1 along with their consistency (alpha) coefficients.

Test-retest reliability after 2–3 days averaged .76 for the five subscales. Concurrent and discriminant validity analyses indicated that BASIS-32 ratings successfully discriminated among patients still hospitalized 6 months after admission from those living in the community, patients working at follow-up from those who were not, and patients with particular diagnoses. Further analyses revealed that several BASIS-32 subscales correlated significantly with corresponding subscales of the SCL-90-R, and corresponding symptoms documented by utilization review nurses. Follow-up ratings revealed that BASIS-32 is sensitive to changes over time in symptomatology and functioning. (See Eisen et al. 1989b for a complete report.)

BASIS-32 has shown promise as a brief, nonstressful self-report instrument for psychiatric outcome evaluation that fulfills major criteria identified by ex-

TABLE 13–1. Composition and reliability of the five BASIS subscales

Interpersonal relationships alpha = .74	Relationships with family members Getting along with people outside the family Isolation or feeling of loneliness Being able to feel close to others Being realistic about self and others Recognizing and expressing emotions appropriately Developing independence, autonomy Sexual activity or preoccupation
Daily living/ role functioning alpha = .76	Managing day-to-day life Household responsibilities/work/school Leisure time or recreational activities Goals or direction in life Feeling satisfaction with one's life
Depression/ anxiety alpha = .78	Adjusting to major life stresses Lack of self-confidence, feeling bad about self Apathy, lack of interest in things Depression, hopelessness Suicidal feelings or behavior Physical symptoms Fear, anxiety, or panic Confusion, concentration and memory problems
Impulsive/ addictive behavior alpha = .71	Mood swings, unstable moods Uncontrollable, compulsive behavior Drinking alcoholic beverages Taking illegal drugs, misusing drugs Trouble controlling temper, outbursts of anger, Impulsive, illegal, or reckless behavior
Psychosis alpha = .65	Disturbing or unreal thoughts or beliefs Hearing voices, seeing things Manic, bizarre behavior

Source. Eisen et al. (1989b).

perts in the field. It has recently been used by the Central Neuropsychiatric Hospital Association Research Task Force in a collaborative outcome study involving seven private psychiatric hospitals and approximately 800 patients and is included in the protocol of a current National Association of Private Psychiatric Hospitals outcome study as well.

The next section will focus on the patient's perspective as a consumer of psychiatric care, and satisfaction with mental health services as a component of treatment outcome.

Self-Reports in Satisfaction Studies

Rationale for Assessment

Self-reports in outcome research allow the patient's viewpoint in evaluating his own progress, whereas the distinguishing feature of satisfaction research is that it allows for the patient's viewpoint in evaluating the treatment received. The importance of assessing patient satisfaction with health care is now widely recognized, based on the premise that feedback from the service recipient provides an essential perspective in the evaluation of treatment (Kalman 1983; Larsen et al. 1979; Lebow 1982a; Loff et al. 1987).

A commitment to consumerism and accountability in the last two decades has resulted in the pursuit of satisfaction studies as a focus for professional inquiry. Much of the earlier impetus came from legislative mandates to include the patient in the evaluative process in publicly funded programs. Emphasizing equally valid clinical and therapeutic reasons for making patient satisfaction an area of study, Kalman identifies the potential for improving 1) patient compliance with treatment; 2) utilization of services; 3) design of programs; and 4) ultimately, treatment outcome. A major component of satisfaction research is the feedback loop, or reporting of results to clinical and administrative staff for their use in treatment and program planning. A number of authors have demonstrated positive effects from program decisions that were influenced by attention to the patient's perspective (Andrews et al. 1986; Cope et al. 1986; Yamamoto et al. 1984).

Methodological Issues

A major problem identified by investigators has been that of definition. Kalman has defined satisfaction as a composite of many variables. "An individual's expectations, experiences, personality, attitudes, psychodynamics, perceptions, and philosophy all act in concert to determine the state of mind that researchers label 'satisfaction'" (p. 48). Kiesler (1983), reasoning that methodological and conceptual issues arise because previous research on patient satisfaction has not been driven by theory, proposed a more informed use of attitude change and attitude measurement technology. From still another perspective, behaviorists introduce behavioral indices to the measurement of satisfaction (e.g., "Would you return to this hospital if you needed to?" or "Would you recommend this hospital to others?"). Others argue that satisfaction should be defined as the extent to which expectations regarding services are later fulfilled (Larsen et al. 1979).

The lack of a standard methodology for its measurement, problems in obtaining random samples, and the absence of normative data are among other challenges faced by investigators who wish to refine their study methods and techniques (Conte et al. 1989; Sishta et al. 1986). The methods commonly used to measure satisfaction are personal interviews, letters from patients, telephone surveys, and questionnaires. Kalman (1983) also noted the use of such instruments as the Ward Atmosphere Scale (Moos and Houts 1968), the Perception of Ward Instrument (Ellsworth and Maroney 1972), and the Ward Climate Inventory (Spiegel and Younger 1972) by investigators focusing on methodologies to identify patient perspectives on their treatment environments.

The lack of a standard satisfaction scale motivated Larsen and colleagues (1979) to construct an empirically based scale with psychometric qualities that had the potential to provide meaningful comparisons across programs (Client Satisfaction Questionnaire, CSQ). An 8-item scale with high internal consistency, the CSQ has been widely used for evaluation of *general* satisfaction. Many evaluators choose to include additional structured or open-ended items to assess *more specific* aspects of treatment, which might otherwise be masked. For example, in a review of 28 studies assessing psychiatric patients' attitudes toward hospital staff, Weinstein (1981) noted wide variation in the assessment of specific staff members that was not evident when looking at the average staff rating of favorableness. Similarly, Eisen and Grob (1982b) identified a specific aspect of communication (i.e., information received regarding treatment and progress) with which patients were dissatisfied; other aspects of communication were viewed more favorably.

Unsolicited data are also useful for consideration—for example, verbal or written communications about the treatment experience. A content analysis of letters from patients and family members who had voluntarily offered feedback to the hospital reflected common reactions and concerns (Eisen and Grob 1979). Specific areas of satisfaction and dissatisfaction were highly consistent with findings from a structured measure used in a follow-up investigation involving 712 former patients and 753 relatives (Grob et al. 1978).

Many of the challenges faced by evaluators of treatment outcome also apply to the assessment of satisfaction. One of these is the possibility of sampling bias resulting from selection in patients contacted and in patients responding. Studies undertaken while the patient is still hospitalized may achieve more representative samples; post-discharge surveys risk attrition because of patients who have left prematurely and/or who are less improved. Lebow (1982a) counseled that potential distortion from selective attrition must be considered in carrying out any study and suggested that studies must test for differences in treatment characteristics (e.g., early termination) and outcome rather than demography, which does not appear to seriously discriminate between responder and nonresponder.

Distortion arising from the respondents' wish to maintain social desirability is another potential problem for satisfaction studies as well as outcome measurement (Larsen et al. 1979; Lebow 1982b; Urquhart et al. 1986–1987). Consistent with other evaluators (Dowds and Fontana 1978; Glenn 1978), we have found that structured questionnaires tend to elicit relatively high degrees of satisfaction from respondents (Eisen and Grob 1982b; Grob et al. 1978, 1982). Unobtrusive measures of satisfaction (e.g., use of specific services and regularity of attendance); minor adaptations in procedure (e.g., inclusion of open-ended sections); a guarantee of anonymity to the respondent; and the use of data gatherers who are independent of the treatment services all help to reduce problems resulting from reactivity (Piersma 1983).

In his comprehensive and critical review of satisfaction studies, Lebow (1982a) highlighted their inherent value yet problematic nature: "Both the criticisms of consumer satisfaction data and the refutations of these criticisms have merit" (p. 255). Validity problems, the tendency toward halo responses, and the "bias" of the patient/consumer are among the critical arguments offered for minimizing the importance of satisfaction data. Counterarguments supporting the value of satisfaction research are also offered. For example, validation can be improved to a point of reasonable confidence, and better psychometric scale and interview construction allow results that are functional. Also, as was pointed out previously in this chapter, differences among patient, clinician, and rater judgments are as likely to arise from differences in point of view or from distortion by clinician or rater as from patient distortion.

Satisfaction and Outcome

In his summary of study results exploring the complex relationship between patient satisfaction and outcome, Lebow (1982b) concluded that a pattern of findings worthy of note is emerging. Although there is considerable overlap between self-reports of global outcome and general satisfaction of services, when outcome is more specifically assessed, as with a symptom checklist, distinctions appear. The timing of the satisfaction evaluation is also an important consideration, with greater overlap appearing late in treatment. In some instances, outcome ratings are reported to be more positive than satisfaction assessments, whereas in others, the reverse is found.

Larsen and colleagues (1979) reported a modest relationship between therapy gain and satisfaction at a 4-week follow-up, which suggests that service recipients may be able to differentiate between satisfaction with services and gain from treatment. However, satisfaction ratings correlated with early treatment dropout, indicating that satisfaction may be a useful variable in a set of dropout predictors.

Our own work supports the view that treatment outcome and satisfaction are not strongly correlated (Eisen and Grob 1982b; Grob et al. 1978). Low but statistically significant correlations between improvement and satisfaction suggest that although there is some tendency for those who are doing well to be more satisfied with the care received, satisfaction cannot be predicted very accurately from knowledge of a patient's improvement or level of functioning. Despite widely varying methodologies and instruments employed in different studies of patient satisfaction, modest correlations of satisfaction and treatment outcome have been consistent across many types of facilities and sample populations. When results are replicated despite such differences, their validity is greatly strengthened. Summing up the state of the art, Garfield (1983) proposed that more systematic studies of consumer satisfaction as it relates to therapeutic outcome and other variables would serve to enhance our knowledge of the therapeutic process.

Conclusion

In recent years, consumer input has received increasing recognition and attention in the evaluation of treatment outcome and psychiatric services. The rationale for this accountability approach derives from an understanding that the recipients of services are responsive and sensitive to a process that involves them in a critique of their total experience. The inclusion of patients in this process enhances our ability to broaden the empirical base of our understanding of the therapeutic intervention. Although we have focused in this chapter on the patient's perspective, we do not minimize the importance and value of other views, including those of clinicians, independent raters, and family members. All of these provide unique contributions to the evaluative process. With this in mind, the goal of a true collaboration between the clinician and the patient in the planning and delivery of services may be better realized.

References

American Psychiatric Press: Diagnostic and Statistical Manual of Mental Disorders, 3rd Edition. Washington, DC, American Psychiatric Association, 1980

American Psychiatric Press: Diagnostic and Statistical Manual of Mental Disorders, 3rd Edition, Revised. Washington, DC, American Psychiatric Association, 1987

Andrews S, Leavy A, DeChillo N, et al: Patient-therapist mismatch: We would rather switch than fight. Hosp Community Psychiatry 37(9):918–922, 1986

Battle CC, Imber SD, Hoehn-Saric R, et al: Target complaints as criteria of improvement. Am J Psychother 20:184–192, 1966

Becker J: Depression: Theory and Research. New York, John Wiley, 1974, pp 24–27

Bowers KS: The psychology of subtle control: An attributional analysis of behavioral persistence. Can J Behav Sci 7:78–95, 1975

Boyle GJ: Self-report measures of depression: Some psychometric considerations. Br J Clin Psychol 24:45–59, 1985

Broverman IK, Broverman DM, Clarkson FE, et al: Sex-role stereotypes and clinical judgments of mental health. J Consult Psychol 34:1–7, 1970

Burnes AJ, Roen SR: Social roles and adaptation to the community. Community Ment Health J 3:153–158, 1967

Byerly FC, Carlson WA: Comparison among inpatients, outpatients, and normals on three self-report depression inventories. J Clin Psychol 38(4):797–804, 1982

Carroll BJ, Fielding FJ, Blashki TG: Depression rating scales: A critical review. Arch Gen Psych 28:361–366, 1973

Castrogiovanni P, Maremmani I, Deltito JA: Discordance of self ratings versus observer ratings in the improvement of depression: Role of locus of control and aggressive behavior. Compr Psychiatry 39(3):231–235, 1989

Chesney AP, Larson D, Brown K, et al: A comparison of patient self-report and physicians' observations in a psychiatric outpatient clinic. J Psychiat Res 16(3):173–182, 1981

Ciarlo JA, Reihman J: The Denver Community Mental Health Questionnaire: Development of a multi-dimensional program evaluation instrument, in Program Evaluation for Mental Health: Methods, Strategies, and Participants. Edited by Coursey R, Spector G, Murrell S, Hunt B. New York, Grune & Stratton, 1977, pp 131–167

Ciarlo JA, Brown TR, Edwards DW, et al: Assessing mental health treatment outcome measurement techniques. National Institute of Mental Health Series FN No. 9 (DHHS Publ No ADM-86-1301). Washington, DC, U.S. Government Printing Office, 1986

Clark AW: The Personality and Social Network Adjustment Scale: Its use in evaluation of treatment in a therapeutic community. Human Relations 21:85–95, 1968

Conte HR, Plutchik R, Picard S, et al: Self-report measures as predictors of psychotherapy outcome. Compr Psychiatry 29(4):355–360, 1988

Conte HR, Plutchik R, Buckley P, et al: Outpatients view their psychiatric treatment. Hosp Community Psychiatry 40(6):641–643, 1989

Cooper P, Osborn M, Gath D, et al: Evaluation of a modified self-report measure of social adjustment. Br J Psychiatry 141:68–75, 1982

Cope DW, Linn LS, Leake BD, et al: Modification of residents' behavior by preceptor feedback of patient satisfaction. J Gen Intern Med 1(6):394–398, 1986

Crook T, Hogarty GE, Ulrich RF: Inter-rater reliability of informants' ratings: Katz Adjustment Scales R Form. Psychol Rep 47:427–432, 1980

Crowne DP, Marlowe D: The Approval Motive: Studies in Evaluative Dependence. New York, John Wiley, 1964

Derogatis LR: SCL-90: Administration, scoring and procedures manual for the R (Revised) version. Baltimore, Clinical Psychometrics Research, 1977

Derogatis LR, Lipman RS, Covi L: SCL-90: An outpatient psychiatric rating scale—Preliminary report. Psychopharmacol Bull 9(1):13–17, 1973

Dinning WD, Evans RG: Discriminant and convergent validity of the SCL-90 in psychiatric inpatients. J Pers Assess 41:304–310, 1977

Dowds BN, Fontana AF: Patients' and therapists' expectations and evaluations of hospital treatment: Satisfactions and disappointments. Compr Psychiatry 19:491–499, 1978

Eisen SV, Grob MC: Assessing consumer satisfaction from letters to the hospital. Hosp Community Psychiatry 30(5):344–347, 1979

Eisen SV, Grob MC: Clients' rehabilitation goals and outcome. Psychol Rep 50:763–767, 1982a

Eisen SV, Grob MC: Measuring discharged patients' satisfaction with care at a private psychiatric hospital. Hosp Community Psychiatry 33(3):227–228, 1982b

Eisen SV, Grob MC, Klein AA: BASIS: The development of a self-report measure for psychiatric inpatient evaluation. Psychiatric Hospital 17(4):165–171, 1986

Eisen SV, Grob MC, Dill DD: Substance abuse in an inpatient psychiatric population. McLean Hospital Journal XIV:1–22, 1989a

Eisen SV, Dill DD, Grob MC: BASIS-32: A self-report measure for evaluating patient progress. McLean Hospital Evaluative Service Unit Report No. 77, 1989b

Eisenthal S, Lazare A: Specificity of patients' requests in the initial interview. Psychol Rep 38:739–748, 1976

Eisenthal S, Lazare A: Expression of patients' requests in the initial interview. Psychol Rep 40:131–138, 1977

Eisenthal S, Emery R, Lazare A, et al: "Adherence" and the negotiated approach to patienthood. Arch Gen Psychiatry 36:393–398, 1979

Ellsworth RB: Utilizing consumer input in evaluating mental health services. Paper presented at the Conference on the Impact of Program Evaluation on Mental Health Care. Loyola University, Chicago, January 1977

Ellsworth R, Maroney R: Characteristics of psychiatric programs and their effects on patients' adjustment. J Consult Clin Psychol 39:436–447, 1972

Ellsworth RB, Foster L, Childers B, et al: Hospital and community adjustment as perceived by psychiatric patients, their families and staff. Journal of Consulting and Clinical Psychology Monograph Supplement 32(5):1041, 1968

Erickson RF: Outcome studies in mental hospitals: A review. Psychol Bull 82(4):519–540, 1975

Fawcett J, Clark DC, Scheftner WA, et al: Assessing anhedonia in psychiatric patients. Arch Gen Psychiatry 40:79–84, 1983

Garfield SL: Some comments on consumer satisfaction in behavior therapy. Behavior Therapy 14:237–241, 1983

Glenn RN: Measuring patients' opinions about hospitalization using the Client Satisfaction Scale. Hosp Community Psychiatry 29:188–190, 1978

Goodstein LD: Review of The Self-Rating Depression Scale, in Personality Tests and Reviews II. Edited by Buros OK. Highland Park, NJ, Gryphon, 1975, pp 537–538

Griest J, Klein M, Van Cura L: A computer interview for psychiatric patient target symptoms. Arch Gen Psychiatry 2(2):247–253, 1973

Grob MC, Eisen SV, Berman JS: Three years of follow-up monitoring: Perspectives of formerly hospitalized patients and their families. Compr Psychiatry 19(6):491–499, 1978

Grob MC, Eisen SV, Edinburg GM: Clinical social work with young adult inpatients: Perspectives of patients, parents and clinicians. Soc Work Health Care 8(2):1–9, 1982

Hargreaves WA, Attkisson CC, Sorensen JE (eds): Resource materials for Community Mental Health Program Evaluation, 2nd Edition (DHEW Publ No ADM-77-328). Washington, DC, U.S. Department of Health, Education, and Welfare Public Health Service, Alcohol, Drug Abuse, and Mental Health Administration, 1977, pp 243–254

Harvey PD, Neale JM: Comments on innovations in the assessment of thought disorder. Schizophr Bull 15:2–3, 1989

Hathaway SR, McKinley JC: Construction of the schedule. In Basic Readings on the MMPI in Psychology and Medicine. Edited by Welsh GS, Dahlstrom WG. Minneapolis: University of Minnesota Press, 1956, pp 60–63

Hesselbrock N, Babor T, Hesselbrock V, et al: Never believe an alcoholic? On the validity of self-report measures of alcohol dependence and related constructs. Int J Addict 18(5):593–609, 1983

Hogarty GE, Katz MM: Norms of adjustment and social behavior. Arch Gen Psychiatry 25:470–480, 1971

Ihilevich D, Gleser GW, Gritter GW, et al: Measuring program outcome: The progress evaluation scales. Evaluation Review 5(4):451–477, 1981

Kalman TP: An overview of patient satisfaction with psychiatric treatment. Hosp Community Psychiatry 34(1):48–54, 1983

Kane RA, Kane RL, Arnold S: Measuring social functioning in mental health studies: Concepts and instruments. National Institute of Mental Health Series DN No. 5 (DHHS Publ No ADM-85-1384). Washington, DC, U.S. Government Printing Office, 1985

Katz MM, Lyerly SB: Methods for measuring adjustment and social behavior in the community: I. Rationale, description, discriminative validity, and scale development. Psychol Rep Mono 13:503–535, 1963

Kearns NP, Cruickshank CA, McGuigan JK, et al: A comparison of depression rating scales. Br J Psychiatry 141:45–49, 1982

Kiesler CA: Social psychological issues in studying consumer satisfaction with behavior therapy. Behavior Therapy 14:225–236, 1983

Kiresuk T, Sherman R: Goal attainment scaling: A general method for evaluating comprehensive community mental health programs. Comm Ment Health J 4:443–453, 1968

Klein DN, Dickstein S, Taylor EB, et al: Identifying chronic affective disorders in outpatients: Validation of the General Behavior Inventory. J Consult Clin Psychol 57(1):106–111, 1989

Kopel S, Arkowitz H: The role of attribution and self-perception in behavior change: Implications for behavior therapy. Genetic Psychology Monographs 92:175–212, 1975

Larsen D, Attkisson C, Hargreaves W et al.: Assessment of client/patient satisfaction: Development of a general scale. Evaluation and Program Planning 2:197–207, 1979

Lebow J: Consumer satisfaction with mental health treatment. Psychol Bull 91(2):244–259, 1982a

Lebow J: Models for evaluating services at community mental health centers. Hosp Community Psychiatry 33(12):1010–1014, 1982b

Lee DJ, DeFrank RS: Interrelationships among self-reported alcohol intake, physiological indices and alcoholism screening measures. J Stud Alcohol 49(6):532–527, 1988

Levitt JL, Reid WJ: Rapid-assessment instruments for practice. Social Work Research & Abstracts 17:13–19, 1981

Loff CD, Trigg LJ, Cassels C: An evaluation of consumer satisfaction in a child psychiatric service: Viewpoints of patients and parents. Am J Orthopsychiatry 57(1):132–134, 1987

Longabaugh R, Fowler R, Stout R, et al: Validation of a problem-focused nomenclature. Arch Gen Psychiatry 40:453–461, 1983

Maisto SA, Sobell LC, Sobell MB: Comparison of alcoholics' self-reports of drinking behavior with reports of collateral informants. J Consult Clin Psychol 47(1):106–112, 1979

May PRA, Tuma AH: Choice of criteria for the assessment of treatment outcome. J Psychiatr Res 2:199–209, 1964

McCarty T, Waring EM, Neufeld R, et al: Innovations in the assessment of thought disorder. Schizophr Bull 15:1–2, 1989

McCrady BS, Paolino TJ, Longabaugh R: Correspondence between reports of problem drinkers and spouses on drinking behavior and impairment. J Stud Alcohol 29(7):1252–1257, 1978

McNair DM, Lorr M, Droppleman LF: Profile of Mood States Manual. San Diego, Educational and Industrial Testing Service, 1971

Mellsop G, Peace J, Fernando T: Pre-admission adaptive functioning as a measure of prognosis in psychiatric inpatients. Aust N Z J Psychiatry 21:539–544, 1987

Mintz J, Kiesler DJ: Individualized measures of psychotherapy outcome. In Handbook of Research Methods in Clinical Psychology. Edited by Kendall P, Butcher JN. New York, Wiley, 1982, pp 491–534

Moos RH, Houts PS: Assessment of the social atmospheres of psychiatric wards. J Abnorm Psychol 73:595–604, 1968

Park LC, Uhlenhuth EH, Lipman RS, et al: A comparison of doctor and patient improvement ratings in a drug (meprobromate) trial. Br J Psychiatry 3:535–540, 1965

Piersma HL: Program evaluation using a patient opinion survey: One hospital's experience. The Psychiatric Hospital 14(3):171–176, 1983

Prusoff BA, Klerman GL, Paykel ES: Concordance between clinical assessments and patients' self-report in depression. Arch Gen Psychiatry 26:546–552, 1972

Sappington AA, Michaux MH: Prognostic patterns in self-report, relative report, and professional evaluation measures for hospitalized and day-care patients. J Consult Clin Psychol 43(6):904–910, 1975

Schaefer A, Brown J, Watson CG, et al.: Brief reports: Comparison of the validities of the Beck, Zung, and MMPI Depression Scales. J Consult Clin Psychol 53(3):415–418, 1985

Shrauger JS, Osberg TM: The relative accuracy of self-predictions and judgments by others in psychological assessment. Psychol Bull 90(2):322–351, 1981

Sishta SK, Rinco S, Sullivan JC: Clients' satisfaction survey in a psychiatric inpatient population attached to a general hospital. Can J Psychiatry 32(2):123–128, 1986

Sobell LC, Sobell MB: Validity of self-reports in three populations of alcoholics. J Consult Clin Psychol 46(5):901–907, 1978

Sobell LC, Sobell MB, Riley DM, et al.: The reliability of alcohol abusers' self-reports of drinking and life events that occurred in the distant past. J Stud Alcohol 49(3):225–232, 1988

Spiegel D, Younger JB: Ward climate and community stay of psychiatric patients. J Consult Clin Psychol 39:62–69, 1972

Spitzer RL, Endicott J, Fleiss JL, et al.: The Psychiatric Status Schedule: A technique for evaluating psychopathology of impairment of role functioning. Arch Gen Psychiatry 23:41–55, 1970

Stevenson J, McCullough L, Stout R, et al: The development of an individualized, problem-oriented psychiatric outcome measure. Evaluation & the Health Professions 12(2):134–158, 1989

Turner RM, McGovern M, Sandrock D: A multiple perspective analysis of schizophrenics' symptoms and community functioning. Am J Comm Psychol 11(5):593–607, 1983

Urquhart B, Bulow B, Sweeney J, et al.: Increased specificity in measuring satisfaction. Psychiatr Q 58(2):128–134, 1986–1987

Wallace CJ: Functional assessment in rehabilitation. Schizophr Bull 12(4):604–631, 1986

Waskow IE, Parloff MG (eds): Psychotherapy change measures: Report of the Clinical Research Branch Outcome Measures Project (DHEW Publ No ADM-74-120). Washington, DC, U.S. Government Printing Office, 1975

Weinstein RM: Mental patients' attitudes toward hospital staff. A review of quantitative research. Arch Gen Psychiatry 38:483–489, 1981

Weiss RD, Griffin ML, Mirin SM: Diagnosing major depression in cocaine abusers: The use of depression rating scales. Psychiatry Res 28:335–343, 1989

Weissman MM: The assessment of social adjustment: A review of techniques. Arch Gen Psychiatry 32:357–365, 1975

Weissman MM, Bothwell S: Assessment of social adjustment by patient self-report. Arch Gen Psychiatry 33:1111–1115, 1976

Weissman MM, Prusoff BA, Thompson WD, et al.: Social adjustment by self-report in community sample and in psychiatric outpatients. J Nerv Ment Dis 166(5):317–326, 1978

Weissman MM, Sholomskas D, John K: The assessment of social adjustment. Arch Gen Psychiatry 38:1250–1258, 1981

Willer B, Biggin P: Comparison of rehospitalized and non-hospitalized psychiatric patients on community adjustment: Self-assessment Guide. Psychiatry 39:239–244, 1976

Winokur A, Guthrie MG, Rickels K, et al: Extent of agreement between patient and physician ratings of emotional distress. Psychosomatics 23(11):1135–1146, 1982

Yamamoto J, Acosta FX, Evans LA, et al.: Orienting therapists about patients' needs to increase patient satisfaction. Am J Psychiatry 141(2):274–277, 1984

Zimmerman M, Coryell W: The Inventory to Diagnose Depression (IDD): A self-report scale to diagnose major depressive disorder. J Consult Clin Psychol 55(1):55–59, 1987

Zimmerman M, Coryell W: The validity of a self-report questionnaire for diagnosing Major Depressive Disorder. Arch Gen Psychiatry 45:738–740, 1988

Zimmerman M, Coryell W, Corenthal C, et al.: A self-report scale to diagnose Major Depressive Disorder. Arch Gen Psychiatry 43:1076–1081, 1986

❖ 14 ❖   Follow-up Study Methodology: The Menninger Project and a Proposed Ideal Study

Lolafaye Coyne, Ph.D.

In the last 30 years, a number of psychiatric institutions have conducted follow-up studies, many of which have been focused on a specific diagnosis. McGlashan (1988) reported on 12 follow-up studies of patient populations that were either exclusively or partly schizophrenic. Among other studies are two conducted at McLean Hospital and one at the Austen Riggs Center.

Only 2 of the 14 studies were prospective: the second Massachusetts Mental Health Center study (Vaillant 1978) and the long-term follow-up study of a subgroup of the Washington International Pilot Study of Schizophrenia cohort (Carpenter et al. 1987). Although the Boston State Hospital study (Gardos et al. 1982a, 1982b) was retrospective, a considerable amount of prospective data were available from an earlier drug study of which these subjects were a part. Five of the studies followed only one cohort of patients: the two Alberta Hospital studies (Bland et al. 1976; Bland and Orn 1978); the Boston State Hospital study; the second McLean Hospital study (Pope et al. 1983); and the Washington International Pilot Study (Carpenter et al. 1987). Eleven of the 14 studies had a personal interview with the patient as one source of data—in several instances, the only source.

Several of the studies collected data from personal or phone interviews with patients, relatives, and/or treaters. In the Phipps Clinic study, Stephens and colleagues (Stephens 1970, 1978; Stephens and Astrup 1963, 1965) obtained data from letters, phone interviews, and personal interviews with patients, relatives, and hospitals. The study at McLean Hospital (Grob et al. 1978) and the Austen Riggs study (Plakun et al. 1985) used mailed questionnaires sent to patients and relatives (Grob et al. 1978) or to patients (Plakun et al. 1985). Five studies included patients other than those who were schizophrenic: two studies at McLean Hospital (Grob et al. 1978; Pope et al. 1983); one study at the Austen Riggs Center (Plakun et al. 1985); the Iowa 500 follow-up study (Clancy

237

et al. 1974; Morrison et al. 1972; Tsuang and Winokur 1975; Tsuang et al. 1979); and the Chestnut Lodge study conducted by McGlashan (1984a, 1984b). The Iowa 500 follow-up study introduced new methodology into follow-up studies—for example, the inclusion of several diagnostic groups as well as a group of surgical controls. The McGlashan study included seven diagnostic groups, compared self-report with data obtained from a semistructured personal interview, and in general pioneered much of present-day follow-up methodology.

In this chapter, I will describe the Menninger Adult Hospital Ongoing Follow-up Project and present a proposed ideal outcome study. This ideal outcome study is based in part on a review of the follow-up literature listed previously and in part on experience with the Menninger Ongoing Follow-up Project. Finally, I will discuss design and statistical problems that are likely to be shared by all outcome studies.

The Menninger Adult Hospital Ongoing Follow-up Project

Currently, we begin our study with an assessment at discharge of all patients from the long-term units and one short-term unit who give informed consent to participate. Assessment is by a semistructured interview conducted in person in the week prior to discharge, and, in a few instances, by phone shortly after discharge. The interview includes questions to provide information from which the Brief Psychiatric Rating Scale (BPRS; Overall and Gorham 1962), the Global Assessment Scale (GAS; Endicott et al. 1976), and a Therapeutic Alliance Scale (Allen 1985) developed at The Menninger Clinic can be rated. The interviewer takes careful notes on the interview and rates these instruments. An independent rater also rates them on the basis of the interviewer's notes. Interviewers and independent raters are practicing clinicians but cannot be the patient's treaters (either on-floor or off-floor). The project staff are a multidisciplinary team, including social workers, psychologists, nurses, vocational counselors, and psychiatrists.*

Raters have been trained to a level of adequate reliability through participation in a number of reliability studies. If the two raters differ by more than one point on the BPRS and the Therapeutic Alliance Scale, or if their ratings fall in different bands on the GAS, they are required to reach a consensus rating based on a discussion of the evidence for their ratings. These consensus ratings are made in a regular project meeting, and the discussion around them serves to

---

* Current project staff are: Lolafaye Coyne, Ph.D.; Carolyn Grame, M.S.S.W., Ph.D.; David Deering, Ed.D., R.N.; Melissa Smith, Ph.D.; Thomas E. Rooks, M.S.N., R.N.; Debra Langworthy, M.N., R.N.; Morris Taylor, M.S.; Glenda Hannings, R.N.; and Herbert E. Spohn, Ph.D.

mitigate rater drift over time. When consensus ratings are not required, the average of the two ratings is used.

In addition to the assessment of symptoms, overall functioning, and therapeutic alliance at discharge, a section of the interview assesses patient satisfaction. Patients make four 4-point satisfaction ratings: "Have the services helped you to deal with your problems? Did you get the kind of service you wanted? How would you rate the quality of service? How satisfied are you with the service?" Other questions deal with satisfaction with specific components of the treatment. There are also questions as to whether the treatment was worth the time and/or the money and if patients would return for treatment or recommend our treatment to a friend or relative. Patients are asked where they heard about The Menninger Clinic and how they made the decision to come here.

The first follow-up assessment is at 1 year post-discharge. Every effort is made to obtain a 1-year follow-up assessment on the cohort of patients identified at discharge. Permission to contact the patient at 1 year post-discharge is obtained during the discharge interview. Patients are asked to provide changes of address following discharge but are free to refuse participation at 1-year follow-up. In addition to the original cohort assessed at discharge, patients who declined to participate at discharge are contacted at 1 year post-discharge and asked to give informed consent to participate. Although the main goal of the project is to follow the same cohort of patients from discharge through several follow-up points, a secondary goal is to obtain information on as many patients as possible following discharge.

The 1-year follow-up assessment is again based on a semistructured interview but is conducted by phone, with a few exceptions for those patients who are in the Partial Hospitalization Services or living in Topeka. The same questions are asked to provide information from which the Brief Psychiatric Rating Scale and the Global Assessment Scale can be rated. Other questions are added to assess the Strauss-Carpenter General Adjustment Scales (Strauss and Carpenter 1972, 1974; Alcohol and Drug Abuse, Work Adjustment, Dependence/Independence, Usefully Employed, and Personal-Social Relations); our revision of the Dorney Role Functioning Scales (Dorney 1982; Work Productivity, Independent Living, Immediate Social Network Relations, and Extended Social Network Relations); and a Follow-Up Adjustment Scale (Harty et al. 1981) developed at The Menninger Clinic. A detailed environmental assessment is obtained, including information on further treatment, participation in aftercare programs, jobs, further education, home management, suicide attempts, substance abuse, and problems involving the police. A smaller subset of questions dealing with treatment satisfaction is also included. Patient satisfaction ratings are not included at the follow-up points. The same procedures, including a semistructured interview and scales to be rated, are repeated at a 5-year post-discharge follow-up.

As yet, we have not been able to do an admission assessment that we think is highly desirable. We plan to add this as soon as we can acquire adequate personnel and resources. In the meantime, we can refer to an extensive hospital data base (Patient Entry Data and Treatment Data at Discharge), which has been collected for many years. This data base is collected from medical records by trained research assistants who are blind to outcome. Data include demographic variables (such as age, sex, marital status, rural/urban background); chronicity/severity variables (such as precipitating factors, age of first treatment contact, age of first hospitalization, number of prior hospitalizations, total length of prior hospitalization); prior work history; prior educational level; and diagnosis. These variables can serve to define the patient population under study and to provide potential prognostic variables. They may be used to define groups to be contrasted on follow-up outcome. However, it is quite possible that these groups will not be equivalent on the criterion variables at admission. In this case, the absence of an admission assessment is a definite limitation.

Because one of the difficulties in sequential assessments of the same cohort is nonparticipation, we are introducing an additional component in our project. We have developed questionnaires that parallel the semistructured interviews. These are to be sent to all patients who did not participate at discharge or follow-up, except for those who refused either follow-up assessment. The questionnaire is designed to provide information from which the same ratings on the various scales can be made by clinical raters. The data obtained from the questionnaire will be kept separately from data obtained by in-person or phone interview, and these data will be summarized and presented as a different data source.

An important component of our project is that of program evaluation. In this context, group summaries of both quantitative ratings and qualitative information are fed back periodically to each treatment unit at staff meetings. Data summarized for long-term and short-term cohorts are presented to the hospital director and administrator. This information includes patients' perceptions of the usefulness of various treatment components; suggestions for improved treatment; and information about post-discharge work, education, and treatment. Periodic presentations of both quantitative and qualitative data are also made at hospital education meetings and at various national meetings. Publications in clinical journals are under way.

Our 7 years of ongoing follow-up have revealed problems, the most salient of which is the problem of locating people. The restrictions entailed by informed consent and confidentiality procedures make it difficult to contact relatives, friends, and other sources in trying to locate the patients who have not provided current addresses to the hospital. Although this problem might be partially alleviated by obtaining consent from patients at the discharge interview to contact relatives or friends whom they nominate, this might decrease the patients' willingness to participate in further follow-up assessments. A related problem is the difficulty in getting repeated assessments from the same patient. We find patients may be willing to participate at discharge and not at follow-up or may not be willing at discharge and willing at the follow-up points. The difficulty of getting data from the same patients across a number of assessment points seriously jeopardizes the consistency of the data. Another problem is getting sufficiently detailed information, particularly concerning rehospitalizations following treatment—number of hospitalizations, length of each, and kind of hospital. Memory often does not permit the patient to report the amount of detail that is desired. Similar memory problems may occur about number of jobs and other details of employment history.

Obtaining informed consent is consistently a problem to some extent in follow-up studies. If informed consent is sought separately at each follow-up point, there may be major difficulties in getting patients who agree to participate to mail back their informed consent forms. We do not conduct a follow-up interview if we do not have the signed informed consent form in hand. A special problem exists for patients who are discharges against medical advice (AMA) and patients whose discharges take place so quickly that it is not possible to interview them in the week before discharge. In these instances, we interview the patient by phone shortly after discharge. For both of these groups, we find lower rates of locating the patient and obtaining permission for the interview. We have particular difficulty with those patients with AMA discharges. This is because we have chosen not to interview the patient in the week prior to discharge, lest this interfere with the patient's treatment around the issue of leaving. Patients who were AMA discharges are often difficult to locate and even more difficult to get to consent to participate. This causes a problem in representativeness. In one study, we compared those patients on whom we had at least one interview with those whom we were not able to interview at all. The few significant differences that were found in analyzing a large number of hospital data base variables could largely be attributed to the fact that we had interviewed very few AMA discharges. This continues to be a problem, and as yet, we have not found any workable solution.

A Proposed Ideal Outcome Study

What follow are recommendations about the kind of outcome study that our hospitals should begin to do. These recommendations come from review of the literature on follow-up studies and from personal experience with the Menninger Ongoing Follow-up Project.

The cohort and assessment points.   First, the study should sequentially follow the same cohort of patients across time by means of serial assessments. At a minimum, there should be a discharge assessment and assessments at several post-discharge follow-up points. The discharge assessment should provide the following: 1) the identification of the cohort, 2) a baseline at the end of treatment, 3) an opportunity to obtain informed consent for contact at later follow-up points, and 4) an opportunity to request that the patient report changes in address after discharge. Post-discharge follow-up points should include 1 year, 3 years or 5 years, and 10 years post-discharge. Ideally, additional assessments would continue even beyond 10 years. An alternative is to time the follow-up assessments from admission instead of discharge. Post-admission assessments provide standard comparison points that are the same for all patients regardless of the length of their treatment. One or more such post-admission assessments may be quite useful when patients with widely varying lengths of treatment are included in the cohort. A possible compromise might be to include one follow-up assessment post-admission, perhaps replacing the 1-year or 3-year post-discharge follow-up.

Many of the reported follow-up studies have been done on different cohorts of subjects, with each cohort being based on a different time since discharge. Although these studies have yielded useful information with regard to both methodology and outcome, this cross-sectional approach has confounded data and findings with sample differences and treatment differences that occur over time. In some of our studies, characteristics for samples that are separated by 8 years have changed considerably. The patient population tended to get older or younger, and the diagnostic distribution varied as the *Diagnostic and Statistical Manual of Mental Disorders* (American Psychiatric Association 1980, 1987) changed and as certain diagnoses become more or less prominent. When different samples at different times post-discharge are compared, nonequivalency in patient characteristics, treatments, and so on creates serious problems for statistical analysis and even more so for interpretation of results. The most legitimate and meaningful way to make comparisons of patient outcome over years following discharge is to follow the same cohort of patients over time, assessing them serially.

Baseline admission data.   At a minimum, baseline data for admission and preadmission should be collected from medical records. These data should include demographic, clinical, and environmental variables that are broad enough in scope to provide a good definition of the cohort assessed at discharge and follow-up. Variables should include admission age, sex, marital status, work prior to admission, educational level at admission, rural/urban background, age of onset, age of first hospitalization, years between age of onset and admission, number of prior hospitalizations, total length of prior hospitalizations, prior outpatient treatment, prior use of psychotropic medication, precipitating factors, and premorbid adjustment (McGlashan et al. 1988). Such variables describe the cohort and serve as prognostic or predictor variables to relate to outcome at discharge and at follow-up. An important use of such baseline data is to compare nonresponders, refusers, and responders to ascertain the amount and kind of bias, if any, in the study sample.

These variables should be collected by trained research assistants or clinicians who have demonstrated acceptable reliability in systematic reliability studies and who are blind to outcome. The amount of missing data on each of the variables should be recorded, and the missing data rates should be cited in any publications or reports. Also, researchers should report on how missing data were handled in statistical analyses.

Nonresponding.   Nonresponding is a major problem in any outcome study, but there are no guaranteed solutions. Various methods have been tried with phone follow-up interviews, including repeated attempts at phone calls, calls at night after working hours, and requests of patients at discharge asking for the most convenient time to call. Mailing questionnaires to those who have not kept their phone appointments, or who have not participated for other reasons than refusal, may also help.

Diagnoses.   It is highly desirable that operational criteria be used for diagnoses. However, it is often difficult to impose an expensive and time-consuming research diagnostic interview onto a clinical system for the purpose of an outcome study. At a minimum, DSM-III-R should be used, and the specific criteria that have been met for each diagnosis should be recorded. The diagnostic assessment, whether done by a research interview or as part of regular clinical practice, should be done by persons other than those who assess outcome. Another important requirement is that both Axis I and Axis II diagnoses as well as multiple diagnoses on the same axis be recorded, because comorbidity is an important prognostic variable and one that distinguishes subgroups within the cohort.

Admission assessment.   If subgroups within the cohort are to be compared on outcome and they are likely not equivalent at admission (e.g., different diagnostic groups), it becomes essential that the study begin with an admission assessment. This is especially true when the outcome measures are rating scales, either self-report or independently rated. This kind of outcome study is a prospective study. The cohort to be serially assessed is identified at admission, and informed consent about being contacted at discharge and follow-up is obtained at that time. The patient is always free to refuse to participate at any later assessment point.

However, if follow-up outcome measures consist of objective data such as employment, further treatment, further education, legal problems, suicide attempts, and so on, then baseline chart data collected at admission can probably provide an initial level against which to compare this kind of outcome data.

If kinds of treatment are to be compared, a randomized clinical trials design or some promising quasi-experimental design should be used.

Assessment method. The suggested method of assessment is a semi-structured interview conducted by a clinician in person at discharge and by phone at the follow-up points. The clinician must not be the treater and should be blind to diagnosis. However, the clinician-interviewer should have enough information about the patient so that mistakes will not be made in the interview because of lack of information. The interviewer should know any unusual circumstances regarding the patient, the family, and the hospitalization, as well as the symptoms and issues that were salient in the treatment. The semistructured interview assures that all of the necessary areas are included in the interview. This format leaves the clinician free to use clinical skill to stop asking questions in an area when it is sufficiently covered and to add further probe questions when more information is necessary.

Clinically trained interviewers also know how to act appropriately when they believe patients are a risk to themselves or to others. Clinicians can tactfully suggest to such patients that they talk with a current treater or with a treater from the past hospitalization if they are not currently in treatment. In extreme cases, the clinician-interviewer may think it necessary to suggest to the hospital administration that a former treater get in touch with the patient.

Clinician interviews may be supplemented by a limited number of self-report measures to be filled out by the patient. Those selected should focus on areas where the direct perspective of the patient may corroborate (or perhaps even more important, disagree with) the clinician's perspective.

If rating scales other than patient self-report are to be used as outcome measures, the interviewer should also be a rater. A second independent rater who rates from audiotapes or handwritten notes or from listening in on the original interview or phone call adds validity beyond that of a single rater's ratings. All raters should be trained to demonstrated reliability on all scales. In the actual study, when the difference between the two ratings exceeds a certain magnitude defined in advance for each scale, the two raters should meet and reach a consensus rating. This technique guards against overlooking data. It is particularly useful when the two raters are from different disciplines, with different educational backgrounds and experiences. In this instance, the raters may focus on different information, and the pooling of all information may yield a more valid rating than either of the individual ratings alone.

Outcome measures. Outcome should be both multidimensional and multiperspective. Outcome measures should include at least symptom status, a measure of general functioning, and measures of role functioning (e.g., work, independent living, and immediate and extended social relationships). Outcome measures should not neglect "real life" variables that are important to families, insurance companies, and other groups, such as what the patient's occupation is, whether the patient has returned to previous work level, or whether the patient has reached potential with regard to work. Work assessments should also include home management, care of children, and so on for those who are not employed outside of the home. Other "real life" variables that should be included are further education (specifying whether it is part-time or full-time and leading toward a degree or not) and further treatment, both outpatient and inpatient. Information on further treatment should be collected in considerable detail— not only number of rehospitalizations, but the length of each and some indication, if possible, of the time in the community between hospitalizations. Rehospitalization has been used as an outcome variable in a number of follow-up studies. Often these data are based only on the hospital under study, and this probably leads to underestimates of the number of rehospitalizations. Certainly, in a follow-up interview or a mailed questionnaire, information should be sought about rehospitalizations in other hospitals and in as much detail as possible. Other variables should include substance abuse, number of suicide attempts and lethality, if possible, and number and severity of legal problems, with details about the kinds of problems. Definitions of these variables should be operationalized at the beginning of the study so that the interviewer can obtain adequate information and guidelines for coding these variables should be provided. Coding information after it has been collected without such guidelines can be time-consuming and frustrating and may yield data that are not as detailed or as valid.

Patient satisfaction can be a useful outcome variable, particularly at discharge. Although overall patient satisfaction ratings tend to be biased upward, more specific ratings about individual components of treatment can be quite informative, particularly if this information is to be fed back to the treating staff. Open-ended questions should include asking patients for suggestions about improving treatment and identifying treatment components that were particularly helpful or not helpful. It is also useful to ask if the patient thought that the treatment was worth the time and the money and if he or she would return to the hospital in question or would recommend treatment there for a relative or friend. We find it quite useful to ask how patients found out about our hospital and how they made the decision to come here. Although these kinds of questions are most useful at discharge, abbreviated portions can be repeated at follow-up, particularly the first follow-up. Change in opinions about treatment and specific components after discharge can be quite interesting.

Outcome should be multiperspective, including data from at least the patient and a significant other. This could be expanded to include other treaters and friends. Use of significant others, other treaters, and even hospital records becomes particularly important in the case of deceased patients. If deceased patients are not included in the study, the sample may be biased. Past studies have not agreed as to the direction of the bias, with some finding that deceased subjects had appeared more healthy and others finding the opposite. In any event, deceased patients should be included in the cohort to which they belonged, and every effort should be made to collect adequate data on them.

Design and Statistical Issues

Even with the best designs, and especially with designs that are not ideal, a number of statistical and design problems need to be addressed.

Power. Probably the most frequent flaw in outcome studies is that of inadequate power to detect the size of effect that might be anticipated in such studies. This problem is more salient in studies that compare groups; but even in serial assessments of the same cohort, if there is considerable attrition, the final sample size may be inadequate to detect moderate or less change. When comparison groups are contrasted, no more than a moderate effect might reasonably be anticipated.

Cohen (1962) surveyed all articles using statistical tests of hypotheses that were published in one year of the *Journal of Abnormal and Social Psychology*. There were 70 articles using 2,000 statistical tests, and the median power to detect a moderate size effect was only .48. This means that in half of those tests of significance, there was less than a fifty-fifty chance of detecting a real moderate size difference.

Bartko and colleagues (1988) suggested that any study that reports nonsignificant results should cite the power that was achieved in the tests yielding those results. Many studies report nonsignificant results and, unfortunately, interpret them as showing "no differences" when the power was inadequate to detect a real difference.

Attrition. The most prominent problem in outcome studies with sequential assessments is that of attrition. First, attrition produces a loss in power, because analyses comparing a set of subjects over time are based on only those subjects for whom data are complete.*

Second, attrition produces a lack of representativeness in the final sample. Selection biases are prone to operate, and it is not always certain in which direction the biases lie. Less healthy patients drop out of the study, but it is also

---

* There are some longitudinal designs that can handle small amounts of missing data but not the amount that often is present in such studies. Estimation of missing data often assumes randomly missing data, which is usually not the case. For dichotomous outcome data, Life Table or Survival Analysis is an appropriate univariate analysis.

possible that patients who become increasingly healthy do not want to participate in further follow-up assessments. Also, attrition destroys the randomness of initial random assignment to comparison groups.

Representativeness of the final sample should be investigated. Baseline medical records data permit those who completed the study to be contrasted with those who did not complete the study or with those who refused to participate.

Proper interpretation of nonsignificant results. Given that an outcome study had adequate power to detect at least a moderate size effect, a nonsignificant result should be interpreted as "we were unable to find evidence of a significant difference between the groups (or a significant change)." In the case of a nonsignificant statistical test, it is important to remember that the absence of evidence is not evidence of absence.

In the NIMH Treatment of Depression Collaborative Research Report (Elkin et al. 1989), the statement concerning nonsignificant results offers an excellent example of how they should be reported:

> Thus there is no evidence . . . that either of the psychotherapies was inferior to the standard reference treatment at termination of treatment on measures of depressive symptoms or general functioning. These statistical analyses do not, of course, permit the inference that the psychotherapies and the standard reference treatment were "equal" in effectiveness. However, since we had satisfactory power in these analyses for detecting large effect size differences between pairs of treatments . . . , it is unlikely that very large or important differences were missed. (p. 977)

Replication. As various studies have pointed out (Bartko et al. 1988; Nunnally 1967), many statistical methods such as multiple discriminant analysis, factor analysis, and so on use all measurement variance in the data set as though it were valid variance. Ignoring the presence of random error variance in the data may capitalize on chance and thus produce spurious results. Replication is necessary to help rule out spuriousness. There are statistical means of replication within a single study, including jackknifing (which may be applied to smaller samples) and split sample techniques (which require large samples). These techniques are usually available in standard computer program packages and should be used whenever possible.

One of the "rules" in hypothesis testing is that statistically significant findings should be replicated in at least one other sample under the same experimental conditions before confidence can be placed in their validity. For those doing ongoing follow-up studies such as the Menninger Ongoing Follow-up Project (where all patients who agree to participate are followed), when an adequate sample size has been attained, statistical analyses are run. Because follow-up is ongoing, another sample is begun. This procedure can produce, albeit over a number of years, several replication samples. If ample baseline data are collected, differences between samples can be examined and the extent of replication of findings can be ascertained.

Multivariate analysis. If outcome should be multidimensional and multiperspective—and most outcome studies do use more than one test score or rating, and often more than one respondent—the result is a multivariate design. It is important to recognize that if the design is multivariate, repeated application of univariate statistical tests is not appropriate. Repeated statistical tests, one variable at a time, produce inflated Type I error—that is, too many significant results as well as individual results that are too significant. The appropriate course is to use multivariate statistical tests. Multivariate tests do not inflate the Type I error. In addition, they take into account the intercorrelations among the outcome variables, and it is likely that outcome variables are relatively highly intercorrelated. If a "reasonable" number of variables are included in a multivariate analysis, the power is not appreciably reduced over that of univariate analysis.

Although multivariate analyses of variance that compare groups on a set of outcome variables are appearing quite frequently in outcome literature now, one difficulty seems to arise in deciding which of the variables contributed to the overall multivariate significance. The appropriate way to determine this contribution is by use of the discriminant function coefficients that are provided in standard MANOVA computer programs. Lyle Jones (1966) illustrated how this may be done. Another useful procedure is Roy-Bargmann step-down analysis, which is often provided in MANOVA computer programs. In this procedure, the order in which the variables are to be analyzed is specified. The significance for the first variable entered is computed, and then the significance for the second variable partialling out the first, for the third partialling out the first and second, and so on. This permits the investigator to test hypotheses regarding the significance of particular variables given that other variables have already been entered.

There are multivariate designs not only for comparison of groups but for testing change in one group over a series of assessments (Hotelling T^2) and for the comparison of groups with repeated measures over time (multivariate profile analysis [Morrison 1967]). Traditional univariate repeated measures of independent groups analysis of variance has among its assumptions homogeneous intercorrelations among the repeated measures, an assumption that is rarely met. Although there are corrections that are to be made to the degrees of freedom (e.g., Geisser-Greenhouse corrections; Greenhouse and Geisser 1959), a more effective procedure is multivariate profile analysis that does not assume homogeneous intercorrelations but uses the actual intercorrelations instead. Autocorrelated assessments over time, a common correlational pattern in outcome data, can be handled explicitly by this analysis.

A further complication in multivariate design is "doubly multivariate" data—data that are longitudinal (because there are assessments for more than one time point) as well as cross-sectional (because there is more than one variable assessed at each point in time). There may be independent groups being compared as well. Multivariate analysis of variance can handle these, although it is desirable to reduce the number of variables in an analysis by factor analysis or by hypotheses to make the interpretation of results less formidable.

Number of outcome variables.   Although multivariate analysis is appropriate to handle multidimensional, multiperspective designs, it is not a panacea that allows inclusion of every variable that could possibly represent outcome. As Bartko and colleagues (1988) pointed out, "it is . . . crucial that main hypotheses be defined in advance and highly selected measurement variables be used in confirmatory analysis" (p. 581). In other words, it is better to hypothesize than to hunt for significant results in a very large number of variables. Other approaches include factor analysis to reduce the number of variables for further analyses, which at the same time yields higher conceptual level variables (factors) that may permit more meaningful findings. In univariate analyses, particularly correlation matrices, the use of the Bonferroni correction is mandatory when large numbers of variables are analyzed. The Bartko paper and Grove and Andreasen (1982) provide discussion of the rationale and procedures for applying Bonferroni corrections.

Reliability training and reliability studies.   Even though an outcome study is using rating scales or other instruments with published reliability, this implies only that it is possible to obtain reliability with these instruments and does not necessarily imply that reliability will be obtained within a particular study. It is essential that the raters in an outcome study receive reliability training and demonstrate adequate reliability, and it is desirable that the actual study raters achieve reliability for the setting and instruments in question.

It is important to note that chart data are not collected with perfect reliability. In reliability studies of baseline variables collected from medical records, Canfield and colleagues (1986) showed that these are not all collected reliably and that there is considerable variability in their reliability.

The lack of equivalent comparison groups at baseline.   One of the most formidable problems for statistical analyses that contrast comparison groups on sequential assessments across time is that of significant baseline differences among the groups. Comparison of the profiles representing change requires that the groups start at nonsignificantly different levels. The most commonly used "solution" is analysis of covariance using the baseline assessment as covariate. However, analysis of covariance has among its assumptions 1) random assignment to the groups being compared and 2) homogeneity of regression between the covariate(s) and the dependent (outcome) variables among the groups. In many outcome studies, the groups being contrasted have not been randomly assigned, and in those few where random assignment was used, attrition over time has probably resulted in a lack of randomness in the groups being compared.

Also, heterogeneity of regression between the covariates and the dependent variables among the groups is a common finding. There is no ideal solution for this problem. Perhaps the best is stratification across the groups on the baseline level of the outcome variable. This requires the group sample sizes to be large enough to permit at least two strata on the baseline assessment. This procedure may force the analysis to be univariate rather than the more appropriate multivariate analysis, although in some instances stratification on the baseline level of one outcome variable may take care of significant baseline differences on other highly intercorrelated outcome variables. This is a problem that looks to new designs and statistical methodology for improved solutions in the future.

Baseline level as the best predictor of follow-up outcome. A very familiar problem in outcome studies is the "rich get richer" phenomenon. Repeatedly, studies have found that the best predictor of an outcome variable at discharge or follow-up is the baseline level of that variable. In fact, once the variance accounted for by baseline level has been removed, other predictors have very little change variance left to account for. An even more difficult situation exists when other predictor variables are intercorrelated with the baseline level of the variable in question. Although statistical techniques exist for the removal of the variance accounted for by the baseline level of a given variable, the restriction of the amount of change variance remaining for other predictors cannot be overcome by statistical methodology. The best approach is a judicious selection of relatively independent outcome variables that are also sensitive to change.

High intercorrelations among the outcome variables. Another recurring problem in outcome studies is what we called in an earlier study the "glob at follow-up." That is, after what we had hoped to be a judicious selection of important outcome variables, we found, to our disappointment, that the outcome variables at discharge, and even more so at follow-up, were highly intercorrelated and when subjected to factor analysis yielded one general factor. Thus, we lost our outcome profile and the possibility of differentiation of outcomes by means of different variables. Although this could point to global change rather than differentiated change, it more likely points to assessment problems, such as halo effect and other response sets. In a follow-up study of adolescents, we found one general factor at follow-up for the parents' assessments of 10 different outcome variables, but three quite meaningful, differentiated factors for the patients' assessments. Perhaps the amount of relevant information available to the respondent may also play a part.

Clinical significance.   Although statistical significance is an appropriate goal in outcome studies, the ultimate desire is to be able to say something beyond statistical significance. Outcome studies are conducted because of an interest in clinical outcome, and the wish is to show some clear practical difference favoring one group over another or a change in one or more groups that has clinical implications. This information is not provided by statistical significance alone. Statistical significance is a *necessary* condition for clinical significance. If statistical significance is not attained, it is not appropriate to ask about clinical significance; but if statistical significance is attained, then questions about clinical significance are of great interest. Although these questions are being pursued by statistical methodologists, as yet there is no standard procedure or measurement strategy to assess clinical significance that is uniformly used. There are several candidates (e.g., Christensen and Mendoza 1986; Jacobson and Revenstorf 1988), but none have won universal support. We can only hope that new methodology will be developed in the near future to help answer this extremely important question.

References

Allen JG: Therapeutic alliance: collaboration in hospital treatment (Copyright © 1985 The Menninger Foundation). (Scale available from The Menninger Foundation, Box 829, Topeka, KS 66601.)

American Psychiatric Association: Diagnostic and Statistical Manual of Mental Disorders, 3rd Edition. Washington, DC, American Psychiatric Association, 1980

American Psychiatric Association: Diagnostic and Statistical Manual of Mental Disorders, 3rd Edition, Revised. Washington, DC, American Psychiatric Association, 1987

Bartko JJ, Carpenter WT Jr., McGlashan TH: Statistical issues in long-term followup studies. Schizophr Bull 14:575–587, 1988

Bland RC, Parker JH, Orn H: Prognosis in schizophrenia: a ten-year followup of first admissions. Arch Gen Psychiatry 33:949–954, 1976

Bland RC, Orn H: Fourteen-year outcome in early schizophrenia. Acta Psychiatr Scand 58:327–338, 1978

Canfield M, Clarkin J, Coyne L, et al: Reliability of data taken from medical charts. The Psychiatric Hospital 17:173–179, 1986

Carpenter WT Jr., Strauss JS, Pulver AE, et al: The prediction of outcome in schizophrenia: IV. eleven-year follow-up of the Washington IPSS cohort. Unpublished manuscript, 1987

Christensen L, Mendoza JL: A method of assessing change in a single subject: an alteration of the RC index. Behavior Therapy 17:305–308, 1986

Clancy J, Tsuang MT, Norton B, et al: The Iowa 500: a comprehensive study of mania, depression and schizophrenia. The Journal of the Iowa Medical Society 64:394–398, 1974

Cohen J: The statistical power of abnormal-social psychological research: a review. Journal of Abnormal and Social Psychology 65:145–153, 1962

Dorney DC: Setting resource utilization standards in a community mental health center. Quality Review Bulletin 8:1–21, 1982

Elkin I, Shea MT, Watkins JT, et al: National Institute of Mental Health Treatment of Depression Collaborative Research Program, general effectiveness of treatments. Arch Gen Psychiatry 46:971–982, 1989

Endicott J, Spitzer RL, Fleiss JL, et al: The Global Assessment Scale: a procedure for measuring overall severity of psychiatric disturbance. Arch Gen Psychiatry 33:766–771, 1976

Gardos G, Cole JO, LaBrie RA: A twelve-year follow-up study of 124 chronic hospitalized schizophrenics: I. current psychosocial adjustment. Unpublished manuscript, 1982a

Gardos G, Cole JO, LaBrie RA: A twelve-year follow-up study of chronic schizophrenics. Hosp Community Psychiatry 33(12):983–984, 1982b

Greenhouse SW, Geisser S: On methods in the analysis of profile data. Psychometrika 24:95–112, 1959

Grob MC, Eisen SV, Berman, JS: Three years of follow-up monitoring: perspectives of formerly hospitalized patients and their families. Compr Psychiatry 19:491–499, 1978

Grove WM, Andreasen NC: Simultaneous tests of many hypotheses in exploratory research. J Nerv Ment Dis 170:3–8, 1982

Harty M, Cerney M, Colson D, et al: Correlates of change and long-term outcome: an exploratory study of intensively treated hospital patients. Bull Menninger Clin 45:209–228, 1981

Jacobson NS, Revenstorf D: Statistics for assessing the clinical significance of psychotherapy techniques: issues, problems and new developments. Behavioral Assessment 10:133–145, 1988

Jones LV: Analysis of variance in its multivariate developments, in Handbook of Multivariate Experimental Psychology. Edited by Cattell RB. Chicago, Rand McNally, 1966, pp 251–265

McGlashan TH: The Chestnut Lodge follow-up study: I. follow-up methodology and study sample. Arch Gen Psychiatry 41:573–585, 1984a

McGlashan TH: The Chestnut Lodge follow-up study: II. long-term outcome of schizophrenia and the affective disorders. Arch Gen Psychiatry 41:586–601, 1984b

McGlashan TH: A selective review of recent North American long-term followup studies of schizophrenia. Schizophr Bull 14:515–542, 1988

McGlashan TH, Carpenter WT Jr., Bartko JJ: Issues of design and methodology in long-term followup studies. Schizophr Bull 14:569–574, 1988

Morrison DF: Multivariate Statistical Methods. New York, McGraw-Hill, 1967, pp 133–153

Morrison J, Clancy J, Crowe R, et al: The Iowa 500: I. diagnostic validity in mania, depression, schizophrenia. Arch Gen Psychiatry 27:457–461, 1972

Nunnally J: Psychometric Theory. New York, McGraw Hill, 1967, pp 348–423

Overall JE, Gorham DR: The Brief Psychiatric Rating Scale. Psychol Rep 10:799–812, 1962

Plakun EM, Burkhardt PE, Muller JP: 14-year follow-up of borderline and schizotypal personality disorders. Compr Psychiatry 26:448–455, 1985

Pope HG Jr., Jonas JM, Hudson JI, et al: The validity of DSM-III borderline personality disorder: A phenomenologic, family history, treatment response, and long-term follow-up study. Arch Gen Psychiatry 40:23–30, 1983

Stephens JH: Long-term course and prognosis in schizophrenia. Seminars in Psychiatry 2:464–485, 1970

Stephens JH: Long-term prognosis and followup in schizophrenia. Schizophr Bull 4:25–47, 1978

Stephens JH, Astrup C: Prognosis in "process" and "nonprocess" schizophrenia. Am J Psychiatry 119:945–953, 1963

Stephens JH, Astrup C: Treatment of outcome in "process" and "nonprocess" schizophrenics treated by "A" and "B" types of therapists. J Nerv Mental Dis 140:449–456, 1965

Strauss JS, Carpenter WT Jr.: The prediction of outcome in schizophrenia: I. characteristics of outcome. Arch Gen Psychiatry 27:739–746, 1972

Strauss JS, Carpenter WT Jr.: The prediction of outcome in schizophrenia: II. relationships between predictor and outcome variables: a report from the WHO international pilot study of schizophrenia. Arch Gen Psychiatry 31:37–42, 1974

Tsuang MT, Winokur G: The Iowa 500: Field work in a 35-year follow-up of depression, mania, and schizophrenia. Canadian Psychiatric Association Journal 20:359–365, 1975

Tsuang MT, Woolson RF, Fleming JA: Long-term outcome of major psychoses: I. schizophrenia and affective disorders compared with psychiatrically symptom-free surgical conditions. Arch Gen Psychiatry 39:1295–1301, 1979

Vaillant GE: A 10-year followup of remitting schizophrenics. Schizophr Bull 4:78–85, 1978

❖ 15 ❖

Design for a
Quasi-Experimental Study to Test
Length of Stay Prediction Hypotheses

Herbert E. Spohn, Ph.D.
Lolafaye Coyne, Ph.D.

In this chapter, we will be describing the design and methodology of an ongoing multihospital collaborative study aimed at assessing required length of psychiatric hospital treatment. We think this chapter will be of special interest because, within the practical and ethical constraints on the design of prospective studies in private hospital settings, our design is quasi-experimental in nature. That is, absent the freedom to employ random assignment to differing length of stay conditions, we have nonetheless been able to control for factors other than actual length of stay, the independent variable that might influence outcome.

The core of this chapter is devoted to a description of the quasi-experimental design. Additionally, we will deal with problems encountered in establishing satisfactory levels of interrater reliability levels on outcome measures, and also with problems in developing length of stay predictions that are to be derived from ratings on 15 predictor variables based on information available at admission to hospitalization.

Design

As we have already noted, this is a prospective study designed to test hypotheses concerning predicted optimal length of stay versus actual length of stay in terms of outcome during and after hospitalization; hence, major dimensions are actual length of stay and predicted optimal length of stay. For both of these, length of

Among those whose contributions have been of particular importance to the planning of this project at Harding Hospital are George Harding, M.D., Richard Griffin, M.D., and especially Anne Logue, M.A., Project Director. The contributions at the Menninger Hospital of Jon Allen, Ph.D., Donald Colson, Ph.D., and Glen O. Gabbard, M.D., are reflected in their publications cited in the text of this chapter.

stay is categorized into three levels: short-term (up to 5 weeks), intermediate-term (5 weeks to 8 months), and long-term (more than 8 months).

In previous length of stay studies, patients have been randomly assigned to the (actual) length of stay levels (see Glick et al. 1975; Mattes et al. 1977). We chose not to do this for several reasons. First, for both practical and ethical reasons, we cannot randomly assign patients at a private psychiatric hospital to different length of stay conditions. Secondly, we believe that treaters who are assigned to a particular length of stay condition for an experimental study may find these conditions uncongenial to their own convictions concerning the length of treatment optimum for a particular patient. We believe random assignment in this case would represent an experimental imposition that could result in treatment associated with a particular length of stay—one that is not necessarily the treatment that would have been received under *actual* treatment conditions. A consequence of this might be that the "experimental" treatment would not be administered with full conviction on the part of treaters. Thus, in order to make this study possible and to make generalizability to *actual* treatment conditions more likely, we were forced to develop a design that did not require random assignment but would be rigorous enough to be considered a quasi-experimental design.

That design is a collaborative design. It required the participation of private psychiatric hospitals dedicated primarily to short-term (or possibly intermediate-term) treatment and others dedicated to long-term (or possibly intermediate-term) treatment. In order to increase the reliability and generalizability of our findings, we wanted to have enough collaborators to replicate both short-term and long-term as well as intermediate-term stays in several hospitals. However, a number of practical considerations restricted us to one collaborator, Harding Hospital, which is replicating primarily short-term and intermediate-term cells; our own institution has units replicating all three length of stay cells. It will be evident from this that the one unreplicated cell is long-term treatment. We recognize that this fact places limitations on generalizability.

An additional advantage of this collaborative design is the increased ability to obtain the necessary numbers of subjects for the various cells required in the design in a shorter period of time. Additionally, of course, our collaborative design ensures that each patient gets the treatment of choice by a motivated treater.

In the selection of collaborating hospitals, selecting both long-term and short-term hospitals differing in treatment philosophy and treatment programs would have made it possible to examine the interactions of treatment philosophy and treatment program with actual and predicted optimal length of stay. However, quite aside from the practical problems in recruiting collaborators, the implication of two more factors, added to the design for the number of subjects required to complete the study in a timely fashion, made this interesting but not feasible.

In order that the quasi-experimental design using collaborating hospitals yields findings that are sufficiently close to those that would be obtained by random assignment to the various length of stay categories, it is either necessary that the outcome for patients in the various length of stay cells differ only in length of stay and not because of differences in treatment philosophy, treatment programs, and patient population, or it is necessary to systematically vary and assess differences in these potentially confounding factors. Because it was not possible to systematically vary treatment philosophy and treatment programs, we needed to control for these in other ways. (How patient populations were handled will be discussed later in this chapter.) For treatment philosophy, we selected a collaborating hospital with a psychodynamic orientation similar to that of our own institution. The two collaborating institutions refer patients among themselves and have comparable treatment philosophies, although treatment programs may differ to some extent.

We deal with differences in treatment programs by documenting the treatment received by each of the patients participating in the study. Toward this goal, Colson and associates (1988) developed a set of Treatment Variables that are rated by the primary treater and the primary nurse periodically over the course of hospitalization. These Treatment Variables include six example-anchored scales representing more general dimensions of treatment, and a number of individual items assessing the treatment emphasis for each patient. In addition, the researchers developed a set of Family Treatment Variables describing the work with the family (Colson et al. 1990). These scales comprise 12 example-anchored scales that are rated by the primary treater and the patient's social worker periodically during the hospitalization.

Finally, if our assumptions regarding the similarity of treatment philosophy are found not to have been met and the documentation of treatment provided reveals more differences among hospitals than expected, the statistical analysis will, in part, control for these differences. In the statistical analysis (to be described in more detail later), differences among hospitals in mean level on the various outcome measures will be removed from the error terms. Thus, variation in outcome due to hospital differences alone will not penalize our testing of the hypotheses pertaining to length of stay.

The second major dimension is that of predicted optimal length of stay. At admission, a patient will be predicted to be most suitable for short-term, intermediate-term, or long-term length of stay using statistical and clinical procedures. These prediction procedures will be described in more detail in a later section.

Our hypotheses are that those patients for whom short-term treatment is predicted as optimal who receive actual short-term treatment, those for whom intermediate-term treatment is predicted who receive intermediate-term treatment, and those for whom long-term treatment is predicted who receive long-term treatment will have better outcomes than those in other predicted/actual length of stay combinations. That is, we predict that the patients in the diagonal cells of the predicted/actual length of stay matrix will have better outcomes than those of the patients in the off-diagonal cells. Perhaps another way of describing this outcome "matrix" is that when predicted and actual length of stay are congruent, outcome will be better than when predicted and actual treatment received are incongruent.

Obviously, outcome is the basis for testing these hypotheses. We assess outcome at five times: a baseline assessment at admission, once during the course of treatment at 4 weeks post-admission, at discharge whenever that occurs, at 1 year post-discharge, and finally at 18 months post-admission. Together with the baseline admission assessment and the 4 weeks assessment, this latter assessment point will provide comparisons at constant time periods for all patients. The 18 months post-admission assessment is a particularly interesting one for comparison of outcomes for the various actual length of stay cells. For short-term patients, this will be not quite 17 months after their discharge; for intermediate-term patients, 10 months after their discharge; and for long-term patients, possibly only a few months after discharge—or even before discharge. With these five assessment points, we have added a repeated measures factor with five levels to our design.

A key feature of our design is the prediction procedure. We developed and selected a set of scales to assess predictor variables from pre-admission and admission data. These variables were chosen from clinical experience, from a review of the "length of stay" literature, and from a survey conducted with a large sample of clinicians from the Menninger Adult Hospital and Harding Hospital (Allen et al. 1988). In this survey, each clinician was asked to write vignettes describing three patients each for whom short-term, intermediate-term, or long-term hospitalization (as defined in this study) would be optimal.

A striking amount of concordance was found among the variables selected by these three different methods. The first variable, which serves as a contextual variable, is that of diagnosis. Given a diagnosis of schizophrenia, affective disorder, or personality disorder, various combinations of the remaining predictor variables come into play in making the prediction of optimal length of stay. That is, similar profiles of ratings on the predictor variables may lead to differing predictions of optimum length of stay, depending on diagnosis. These predictor variables include usefully employed, personal-social relations, heterosexual relations, highest level of premorbid adaptive functioning, psychosocial stressors, physically destructive behavior, patient alliance/motivation, family role, prior medication response and hospital response, age, sex, number of previous hospitalizations, and treatment status at admission.

In order to make the prediction of length of stay for a particular patient an objective and repeatable method by other clinicians in different hospitals, one of the authors developed the following procedure. All of the predictor variables listed in the last paragraph are assessed on a large and representative sample of discharged patients from the collaborating hospitals. These data are then used to cluster the patients belonging to each diagnostic category into homogeneous groups, groups whose members are similar to each other on the predictor variables. These groups, represented by a mean profile as well as individual case vignettes, will constitute empirical clinical prototypes.

Our initial plan had been to apply a set of criteria or indications for short-, intermediate-, and long-term treatment (Allen et al. 1988) on the basis of the survey of clinicians at the Harding and Menninger hospitals to three sets of cluster analysis-derived clinical prototypes—one set each for schizophrenia, affective disorder, and personality disorder. In this fashion, we hoped to arrive at a set of profiles for which differing length of optimum stay had been predicted. Patients in the study proper are to be classified by statistical procedures into the appropriate empirical clinical prototype, and their length of stay would be determined by the prediction for that prototype made according to joint decision rules.

These clinical prototypes obtained by clustering have important design advantages. First, they are more stable and less idiosyncratic than any individual patient's profile on the predictor variables. Secondly, the fact that patients from different hospitals fall in the same clusters (clinical prototypes) provides evidence of comparability of hospital populations across the collaborating hospitals. This in turn provides the control for the possible patient population difference among hospitals needed for our quasi-experimental design. Finally, clustering of patients within predicted length of stay levels provides a kind of stratification on a set of severity and other *control* variables that could be construed to influence outcome independently of length of stay. It is primarily this procedure that substitutes for random assignment as a means for controlling for confounding variables and constitutes the design as quasi-experimental.

In a later section of this chapter, we will give attention to some of the problems we encountered in arriving at prediction hypotheses by the previously described procedure and how these problems are being solved. However, it should be clear that our revised procedure does not depart substantially from the originally planned procedure and thus has no bearing on the design advantages gained by deriving clinical prototypes by means of clustering.

Thus, we have developed a design with three independent factors, two of crucial importance to the testing hypotheses—Predicted Optimal Length of Stay and Actual Length of Stay—and a nested control factor, Hospital, together with one repeated measures factor, Time of Assessment. Because we have multiple outcome measures (which we will describe later), the statistical analysis will be a multivariate profile analysis that includes subsets of outcome variables in each analysis. The variance component of interest is predicted length of stay (LOS) interacting with actual length of stay and time of assessment (Predicted LOS x Actual LOS x Time). Particular contrasts with the time of assessment factor will be utilized to track differences among length of stay cells across time. The Hospital factor and its interactions with all other factors will not be tested for significance, because the purpose of introducing this factor was to control for hospital differences on outcome and not to compare hospitals.

Outcome Measures and Reliability

The specific nature of our outcome measures plays a critical role in this design, because we will be testing the validity of length of stay hypotheses by predicting differential outcome depending on congruence or incongruence of actual length of stay assignment with hypothetically optimal length of stay assignment. This fact imposed a critical constraint on the selection of outcome measures. In terms of change from admission to discharge and from discharge to follow-up, the outcome measures had to be coordinated with the goals of treatment. To achieve this methodologically important objective, we made selections among a plethora of standard outcome measures. We chose as our two major outcome instruments the Bellak Ego Functions Scales (Bellak et al. 1973) and the Brief Psychiatric Rating Scale (BPRS; Overall and Gorham 1962). As already noted, both hospitals share in a psychodynamic orientation and aim at achieving some degree of personality change. Hence, the Bellak scales were ideally suited to our design. Of course, symptomatic change is also a major goal of treatment at the two hospitals. Hence, we chose the BPRS which, like the Bellak scales, has the virtue of being sensitive to change and of enjoying wide-ranging acceptance in the field as a standard symptom rating scale.

Our thinking about goals and outcome measures went beyond the choice of instruments. We recognized that we needed to define operationally what constituted "optimal hospital treatment benefits." We recognized that hospital treatment at the two hospitals did not aim at "cure." Rather, the goals of treatment are to achieve sufficient gains at discharge so that they could be sustained and enhanced with appropriate post-hospital treatment and environmental support and that with combined hospital and post-hospital adjunctive treatment, the risk of rehospitalization would be substantially reduced. This became our definition of optimal benefits.

In addition to the Bellak scales and the BPRS, we are employing a number of other outcome measures in accordance with the well-established principle in treatment evaluation research that outcome is likely to be multifaceted and that lack of gains in one area may be offset by a positive change in another. Important among these other instruments are scales rated at 1-year follow-up to assess the quality of community adjustment, as well as several self-report measures. Frequency and length of rehospitalization also serve as outcome measures.

Now let us consider the most important aspect of outcome measurement, namely interrater reliability, and dramatize its importance with an example. We know from past experience with the Bellak Ego Functions Scales that expectable change in most of these scales was generally no greater than one scale point. Unless we were able to achieve a very high degree of interrater reliability on the Bellak scales, so small a "true" change might easily be obscured by measurement error.

Our method of achieving a high degree of interrater reliability entailed the following. To begin with, we had determined that we would employ only experienced clinician-raters with a minimum advanced degree at the masters level. We evolved a semistructured interview administered to patients to generate the verbal behavioral data on which ratings could be based. We made a series of videotapes of interviews with consenting psychiatric patients conducted by experienced clinicians. These videotaped interviews were rated in a series of group sessions involving clinician raters at both hospitals. At these sessions, divergence in ratings among raters was discussed until consensus was reached. Conventions to resolve particularly ambiguous patient behavior or response to interview questions were developed and became a part of a rating manual. This procedure was followed by a formal reliability study involving the rating of a series of new videotapes. The results of these studies were analyzed by means of intraclass correlations. We made a number of noteworthy discoveries in this process.

Most important of all, reliability on all of our scales was never sufficiently great to permit the use of only a single rater. All our scales are now rated independently by two raters who reconcile differences by consensus in order to reduce measurement error to levels lower than "true" change values.

One of the surprises we encountered in reliability training was that clinicians more readily achieved agreement on rating scales such as the Bellak Ego Functions Scales, which are defined in broad conceptual terms, than on symptom rating scales such as the BPRS, which are defined in behavioral terms. It soon became apparent that level differences in rating subscales such as "conceptual disorganization" or "motor retardation" among clinician raters were a significant part to the problem. Level differences occur when two clinician raters disagree on the severity level of psychopathology manifested by a given patient. We discovered that underlying this phenomenon were normative parameters among clinicians based on differences in the patient-experience base of the rater. A clinician on a hospital unit with very severely ill patients was likely to rate lower than a clinician on a unit with less severely disturbed patients. We succeeded in alleviating this problem by developing example-anchored scale point definitions (Gabbard et al. 1987), which provided a detailed behavioral description of severity levels.

Optimal Length of Stay Prediction Hypotheses

Previously in this chapter, we hinted that our initial plans to develop prediction hypotheses had encountered some difficulties. We give attention to the nature of these difficulties and to ways in which we have learned to cope with them because we think this may be of interest to others involved in similar efforts, and, perhaps more importantly, because our discoveries make explicit the often intuitive process whereby clinicians arrive at prognostic judgments with respect to length of stay.

As we began to apply the length of stay criteria developed by Allen and colleagues (1988) to the Harding-Menninger clusters, based on similarities in ratings on the 15 predictor variables (i.e., the empirical clinical prototypes), four problems quickly became apparent.

1. Our assumption that the 15 predictor variables would be equivalent turned out to be invalid. Judges gave differential weight to ratings on different variables (e.g., prior response to medication loomed larger than frequency of destructive behavior in making LOS prediction decisions).
2. The criteria for differing length of stay took insufficient account of the level of psychological resources and strengths that patients manifested at admission. On the other hand, judges attempting to apply these criteria imputed considerable importance to this variable.
3. We had paid too little attention to the quality and extent of the social support network available to patients on discharge. Our judges assigned considerable importance to this matter. That is, the presence or absence of a social support network to which the patient could return figured significantly in making optimal length of stay decisions.
4. It had been a given throughout all of our planning that length of stay predictions should be based only on information available at admission. That is, what we were striving toward was a prediction procedure that, if validated, would make it possible very early in the course of hospitaliza-

tion to assign an optimal length of stay. However, what we discovered was that there was considerable variability across patients in the amount of information available for rating on the 15 predictor variables. As a result, not only was there critical information missing in some cases, but the clusters themselves were also to some extent shaped by this fact.

We are now in the process of revising the procedure by which prediction hypotheses will be arrived at in light of the identification of the problems noted here. To begin with, we will rerate the predictor variables on the basis of the full information pertinent to each of the variables. Missing information will be extracted from clinical charts that provide information obtained in the course of treatment, and, particularly, from a diagnostic conference that takes place sometime after admission. We will, however, use only information that cannot be construed to have been conditioned by the treatment process itself. In obtaining data from these sources, we will give a high priority to information about the social support network available to the patient at discharge as well as to strengths and psychological resources that patients bring to treatment.

With this expanded information base in hand, we will recluster on the 15 predictor variables but with differential weights assigned to predictor variable—weights that will reflect clinician judgment-based priorities assigned to different variables in terms of the relative relevance to predicting optimum length of stay. It will be to the new clusters that three senior clinicians from the Harding and the Menninger Hospital will assign optimum length of stay "ratings" employing a decision tree procedure. Individual patients in the study proper will be assigned optimum length of stay predictions corresponding to the cluster into which their predictor variable profile best fits.

It may have become apparent to the reader that in the development of methodology and procedure of the present design, we have very largely been guided by clinical judgment. Notwithstanding that this has posed a number of problems for us—the solutions of which the feasibility of this project is dependent on—we believe that this process has greatly strengthened the project. We say this because by forcing clinicians, in effect, to make explicit the criteria on which they rated patient behavior and verbalizations in the reliability studies, and by sensitizing ourselves to underlying assumptions that clinicians use to make prognostic judgments, we have been able to devise operations that objectify this process. This has permitted a meaningful test of what for all of the clinicians involved are state-of-the-art hypotheses about what characteristics of patients suit them to what length of psychiatric hospital treatment.

Current State of the Project

As we noted at the beginning of this chapter, data gathering at both hospitals has been under way for some time. Because our original intent was to test prediction hypotheses concerning the total patient population of patients accepted for treatment in both hospitals, our only exclusion criterion is to patients with an IQ of less than 70. Upon completion of the prediction procedures, we will be in a position to determine roughly how many more patients must be entered into the research so that we may perform meaningful statistical analyses. It will be obvious from the foregoing that data analysis can begin only when there are adequate and approximately equal numbers of cases in all nine cells of the design.

This brings us to our final point in this chapter. Implementing the design we have described and bringing the project to successful completion is a time-consuming process and one that is fraught with unforeseen problems. We have been fortunate in the support that the leadership of both hospitals has been willing to afford us. However, our results certainly could make a difference in the future course of private psychiatric hospital treatment. Therefore, it is not altogether surprising that the leadership of our two hospitals is impatient with our necessarily slow progress toward completion of the project.

References

Allen J, Scovern A, Logue A, et al: Indications for extended psychiatric hospitalization: a study of clinical opinion. Compr Psychiatry 29:604–612, 1988

Bellak L, Hurvich M, Gediman, HK: Ego Functions in Schizophrenics, Neurotics and Normals. New York, John Wiley, 1973

Colson D, Coyne L, Pollack W: Scales to assess the emphasis of psychiatric hospital treatment. Psychiatry 51:281–290, 1988

Colson D, Grame C, Coyne L: Scales to assess the emphasis of family intervention accompanying psychiatric hospitalization. Bull Menninger Clin 54:368–383, 1990

Gabbard GO, Kennedy LL, Coyne L, et al: Interrater reliability in the use of the Brief Psychiatric Rating Scale. Bull Menninger Clin 51:519–531, 1987

Glick ID, Hargreaves WA, Raskin M, et al: Short versus long hospitalization: a prospective controlled study, II: results for schizophrenic inpatients. Am J Psychiatry 132:385–390, 1975

Mattes JA, Rosen B, Klein DF: Comparison of the clinical effectiveness of "short" versus "long" stay psychiatric hospitalization, II: results of a three-year posthospital follow-up. J Nerv Ment Dis 165:387–394, 1977

Overall JE, Gorham DR: The Brief Psychiatric Rating Scale. Psychol Rep 10:799–812, 1962

❖ 16 ❖ Quality Assurance and Treatment Outcome: A Medical Perspective

Benjamin Liptzin, M.D.

Introduction

In recent years, increasing attention has been paid to issues of accountability in health care generally, including mental health care. This is partly because of the rapidly rising costs of health care, with prices for hospital and medical services rising faster than other consumer prices and with health care expenditures accounting for an increasing share of the Gross National Product of the United States. This has led to a variety of attempts to slow down these increases by changing the reimbursement system: the use of prospective payments by diagnosis to hospitals (DRGs); a Resource Based Relative Value Scale for physician's fees; and the restructuring of the care delivery system using health maintenance organizations (HMOs) and preferred provider organizations (PPOs). These attempts to reduce costs have in turn raised questions about the effects on patients and providers (Clifford 1989; Liptzin 1989), including questions as to the quality of care provided. In response, professional review organizations (PROs), which are federally funded to review the care of Medicare patients, now focus more on quality concerns and less on controlling utilization than their predecessors, professional standards review organizations (PSROs). A recent Institute of Medicine committee has recommended that PROs be explicitly refocused as "Medicare Quality Review Organizations" (Lohr and Schroeder 1990).

The emphasis on quality of care is also stimulated by the rapidly rising costs of professional liability insurance and the publicity given to multimillion-dollar damage awards. Attorneys argue that the tort liability system is an essential mechanism for monitoring the quality of care and providing compensation for the victims of substandard or negligent care. Physicians argue that the present

The author thanks Mayree Libby and Helen Tavares for their review and comments on this paper.

tort system leads to the practice of defensive medicine, punishes good doctors for bad outcomes rather than bad care, and does not equitably compensate those who have suffered bad outcomes. The development of practice guidelines by medical specialty organizations is one attempt to try to improve the quality of care and reduce the number of malpractice lawsuits. Quality assurance activities in hospitals are also closely tied to risk management and risk reduction programs.

One final impetus to a focus on quality is the general societal demand for more accountability and less automatic trust in the competence of institutions, whether they are governmental, religious, or professional. This has led to consumer demands for more information about the risks and benefits of treatment and expanded legal requirements for informed consent by patients prior to treatment. In addition, more attention is being paid to patient satisfaction with care and not just the technical outcome of care. Society has changed a great deal from the days when the television star of "Father Knows Best" was transformed into the caring and competent "Doctor Knows Best" of "Marcus Welby, M.D." Physicians have to justify and explain everything they do.

What is Quality?

With all the emphasis on quality of care, how is it defined and measured? The *Joint Commission Guide to Quality Assurance* suggests that different parties may have different views of quality (Fromberg 1988). Consumers value responsiveness to perceived care needs; level of communication, concern, and courtesy; degree of symptom relief; and level of functional improvement. Practitioners value the degree to which care meets the current technical state of the art and the freedom to act in the full interest of the patient. Purchasers of health care value the efficient use of funds, the appropriate use of health care resources, and the maximum possible contribution of health care to reduction in lost productivity.

Another definition comes from the Council on Medical Service of the American Medical Association, which characterized care of high quality as that which consistently contributes to the maintenance or improvement of health and well being (Council on Medical Service 1988). Their report goes on to explain:

> This definition recognizes that, when other variables which could affect outcome—such as patient age, sex, living environment, attitude toward illness, health history, severity of illness, and natural history of the disease—are adequately measured and accounted for, patient outcome reflects the degree of effectiveness with which health professionals combine their own skill and compassion with the use of technology for the patient's benefit. It encompasses both

the effects of care on the patient and the proficiency with which such care is provided. Also implicit in the definition is the need to develop more meaningful criteria as to what constitutes a "favorable" outcome. (pp. 2–3)

They point out that other essential elements characterize care of high quality:

Such care should:
- Emphasize health promotion, disease and disability prevention, and early detection and treatment.
- Be provided in a timely manner, without inappropriate delay, interruption, premature termination or prolongation of treatment.
- Seek the patient's cooperation and participation in the decisions and process of his/her treatment.
- Be based on accepted principles of medical science, and the skillful and appropriate use of other health professionals and technology.
- Be provided with sensitivity to the stress and anxiety that illness can cause, and with concern for the patient's and family's overall welfare.
- Use technology and other resources efficiently to achieve the treatment goal.
- Be sufficiently documented in the patient's medical record to allow continuity of care and peer evaluation. (p. 3)

Clearly, any attempt to measure or improve the quality of care must take into account the outcomes of care. Other papers cited herein describe methodologies for measuring treatment outcome from different perspectives and summarize the results of treatment outcome studies for different age and diagnostic groupings. In this chapter, I will describe psychiatric quality assurance activities with a special emphasis on psychiatric hospitals. This will include attention to the outcomes of care as well as the process by which care is delivered. The perspective here is a medical one; Chapter 17 provides a nursing perspective.

Psychiatric Quality Assurance Activities

In an earlier paper (Liptzin 1974), I suggested that peer review in psychiatry would be difficult because of inadequate records, lack of agreement on diagnosis, wide variations in criteria for hospitalization and discharge, the complex nature of the psychotherapy treatment process, and problems in fitting all mental health care to the "medical model." Since that time, a great deal of work has been done in psychiatric peer review, some of which is summarized in Hamilton (1985). Other recent reviews of quality assurance in mental health include Mattson (1984), Stricker and Rodriguez (1988), Zusman (1988), and Fauman (1989).

One result of the increased scrutiny of psychiatric care is a heightened awareness of the importance of the written record in carefully documenting the care provided to patients. Van Vort and Mattson (1989) suggested that clinicians need to ensure that records are clinically pertinent and useful for communication rather than just as a legal document to satisfy requirements for accountability.

Another approach to improving documentation was the development of a multidisciplinary treatment-planning form at the New York Hospital, Westchester Division (Munich 1990) with a system for monitoring charts (Munich et al. 1990). This form was specifically developed for seriously and persistently ill patients who require more than a minimal hospital stay. According to Munich, the form helps to integrate treatment planning and to communicate more clearly, and it provides a more complete current picture of the patient's status and treatment for use by clinicians and outside reviewers.

Much of the emphasis on improved documentation comes from the demands of managed care reviewers who insist on evidence that hospitalization is necessary, that active treatment is going on, and that there is active discharge planning. Prunier and Buongiorno (1989) suggested standard criteria for admission to acute inpatient psychiatric facilities: "1) Imminent danger to oneself or others, 2) Symptoms of sufficient severity to acutely impair one's activities of daily life (ADLs), 3) Impulsive or assaultive behavior, and 4) Impending delirium tremens and/or management of other withdrawal states" (p. 279). They also suggest that the criteria for continued stay include severity of illness and intensity of treatment required. Melnick and Lyter (1987) have pointed out that the increase in concurrent review of psychiatric inpatient care has led to an expansion of hospital utilization review and quality assurance departments, greater nonclinical demands on physicians, and interruptions or uncertainty about ongoing treatment. Sederer (1987) has suggested that professionals need to understand the basic elements of utilization review, quality assurance, and peer review in order to cope with current trends. Phillips (1989) has offered guidelines for the peer review of chemical dependence treatment.

As noted previously, medical specialty organizations are in the process of developing practice guidelines. Often these are developed by "experts," but to be useful they must also reflect the views of practitioners. There was a firestorm of protest when the American Psychiatric Association first proposed developing a manual of "Treatments of Psychiatric Disorders" (American Psychiatric Association 1989). It was critical that this manual allow for wide variations in treatment and not be prescriptive.

Another approach to treatment guidelines involves surveys of practicing psychiatrists. As part of a quality assurance project, a random sample of Australian psychiatrists was asked their views on the treatment of depression (Armstrong and Andrews 1986) and of schizophrenia (Andrews et al. 1986).

Quality Assurance Activities in Psychiatric Hospitals

Although most quality assurance programs look at particular patient groups or treatments, some include a program evaluation component. For example, Collins and colleagues (1984) studied the ward characteristics of effective psychiatric programs within the Veterans Administration (VA). They found that wards that performed best on measures of patient post-hospital adjustment were characterized by the following: staff who perceived less order and organization on the ward; nursing staffs with fewer shift rotations; fewer socially passive patients; more neurotic patients who were not on antipsychotic drugs at discharge; and use of lower dosages of the minor tranquilizers. Other types of program outcome studies have been summarized in the Collins article.

Another approach to quality assurance involves the review of patient incidents. Way and colleagues (1985) described the development of an efficient inpatient incident reporting system for the psychiatric centers operated by the New York State Office of Mental Health. They implemented a two-tiered incident system with abbreviated reporting requirements for minor incidents but full documentation, investigation, and review of serious incidents. They found that paperwork was significantly reduced despite a net increase in the total number of incidents reported. Staff were enthusiastic about the changes and thought the new procedures made it easier to discover incident trends and to identify and correct problems.

A problem identified by the New York State Commission on Quality of Care for the Mentally Disabled was that of patient idleness (Sundram 1987). Sundram recommended that state psychiatric centers make efforts to maintain a rhythm of normal life and to avoid letting patients get used to routines of idleness and lethargy. He also proposed that increasing the level of activities and programs might serve to reduce patient abuse and patient assault. Another study looked at incidents of disruptive patient behavior at the VA Medical Center in Hampton, Virginia (Eisenberg and Tierney 1985). The researchers identified patterns of disruptive behavior and made recommendations for preventing the problems.

A specific example of a serious patient incident is that of suicidal behavior. Kibbee (1988) compared two groups of patients admitted to the Brattleboro Retreat who were identified as potentially suicidal on admission. Patients who were placed on suicidal precautions had careful assessments of suicidal ideation in their charts; patients not placed on precautions did not have adequate documentation. A better system for monitoring the care of suicidal patients was subsequently developed. Clements and colleagues (1985) at the University of Rochester reviewed clinical information on nine patients who committed suicide. A suicide prevention task force was formed that made recommendations concerning patient transfers, family therapy, discharge planning, and use of direct markers for assessing suicide risk.

Monitoring of psychotropic drug therapy has been reported from a number of institutions. Cole and Katz (1988) described the drug monitoring done at McLean Hospital and pointed out that there would be needless logistical difficulties and expense unless the pharmacy was computerized. At the Erie County Medical Center, Molnar and Feeney (1985) developed a computer-assisted review process once medication records were abstracted from the patient records. This system made better use of the physician-reviewer's time and provided useful feedback to clinicians on their prescribing practices. Craig and Mehta (1984) described an automated drug exception review system at Rockland Psychiatric Center. Approximately 25% of all new exceptions pointed out to the clinician by the computer resulted in a change in the order by the physician. Van Vort (1988) has suggested that there may be ethical problems raised by reviewing and restricting the use of drugs in the hospital formulary.

Accreditation of Psychiatric Facilities and Quality Assurance

The development of quality assurance programs in psychiatric hospitals is largely the result of standards developed by the Joint Commission on Accreditation of Healthcare Organizations (JCAHO). The JCAHO is a private, nonprofit organization that has been developing standards, surveying hospitals and other health care organizations that voluntarily request a survey, and providing feedback on deficiencies since 1951. It was established by the American College of Surgeons, the American College of Physicians, the American Hospital Association, the American Medical Association, and the Canadian Medical Association as an outgrowth of a voluntary survey program developed by the American College of Surgeons to improve the quality of care in hospitals.

Though still voluntary, the accreditation process took on extra importance after the passage of Medicare and Medicaid legislation in the 1960s. Hospitals that were accredited by the Joint Commission enjoyed "deemed status" and were automatically eligible for reimbursement under these two major payment programs. Nonaccredited hospitals could still apply for eligibility but had to undergo a survey by a state agency and were not likely to be approved. Gaver (1982) stressed the importance of being familiar with accreditation standards because of the financial implications of accreditation and its reflection on the quality of patient care provided at the institution. Coleman and Kirven (1990) emphasized the medical staff's role in quality assurance activities in the Joint Commission standards.

The survey process is not without controversy. Houck (1984) pointed out that standards are rarely subjected to rigorous testing either for efficacy or for cost-effectiveness. Furthermore, the regulatory process is often expensive, inconsistent between agencies, and may create demands for excessive documentation. Barter (1988) suggested that surveys are "nitpicking excursions to control costs" (p. 707). Lieberman and Astrachan (1984) reviewed the history of accreditation of hospital-based psychiatric services and emphasized the importance of mental health professionals taking an active role in shaping the standards of care.

Over the years, these standards have been constantly revised to reflect new approaches to quality assessment. Originally the standards addressed the capacity of the hospital to provide quality care by looking at structural issues, such as the existence of an organized medical staff consisting of licensed physicians and the availability of diagnostic and therapeutic facilities. Standards were then developed for the processes of care, including the content of medical records, pharmacy procedures, and so forth. The quality of care was to be reviewed by the hospital through various committees, including those for tissue review, medical records review, and review of staff credentials.

Different approaches to quality assurance were incorporated into the Joint Commission standards over the years. Revised standards put forth in 1985 emphasized "systematic monitoring and evaluation of important aspects of patient care and service" and not just the previous problem-focused approach. A 10-step monitoring and evaluation process was developed by the Joint Commission:

1. Assign responsibility for the specific duties related to monitoring and evaluation.
2. Delineate scope of care or inventory of clinical activities.
3. Identify important aspects of care which are high-risk, high-volume, and/or problem prone.
4. Identify indicators which are objective and well-defined measurable variables related to the structure, process, or outcome of each important aspect of care.
5. Establish thresholds for evaluation of each indicator, that is, the level at which intensive evaluation is triggered.
6. Collect and organize data pertaining to the indicators.
7. Evaluate care when the threshold is reached to determine whether a problem exists.
8. Take actions to solve problems that are identified.
9. Assess the actions and document improvement.
10. Communicate relevant information to the organization-wide quality assurance program.

Although these steps seem straightforward, many hospitals—including psychiatric hospitals—have had difficulty developing useful clinical indicators. The Joint Commission has established national task forces with the charge of developing clinical indicators in different medical specialties. It is unclear when useful indicators for psychiatric care will be developed as part of that process. In the next section of this chapter, I will discuss the indicators developed at McLean Hospital as part of its overall quality assurance program.

McLean Hospital Quality Assurance Program

McLean Hospital is a 328-bed private, nonprofit psychiatric hospital in Belmont, Massachusetts. McLean was founded in 1811 as the psychiatric asylum for the Massachusetts General Hospital and is a major teaching and research center for Harvard Medical School. The hospital treats patients of all ages and with all types of psychiatric disorders, using the full range of therapeutic modalities in inpatient, outpatient, and residential settings.

The Quality Assurance Department is directed by a nurse with extensive experience in quality assurance, utilization review, and risk management. The coordinator of quality assurance is also a nurse with extensive clinical and supervisory experience, as well as survey and teaching experience for the JCAHO. The utilization review coordinators are nurses with clinical experience who identify problems in the quality of care and flag cases for review by physician advisers.

In 1989, all quality assurance activities at McLean were consolidated under an Assistant General Director of the hospital who had a long-standing academic and professional interest in quality assurance. This gave the program high visibility and involvement in the senior management decision making at the hospital. The organizational placement assured that information about quality of care issues are considered when important programmatic decisions are being discussed. Furthermore, information from quality assurance activities are brought to the attention of the Credentials Committee, whose meetings the Assistant General Director attends.

All hospital quality assurance activities report to an interdisciplinary Patient Care Assessment Committee (PCAC). Particular quality assurance functions are carried out by staff and reported to specific committees, including the Utilization Review, Credentials, Medical Records, Pharmacy, Infection Control, Emergency Medical Care, and Safety Committees. Individual clinical departments (Psychiatry, Psychology, Social Work, Nursing, Rehabilitation Services, Internal Medicine, and Neurology) and clinical services (Ambulatory, Alcohol and Drug Treatment, Child and Adolescent, and Community Residential and Treatment

Services) have their own individual quality assurance committees. Service departments, such as Dietary and Pharmacy, also have their own quality assurance committees. Medical staff monitoring and evaluation consists of Departmental Review conducted by individual departments and services reporting to the PCAC, Medical Records Review including clinical pertinence conducted by the Medical Records Committee, Drug Usage Evaluation, and Pharmacy and Therapeutics Review. The latter two functions are carried out by the Pharmacy Committee in collaboration with the Department of Psychiatry Quality Assurance Committee. All the above activities are summarized annually in a report to the Board of Trustees, who have the ultimate authority for the quality of care provided. The elaborate committee structure and diverse reviews represent an enormous investment of professional effort on quality assurance activities. What evidence is there that it has led to improvements in patient care? Some specific examples of particular QA activities and the benefits that have resulted are presented in the next section.

Examples of Quality Assurance Activities at McLean

A monitor was developed for treatment planning that evaluated patients with a length of stay longer than 6 months on an inpatient unit. The following indicators were identified. Patients with a length of stay of 6 months will have documented the following:

1. Evidence of the continued need for hospital level of care.
2. A comprehensive treatment plan that seems likely to lead to improvement.
3. Discharge criteria.
4. Evidence of benefit from treatment.
5. Timely and active discharge planning.
6. Appropriate consultations initiated and followed up including:
   a. Psychopharmacology consultation.
   b. Psychotherapy consultation.
   c. Comprehensive treatment review with a consultant.

Charts were reviewed on 47 patients who had been in the hospital more than 6 months. In some cases, it was found that discharge planning was complicated, and no suitable halfway house or community residence was yet available. This led to a plan for development of an additional community residence on the grounds of McLean. Other cases were found to be chronically ill and unresponsive despite the best available intensive treatment. Arrangements were being made to transfer those patients to state mental hospitals. Because many of these patients were originally admitted from state facilities, the Admissions Office changed its procedures by requiring a guarantee before accepting such referrals that patients could return to the state facility if they did not respond to treatment at McLean. Some problems in discharge planning were also identified. This led to the development of an Office of Discharge Planning, staffed by a senior staff social worker who provides consultation on patients with difficult disposition problems. The consultation can be requested by the patient's treatment team or by the Utilization Review Department. Over the 18 months this monitor has been in place, the number of patients who have been in the hospital more than 6 months has declined from more than 50 to fewer than 20.

All deaths and other serious incidents (e.g., suicide attempts, assaults) are reviewed by the Executive Committee of the PCAC for problems in their particular care or in the overall system. One review led to a change in policy so that a newly admitted patient could not leave the ward before meeting with the assigned psychiatrist the next morning. Another review recognized the increase in very disturbed patients in the Community Residential Program, and this resulted in increased physician staffing. In another case, it was evident that clinical staff were not aware that certain on-grounds activities (e.g., laboratory tests, educational or activity groups) did not provide individual supervision of patients. This led to a memo and group discussion on the need not only for careful assessment of patients but also for documentation of their ability to attend such unsupervised activities. It was also recognized that patient suicides are always stressful for staff to deal with, even when they have done everything they could to help the desperately distressed individuals who choose suicide as the way out of their misery. A task force developed a set of recommendations to provide assistance to staff who have been directly affected by a patient suicide.

In this review process, all instances of the use of seclusion or physical restraint are logged and tabulated. Individual cases with seclusion or restraint of more than 4 days or of 10 instances in a month are individually reviewed and discussed by the Department of Psychiatry Quality Assurance Committee. Analyses of the data suggested two different patterns of use. Some acutely psychotic patients are restrained early in the course of their hospitalization and then do not require restraint when their clinical condition improves. Other patients with severe characterological problems sometimes lose control and are restrained when their therapy stirs up overwhelming feelings in them, such as when memories of childhood sexual abuse are recovered. These patients may periodically be restrained when their fragile defenses are overwhelmed and they become acutely self-destructive. Seclusion and restraint are procedures that require a physician's order but are generally initiated by nursing staff who interact on a continuous basis with the patient. For that reason, the Nursing Department conducted its own review of seclusion and restraint. It was found that in many cases, prn medication was available but was not offered to patients who were becoming more disturbed. In-service education on crisis prevention and improved communication between nurses and the treating physician were recommended. A task force to examine the use of seclusion and restraint met and concluded that the overall tradition and philosophy of care had to be addressed for the hospital as a whole as well as on individual wards.

A number of drug usage monitors have been developed and implemented (Cole and Katz 1988). For neuroleptic drugs, the risks and benefits of treatment need to be carefully documented in the patient's record, along with some measure (e.g., the Abnormal Involuntary Movement Score [AIMS]) of whether the patient has tardive dyskinesia. Documentation of both these indicators has been problematic, and consideration is being given to including the AIMS in the format for the initial physical exam and in the discharge summary. For anticonvulsant drugs, the rationale for using them needs to be documented along with the risks and benefits. Again, the documentation has been problematic despite reminder notices. The use of anticonvulsants has also been reviewed for monitoring of hematologic and liver function through regular blood tests. The review suggested that most clinicians were following the guidelines for frequency of blood tests but that some were exceeding the recommended guidelines. A study is being carried out to review the recommended guidelines and to determine if changes need to be made.

Examples of other monitors include appropriate use of electroconvulsive therapy, adequacy of treatment plan documentation, adequacy of discharge plans for patients who are readmitted within 2 weeks of discharge, timely documentation of psychotherapy, and appropriate documentation that a consultant's recommendations have been carefully considered. Quality reviews are also incorporated into the ongoing utilization review process and, if serious problems in care are flagged, those are reviewed by the Department of Psychiatry Quality Assurance Committee.

An important challenge for any quality assurance program is to enlist the cooperation of the clinical staff so that they do not feel constantly harassed and criticized. Several strategies may be helpful. First, all monitors and indicators should be discussed with and approved by the medical staff prior to being instituted. This reduces the perception that the Quality Assurance Department is imposing some arbitrary standards on the clinical staff. Second, the results of all quality assurance activities are presented to the medical staff for their review, analysis, and recommendations for needed changes. Third, repeated emphasis is given to the notion that most problems identified are systemic and not a reflection of an individual clinician's deficiencies. Berwick (1989) described this as a continuous monitoring approach rather than one that tries to identify "bad apples." Finally, positive feedback is provided for a job well done and not just criticism for deficiencies identified. This feedback comes from the immediate clinical supervisor who works with the clinician on a daily basis, and not just from the Quality Assurance Department.

Conclusion

Quality assurance activities have taken on increasing importance in psychiatric hospitals. It is critical that it be demonstrated that these activities can actually make a difference in the quality of care provided to patients and their families. The cost of review activities needs to be carefully considered. At a time when there is so much concern about limiting health care expenditures, quality assurance activities should not take away from needed patient care activities. However, as our sophistication in this area develops, it may be possible to identify improvements that can increase quality without increasing costs. In the future, more interdisciplinary quality assurance activities will attempt to address the integration of care.

References

American Psychiatric Association: Treatments of Psychiatric Disorders: A Task Force Report of the American Psychiatric Association. Washington, DC, American Psychiatric Association, 1989

Andrews S, Vaughan K, Harvey R, et al: A survey of practising psychiatrists' views on the treatment of schizophrenia. Br J Psychiatry 149:357–364, 1986

Armstrong MS, Andrews G: A survey of practising psychiatrist's views on treatment of the depressions. Br J Psychiatry 149:742–750, 1986

Barter JT: Accreditation surveys—nitpicking or quality seeking? Hosp Community Psychiatry 39:707, 1988

Berwick DM: Continuous improvement as an ideal in health care. N Engl J Med 320:53–56, 1989

Clements CD, Bonacci D, Yerevanian B, et al: Assessment of suicide risk in patients with personality disorder and major affective diagnosis. QRB 11:150–154, 1985

Clifford J: What DRGs mean to the patient and provider. J Geriatr Psychiatry 22:201–210, 1989

Cole JO, Katz DL: Drug therapy monitoring in a private psychiatric hospital: a consideration of its risks and benefits. McLean Hospital Journal 13:114–157, 1988

Coleman RL, Kirven LJ: The staff psychiatrist and the Joint Commission survey. Hosp Community Psychiatry 41:412–415, 1990

Collins JF, Ellsworth RB, Casey NA, et al: Treatment characteristics of effective psychiatric programs. Hosp Community Psychiatry 35:601–605, 1984

Council on Medical Service: Defining, measuring, assuring quality of care. Chicago,

American Medical Association, 1988

Craig TJ, Mehta RM: Clinician-computer interaction: Automated review of psychotropic drugs. Am J Psychiatry 141:267–270, 1984

Eisenberg MG, Tierney DO: Profiling disruptive patient incidents. QRB 11:245–248, 1985

Fauman MA: Quality assurance monitoring in psychiatry. Am J Psychiatry 146:1121–1130, 1989

Fromberg R: The Joint Commission Guide to Quality Assurance. Chicago, Joint Commission on Accreditation of Healthcare Organizations, 1988

Gaver KD: A guide through the accreditation maze. Hosp Community Psychiatry 33:819–823, 1982

Hamilton JM: Psychiatric Peer Review: Prelude and Promise. Washington, DC, American Psychiatric Press, 1985

Houck JH: Regulation and accreditation: The pros and cons for psychiatric facilities. Hosp Community Psychiatry 35:1201–1204, 1984

Kibbee P: The suicidal patient—An issue for quality assurance and risk management. J Nurs Qual Assur 3:63–71, 1988

Lieberman PB, Astrachan BM: The JCAH and psychiatry: Current issues and implications for practice. Hosp Community Psychiatry 35:1205–1210, 1984

Liptzin B: Quality assurance and psychiatric practice—a review. Am J Psychiatry 131:1374–1377, 1974

Liptzin B: What DRGs mean to the patient and provider—discussion. J Geriatr Psychiatry 22:211–217, 1989

Lohr KN, Schroeder SA: A strategy for quality assurance in Medicare. N Engl J Med 322:707–712, 1990

Mattson MR: Quality assurance—A literature review of a changing field. Hosp Community Psychiatry 35:605–616, 1984

Melnick SD, Lyter LL: The negative impacts of increased concurrent review of psychiatric inpatient care. Hosp Community Psychiatry 38:300–303, 1987

Molnar G, Feeney MG: Computer-assisted review of antipsychotics on acute care units. QRB 11:271–274, 1985

Munich RL: Quality assurance and quality of care: I. Finding the linkages. The Psychiatric Hospital 21:13–24, 1990

Munich RL, Hurley B, Delaney J: Quality assurance and quality of care: II. Monitoring treatment. The Psychiatric Hospital 21: 71–77, 1990

Phillips KL: Chemical dependence treatment review guidelines. Gen Hosp Psychiatry 11:282–287, 1989

Prunier P, Buongiorno PA: Guidelines for acute inpatient psychiatric treatment review. Gen Hosp Psychiatry 11:278–281, 1989

Sederer LI: Utilization review and quality assurance—Staying in the black and working with the Blues. Gen Hosp Psychiatry 9:210–219, 1987

Stricker G, Rodriguez A: Handbook of Quality Assurance in Mental Health. New York, Plenum, 1988

Sundram CJ: Patient idleness in public mental hospitals. Psychiatr Q 58:243–254, 1987

Van Vort WB: Ethics of nonformulary review in psychiatry. Hosp Community Psychiatry

39:1253–1255, 1988

Van Vort W, Mattson MR: A strategy for enhancing the clinical utility of the psychiatric record. Hosp Community Psychiatry 40:407–409, 1989

Way BB, Braff J, Steadman HJ: Constructing an efficient inpatient incident reporting system. Psychiatr Q 57:147–152, 1985

Zusman J: Quality assurance in mental health care. Hosp Community Psychiatry 39:1286–1290, 1988

Quality Assurance and Treatment Outcome: A Psychiatric Nursing Perspective

Elizabeth C. Poster, R.N., Ph.D.

How can we effectively measure the outcomes of nursing care in a psychiatric setting? In this chapter, I describe one model for conducting that activity: the outcome-focused nursing quality assurance program at UCLA's Neuropsychiatric Institute and Hospital (NPI&H), a 188-bed teaching facility with 6 inpatient units providing child, adolescent, adult, and geropsychiatric services. The model is presented within the context of NPI&H's philosophy of nursing care and a discussion of the considerable challenges psychiatric nursing faces in measuring the outcomes of nursing care.

Philosophy of Nursing Care

At the UCLA Neuropsychiatric Hospital and Institute (NPI&H), the professional practice of nursing is defined as the diagnosis and treatment of human responses to actual or potential health problems, consisting of independent, interdependent, and dependent functions. The independent practice of nursing is based on the Johnson Behavioral System Model of Nursing and utilizes the nursing process, which encompasses assessment, diagnosis, planning, intervention, and evaluation (Dee 1987).

The Johnson Behavioral System Model identifies universal patterns of behavior applicable to all individuals. Essential principles of the model include the following components:

1. The individual is conceptualized as a living system in constant interaction with the environment.
2. Specific system tasks are carried out by the individual's eight subsystems (Ingestive, Eliminative, Dependency, Affiliative, Aggressive-Protective, Achievement, Sexual, and Restorative).

3. Balance is maintained when there is an equal distribution of energy among the eight subsystems, and the environment is viewed as all regulatory elements external to the behavioral system, such as biophysical, psychological, and developmental status as well as sociocultural, family, and physical environmental factors.

4. The goal of nursing care is to create an environment that nurtures, protects, and stimulates the behavioral subsystems so that the individual's system balance is maintained or restored.

At the NPI&H, all nursing assessments, nursing care plans (including in-house standard care plans), evaluations, and discharge planning are conducted using this theoretical framework. In addition, nursing diagnoses are being developed that are based on the Johnson Model. To date, 40 Standard Care Plans have been developed that are also based on the Johnson Model.

Assessment as a critical component of the nursing process provides the basis for diagnosis, planning, and implementation of nursing interventions. Systematic and continuous assessment ensures that nursing care goals are congruent with patient and multidisciplinary treatment goals. "Nursing diagnoses describe actual or potential health problems which nurses, by virtue of their education and experience, are capable and licensed to treat" (Gordon 1982, p. 3). Nursing diagnoses are prioritized for planning nursing interventions and determining the criteria for patient outcomes. The nursing plan of care is developed in consultation/collaboration with the patient/family members and multidisciplinary team. It incorporates strategies for maintaining the patient's strengths while modifying identified areas of dysfunction. Discharge planning is incorporated into the plan of care.

Nursing care, founded on respect for human dignity and individual freedom of choice, focuses on two major areas: 1) the patient's effective or ineffective coping mechanisms, and 2) the biophysical, psychological, social, family, ecological, and cultural factors that may affect the behavioral responses of the patient. Nursing interventions assist the patient to maximize his or her potential and achieve behavioral patterns that are functional to the environment and unique to the individual. These nursing interventions include psychotherapeutic modalities, patient-family teaching, behavioral and milieu management, and treatment modalities aimed at patients' physiological responses to health problems. These interventions are also targeted toward family, community, and other health care resources to augment the nursing care and the patient's self-care. Evaluation of nursing care focuses on patient outcomes. Continual evaluation provides information by which nursing interventions are made and modified to achieve the short- and long-term goals of patients.

At the NPI&H, patient care is delivered through a primary nursing care delivery system. Primary nursing is a system organized to maximize continuous and comprehensive delivery of nursing care to patients and their families. Primary nurses are registered nurses accountable for the planning, coordination, and delivery of nursing care to patients from the time of admission to discharge. Psychiatric technicians, licensed vocational nurses, and mental health practitioners in the role of associates assist the primary nurse in carrying out delegated components of nursing care.

Outcome Measurement: The Challenge for Nursing

Although nursing care is a major component of the treatment of all patients admitted for inpatient psychiatric care, evaluating the direct impact of this care is difficult. In most psychiatric settings in which a multidisciplinary team provides multiple interventions, a direct relationship between patient outcome and the quality of care provided by a single discipline is hard to identify and measure. Thus, a major challenge facing psychiatric nursing today is to conduct ongoing research that investigates the relationship between nursing interventions and desired patient outcomes.

Nursing Quality Assurance

Outcome measurement in nursing has a long history beginning with Nightingale and receiving renewed interest in the 1970s as evidenced by the work of several authors (Daubert 1979; Decker et al. 1979; Hegyvary and Haussman 1976; Hilger 1974; Taylor 1974; Zimmer 1974). The emphasis heightened in the 1980s with new national requirements focused on outcomes—requirements proposed by the Joint Commission for the Accreditation of Health Care Organizations (JCAHO), the Health Care Financing Administration (HCFA), the National Association of Private Psychiatric Hospitals (NAPPH), and the Omnibus Reconciliation Act (OBRA) (Marek 1989). In reviewing nursing services, these organizations have defined outcome as "a measurable change in a client's health status related to the receipt of nursing care." The new emphasis on outcomes supersedes former concerns with documentation related to policies and procedures.

Although qualitative methods are valuable in evaluating the outcomes of care, quantitative methods are also needed to measure changes in patient status. Guidelines for selecting an appropriate methodology in nursing quality assurance evaluation have been proposed by Poster and Pelletier (1988). To ensure that patient outcome data are both valid and reliable, standardized evaluation tools should be used. (Lists of currently available instruments and quality assurance studies that identify instruments are available from the author.)

Quality Assurance in Psychiatric Nursing

The selection of the most important outcome indicators for any quality assurance program is a difficult task. In psychiatry and psychiatric nursing, the development of precise, meaningful criteria that describe both negative and positive patient outcomes is especially challenging.

The 1987 JCAHO "Agenda for Change" provides guidelines for the development and use of a standardized set of severity-adjusted clinical indicators to identify and monitor high-volume, high-risk, and problem-prone areas of psychiatric nursing practice (JCAHO 1987, 1988a, 1988b). Their emphasis is on patient outcomes rather than on care delivery (process) or organizational capacity to provide quality care (structure). Although there already exists a small body of research on child, adolescent, and adult psychiatric hospital treatment outcomes, these outcome measures are not easily integrated into an ongoing monitoring and evaluation program (Blotcky et al. 1984; Gossett 1985, 1987; Gossett et al. 1983; Stevenson et al. 1988). The majority of instruments for outcome measurement have been developed through externally funded, time-limited research, and they are not cost-effective for institutional quality assurance programs (Ciarlo 1981; Cook and Shadish 1982; Kirkhart and Morgan 1986).

Despite these difficulties, each institution can identify its own valid indicators with demonstrated relevance to patient outcomes. Choices must be made and priorities set based on the individual institution's resources for monitoring and evaluating selected indicators on an ongoing basis. In choosing outcome indicators, we can turn to those used to measure quality of nursing care in nonpsychiatric settings. These include general measures (physiological status, safety, psychosocial status, mortality, cost of care, patient satisfaction, well-being, quality of life); functional measures (activities of daily living, communication, home maintenance, rehospitalization, frequency of service, goal attainment); and symptom control measures (pain, comfort).

The NPI&H Program for Nursing Quality Assurance

The ongoing evaluation of the professional practice of nursing at NPI&H is accomplished through a number of mechanisms. One is the work of the Nursing Quality Assurance Committee (NQAC). Chaired by the Director of Nursing Research and Education and composed of nurses representing each of the six inpatient units and the hospital's Director of Quality Management, the objectives of this committee are as follows:

- To monitor and evaluate quality of care given by the nursing staff through review and evaluation of documentation in the medical record and other reliable sources of data.

- To identify and assess patient outcomes using objective criteria and/or standards of care as a measure of quality of care.
- To collect, screen, and evaluate information to identify problems having an impact on patient care and clinical performance of nursing staff and to support the identification of opportunities to improve patient care.
- To increase nursing staff competency by using quality assurance study findings that identify nursing activities which are inappropriate, inefficient, and/or ineffective.
- To implement and monitor corrective actions determined by concurrent and retrospective reviews, assessing the effectiveness of the recommendations in improving patient care.
- To use findings of quality assurance activities in the reappraisal/reappointment process.
- To communicate quality assurance findings to nursing staff, other professionals, and administrators, as well as to the Hospital Quality Management Committee and others as appropriate.
- To assure compliance with all JCAHO and other relevant state and federal regulatory agency quality assurance requirements.

NPI&H Outcome Indicators

At the NPI&H, we selected goal attainment and safety as the focus of outcome indicators for our psychiatric nursing quality assurance program. Because patient falls and medication error rates had been monitored for many years, the emphasis on safety represented a natural progression. These two clinical indicators also fit well with JCAHO's recent "high-volume, high-risk, problem-prone schema." In addition, we continued to monitor and evaluate two other outcome indicators: nosocomial infections and patient satisfaction.

Nursing Quality Assurance Committee members developed the following guidelines for collecting data related to goal attainment and based on predicted patient outcomes. Committee members use the Predicted Patient Outcome Data Collection Tool (available from the author) in their concurrent review of patient records at the time of discharge. An established threshold of 80% of the predicted outcomes/goals is expected to be met by discharge. When this level is not met, an in-depth review takes place to determine the reasons. (The 80% level was based on committee members' clinical experience and judgment; no empirical data exist on which to base this decision.) An additional review also takes place whenever a serious negative outcome occurs, such as a suicide attempt or death.

The procedure described herein is standardized so that the following will take place:

1. Each committee member submits three to four data collection tools per month.
2. Each tool analyzes one identified problem that meets the criteria of being either high-risk, problem-prone, or high-volume. These include the following:
   - Aggressive/protective subsystem problem
   - Seclusion/restraint
   - Falls
   - Medication knowledge
   - Suicide potential
   - Eating disorders
   - Electroconvulsive therapy (ECT)
   - Safety, mobility
3. The patient is near discharge.
4. A review of a Standard Care Plan is done whenever possible.
5. Changes in acuity scores between admission and discharge are calculated. Acuity scores are derived from the NPH (Neuropsychiatric Hospital) Patient Classification System (Dee and Randell 1989).

Monitoring predicted patient outcomes has generated a great deal of discussion regarding both the use of measurable terms in the Nursing Care Plan as well as the need to be realistic in predicting outcomes that can be achieved during rather short lengths of stay. Increased inservice education programs, modifications of standard care plans, and changes in documentation procedures have resulted from this emphasis on monitoring and evaluating predicted patient outcomes. The following is an example of how we establish and use predicted patient outcomes to monitor quality of care for individual patients.

Case Example: Adult Inpatient Unit

Mary, a 25-year-old white, single, unemployed student, was admitted to the adult inpatient unit following an overdose of barbiturates. During her 5-week hospitalization, she was diagnosed as having an obsessive-compulsive disorder. Mary had repetitive, recurrent thoughts about God, contamination, and sexuality, which she found unacceptable and a major source of distress. She was also assessed as having suicidal ideation. During her hospitalization, the Standard Care Plan titled "Insufficiency of Aggressive-Protective Subsystem: Suicidal Behavior" was individualized for this patient. Because she met the criteria for high-risk behavior, nursing documentation relating to suicidal ideation was evaluated by the NQAC member.

In reviewing this care plan, it was clear that the seven predicted patient outcomes were met by the date of discharge. In addition, the patient's acuity score had decreased from the date of admission to discharge.

Patient behaviors, described by the Johnson Behavioral System Model as aggressive/protective behaviors, were rated on admission with an acuity score of 3 and included the following:

1. Lacks awareness of potentially hazardous situations.
2. Engages in intense, frequent acting-out behaviors.
3. Fails to protect self in dangerous situations.
4. Selects inappropriate/inadequate response to threat.
5. Lacks awareness of cause and effect.
6. Selects response to threat that contains potential for self-injury of major magnitude.

Patient outcomes at the time of discharge showed improvement in this area of behavior and were given an acuity score of 2. These patient outcomes included the following:

1. Identifies obvious dangers, but not subtle cues of potential harm.
2. Selects indirect verbal/nonverbal response to threat.
3. Selects response to threat that contains potential for self-injury of a minor magnitude.
4. Does not identify or control own reactions to stress consistently or appropriately.

Patient Safety: Fall Outcomes

It is remarkable that research data are not available on the outcome of patient falls in psychiatric settings. Although fall *rates* are common quality of care indicators in hospital quality assurance programs, actual *outcomes* or medical consequences of falls receive little attention. This is particularly surprising because psychiatric patients have a number of high-risk factors, such as labile mental status and behavior, use of medication that affects gait and proprioception, an age group that includes young children and the elderly, and conditions that may alter an individual's awareness of environmental and safety hazards.

At the NPI&H, all patient falls, identified on the hospital's "Unusual Occurrence" report, are reviewed using a coding guide. This coding guide includes elements such as the type of fall, reason for the fall, severity of outcome, treatment post-fall, and location of treatment and medications prescribed as a consequence of the fall (Table 17–1). This process links hospital clinical safety procedures to nursing quality assurance activities. In addition to evaluating severity of patient injury, the review assesses the cost to the patient and the hospital. It also evaluates the appropriateness of diagnostic studies and other "post-fall" measures.

Each incident rated 2 or higher receives a "focused review." The clinical

TABLE 17–1. Patient Fall Outcome—Coding Guide

Type
    1 = Fall from bed
    2 = Fall getting in/out bed
    3 = Fall other than above
    4 = Fall during seizure

Reason for Fall
    1 = Environmental Factors (e.g., wet floor, unstable furniture, play equip.)
    2 = Physiological Patient Characteristics (e.g., mobility, balance or gait problems; sensory impairment; disorientation or confusion; type of medication; substance abuse; orthostasis; dizziness)
    3 = Physical Patient Characteristics (e.g., use of ambulatory assistive devices; ill-fitting shoes; personal safety [running, slipped while playing, slipped in stocking feet])
    4 = None apparent

Severity of Outcome
    0 = None
    1 = Not Consequential (transient non-disabling impairment not requiring medication or medical treatment, c/o pain, redness)
    2 = Consequential (contusions, lacerations, abrasions, broken tooth, minor bleeding edema, bump, disoriented). If consequential, describe.
    3 = Severe (fracture, concussion (with LOC), hemorrhage)
    4 = Death

Treatment
    0 = None
    1 = Observation, Monitoring of V/S, Neuro Signs, X-Ray
    2 = Dressing Only—Icepack
    3 = Dressing Applied
    4 = Sutures, Closed Reduction
    5 = Surgery

Location of Treatment
    1 = Within the Institution
    2 = Transferred to Medical Center/Other Agency (includes diagnostic tests, sutures)

Medications
    0 = No
    1 = Yes (given in response to post-fall symptoms)

nurse manager and/or nursing quality assurance committee members determine whether the fall could have been prevented or if the outcome could have been less harmful to the patient. Through such reviews, we have identified problems such as commodes with ineffective wheel locks, a floor surface on the geropsychiatric unit that required replacement with a nonskid flooring, and the need for use of a "fall-safe monitor" at bedtime for high-risk patients.

Aggregate data of fall outcomes over a 34-month period have been analyzed for patterns and trends. This retrospective cohort study provided evidence that falls are a frequent type of unusual occurrence in the inpatient psychiatric setting and that falls can result in severe patient outcomes (Poster et al. 1991). Knowledge of these rates is essential in providing data that can be utilized in developing meaningful thresholds when monitoring and evaluating falls as part of a psychiatric hospital's comprehensive quality management program.

Patient Safety: Medication Incident Outcomes

For many years, medication incidents have been monitored and evaluated as a clinical indicator in the nursing quality assurance program. "Unusual occurrence" reports provide the major data source for this indicator. Although the error rate for medications (number of errors divided by the number of doses given) has consistently been below 1% over the past 15 years, each incident has the potential for harm to the patient.

To assess the impact of medication incidents, a medication incident patient outcome indicator was added to the nursing quality assurance program. Using a medication incident outcome coding guide, all "unusual occurrences" are now reviewed on a monthly basis. The date, unit, sex of patient, name of drug(s) involved, type of incident, reason for incident, severity of outcome, and comments are analyzed (Table 17–2).

The NQAC determined the threshold for this indicator as follows: *100 percent of medication incidents will have non-consequential patient outcomes.* All incidents resulting in consequential, serious, or critical outcomes receive a focused review by the clinical nurse manager and/or NQAC member. These incidents are reported on Medication Incident Outcome Forms, which are reviewed and analyzed monthly by the NQAC for patterns and trends.

This methodology has resulted in a number of opportunities to improve care. For example, a consequential patient outcome resulted when a patient was given a subcutaneous injection of a medication. Because the nurse's technique was not correct, the patient developed a hematoma. Individualized inservice education enabled that nurse to learn the skill and to use the correct technique thereafter.

Patient Satisfaction

Patient satisfaction as an indicator of quality care reflects the assumption that the consumer is both capable of evaluating nursing care and other services, and that "satisfaction" is an indicator of service effectiveness and quality of care. Although patients' personal reactions to care are tapped by most patient satisfaction questionnaires, such reactions are difficult to convert to measurable terms and even more difficult to interpret with validity (Deiker et al. 1981; Guebaly et al. 1983).

Patient satisfaction in psychiatric settings is even more difficult to assess because of patients' presenting problems, such as inability to deal with affective stimuli, memory deficits, transference issues, distorted views of reality, involuntary admissions, and other acute and chronic affective and cognitive deficits. Also, although the care may be of high quality, unpleasant side effects of medications, limits set on "unacceptable" behaviors, and lack of patient cooperation may give the patient a negative perception of the care received.

However, despite these limitations, it is important to use patient and family feedback in measuring outcomes. Guidelines for the development of "Patient Satisfaction Questionnaires" have been proposed by Rhodes (1986). Determination of the specific components of psychiatric nursing care that will be evaluated by the patient/family member is a critical element in the development process. At the NPI&H, we have successfully used tools such as the Client Satisfaction Questionnaire (CSQ) and Family and Significant Other Satisfaction Questionnaire (F/SSQ) to determine the impact of nursing care on patient/family outcomes (Ryan et al. 1988). For a more thorough discussion of patient satisfaction as an outcome measure in psychiatric settings, see Chapter 13 of this book.

A Focused Outcome Study: Contraband

A focused study provides information about a suspected problem identified through the ongoing monitoring and evaluation of "scanning monitors" (Devert 1985). An example of a patient care problem identified during monthly reviews of unusual occurrences was that of contraband. Potentially dangerous items were being smuggled into the hospital, and this was identified as a serious problem by the nursing staff. These items included over-the-counter medications, illicit drugs, weapons, and potentially hazardous objects such as matches, lighters, and razor blades. Patient contraband falls under the category of a clinical safety issue that, according to JCAHO Risk Management Standards, needs to be identified and prevented (JCAHO 1988c, 1989).

Using an outcome-focused approach, a retrospective review of all Unusual Occurrence Reports over a 28-month period was conducted (Pelletier et al.

TABLE 17–2. Medication Incident Outcome—Coding Guide

Type of Medication Incident
    1 = Wrong patient
    2 = Wrong dosage
    3 = Wrong drug
    4 = Wrong route
    5 = Not given at designated time
    6 = Omitted
    7 = Repeat dosage given
    8 = Unordered medication
    9 = Given after discontinued
    10 = Given after expiration date
    11 = Given more frequently than ordered
    12 = Given before designated start date
    13 = Given without consent
    14 = Other (specify)_____

Reason for Medication Incident
    1 = Transcription omission
    2 = Incorrect I.D. of patient
    3 = Medication record not checked
    4 = Misread med. card
    5 = Transcription error
    6 = Forgot
    7 = Misread medication record
    8 = Expiration date not noted
    9 = Misread label
    10 = Error computing dosage
    11 = Drug not charted after administering
    12 = Change in time schedule
    13 = Consent not obtained
    14 = Pharmacy sent wrong drug
    15 = Swallowing not verified
    16 = Other (specify)_____

Severity of Outcome
    1 = Consequential (observation, monitoring of V/S, neuro signs, cancellation of procedure/lab test)
    2 = Serious (remaining in institution, requiring medication, medical treatment, diagnostic/lab tests)
    3 = Critical (transfer to Medical Center or other hospital for treatment)
    4 = Death

1989). Each incident identified as "confiscation of contraband" was reviewed and analyzed. Data were analyzed according to day and shift of incident; nature and source of contraband; patient's admitting diagnosis, sex, and age; and type of unit. Patient outcomes of these incidents were rated on the following scale:

0 = None

1 = Not Consequential (transient, nondisabling impairment not requiring medication or medical treatment; e.g., complains of pain, redness)

2 = Consequential (contusions, lacerations, abrasions, broken tooth, minor bleeding, edema, bump, disoriented)

3 = Serious (fracture, concussion with loss of consciousness, hemorrhage)

4 = Death

Over a 28-month period, 54 incidents of contraband confiscation were reported with a confiscation rate of .0005 (based on patient bed days). Analysis revealed that the outcome of the contraband possessions during this study period was characterized as "none" in 61% of the cases and "not consequential" in 33% of the incidents. Three incidents (6%) were judged to have had "consequential" outcomes. These were self-inflicted cuts by adult patients using pieces of light bulbs or razor blades. Each incident could have caused serious harm to the patient had the item not been confiscated.

As a result of the findings of this focused study, a number of actions were taken: 1) orientation of all new nursing staff members to the issues and techniques of assessing and confiscating contraband; 2) inclusion of contraband information in the classes related to the prevention and management of assaultive behavior; 3) preparation of a standard letter given to all patients upon admission related to contraband; and 4) the implementation of a new policy and procedure regarding possession, search and disposal of weapons, authorized and unauthorized drugs, and potentially harmful substances/objects.

Conclusion

The current trend in psychiatric nursing research emphasizes studies related to nursing practice interventions and client problems. Research has demonstrated that psychiatric/mental health nursing interventions have a positive effect on the mental health problems of patients. In addition to research studies, quality assurance advancement is a valid research activity for nursing investigation in the 1990s (Flaskerud 1987).

Outcome studies conducted as major components of nursing quality assurance activities can also generate data that help us to evaluate and further substantiate the impact of nursing care on patients. The development of methodologies and measurement tools specific to psychiatric patient outcomes is needed. Nurses must continue to identify direct cause and effect relationships between the process of nursing care and patient outcomes.

References

Blotcky MJ, Dimperio TL, Gossett JT: Follow-up of children treated in psychiatric hospitals: a review of studies. Am J Psychiatry 141:1499–1507, 1984

Ciarlo JA: Final report: the assessment of client/patient outcome techniques for use in mental health programs (National Institute for Mental Health Contract, No. 278-80-0005[DB]). Washington, DC, U.S. Government Printing Office, 1981

Cook T, Shadish W: Metaevaluation: an assessment of the congressionally mandated evaluation system for community mental health centers, in Innovative Approaches to Mental Health Evaluation. Edited by Stahler G, Tash W. New York, Academic, 1982, pp 282–291

Daubert E: Patient classification system and outcome criteria. Nurs Outlook 27:450–454, 1979

Decker F, Stevens L, Vancini M et al.: Using patient outcomes to evaluate community health nursing. Nurs Outlook 27:278–282, 1979

Dee V: Model for professional practice. Los Angeles, UCLA Neuropsychiatric Institute and Hospital. Unpublished paper, publication #113, 1987 (available on request from the author at UCLA Neuropsychiatric Institute and Hospital, 760 Westwood Plaza, Los Angeles, CA 90024)

Dee V, Randell B: NPH Patient Classification System: A theory-based nursing practice model for staffing. UCLA Neuropsychiatric Institute and Hospital. Unpublished paper, 1989 (available on request from the authors at UCLA Neuropsychiatric Institute and Hospital, 760 Westwood Plaza, Los Angeles, CA 90024)

Deiker T, Osborn SM, Distefano JRMK et al: Consumer accreditation: developing a quality assurance patient care evaluation scale. Hosp Community Psychiatry 32:565–567, 1981

Devert C: The Monitoring Sourcebook, Vol 2: Nursing Practice. Chicago, Care Communications, 1985

Flaskerud J: Evaluation of the impact of psychiatric/mental health nursing through research, in Psychiatric/Mental Health Nursing. Edited by Birckhead L. Philadelphia, JB Lippincott, 1987, pp 717–31

Gordon M: Historical perspective: the national group for classification of nursing diagnoses, in Classification of Nursing Diagnoses. Edited by Kim MJ, Moritz DA. New York, McGraw-Hill, 1982, p 3

Gossett JT, Lewis JM, Barnart FD: To Find a Way: The Outcome of Hospital Treatment of Disturbed Adolescents. New York, Brunner/Mazel, 1983

Gossett JT: Psychiatric hospital follow-up study: current findings and future directions. Psychiatric Annals 15:596–601, 1985

Gossett JT: Studies of the outcome of psychiatric hospital treatment, in Current Research in Private Psychiatric Hospitals. Washington, DC, National Association of Private Psychiatric Hospitals, 1987, pp 102–108

Guebaly N, Toew SJ, Leckie A, et al.: On evaluating patient satisfaction: methodological issues. Can J Psychiatry 28:24–29, 1983

Hegyvary S, Haussman R: The real relationship of nursing process and patient outcomes. J Nurs Adm 6:18–21, 1976

Hilger E: Developing nursing outcome criteria. Nurs Clin North Am 9:323–330, 1974

Joint Commission on Accreditation of Health Care Organizations: Agenda for Change Update, Vol 1, No 1. Chicago, Joint Commission on Accreditation of Health Care Organizations, 1987

Joint Commission on Accreditation of Health Care Organizations: Monitoring and Evaluating the Quality and Appropriateness of Care. Chicago, Joint Commission on Accreditation of Health Care Organizations, 1988a

Joint Commission on Accreditation of Health Care Organizations: Agenda for Change Update, Vol 2, No 1. Chicago, Joint Commission on Accreditation of Health Care Organizations, 1988b

Joint Commission on Accreditation of Health Care Organizations: Joint Commission Perspectives 8:9, 1988c

Joint Commission on Accreditation of Health Care Organizations: Accreditation Manual for Hospitals/90. Chicago, Joint Commission on Accreditation of Health Care Organizations, 1989, p 121

Kirkhart KE, Morgan ED: Evaluation in mental health centers. Evaluation Review 10:127–141, 1986

Marek KD: Outcome measurement in nursing. Journal of Nursing Quality Assurance 4:1–9, 1989

Pelletier L, Poster EC, Kay K: Contraband: the hidden risk (a risk management case example). QRB 16(1):9–14, 1989

Poster EC, Pelletier LR: Part II: Quantitative and qualitative approaches to nursing quality assurance program evaluation. Journal of Nursing Quality Assurance 2:63–72, 1988

Poster EC, Pelletier LR, Kay K: A retrospective cohort study of falls in an acute neuropsychiatric setting. Hosp Community Psychiatry (in press)

Rhodes S: Are your customers satisfied? In Hospital Entrepreneurs' Newsletter. Rockville, MD, Aspen Publishers, July 1986, p 2

Ryan J, Poster EC, Auger J, et al: A comparative study of primary and team nursing models in the psychiatric care setting. Arch Psychiatr Nurs 2:3–13, 1988

Stevenson JF, Beattie MC, Clives RR, et al: An outcome monitoring system for psychiatric inpatient care. QRB 14:326–331, 1988

Taylor J: Measuring the outcomes of nursing care. Nurs Clin North Am 9:337–348, 1974

Zimmer M: Guidelines for development of outcome criteria. Nurs Clin North Am 9:317–355, 1974

❖ 18 ❖   Measuring Outcome: A Post-Discharge Assessment Model

John W. Goethe, M.D.
Marcia L. Gerulaitis
Bonnie L. Szarek, R.N.
Judith Weber, M.S.W.

A wide variety of issues must be considered in outcome assessment, including why outcome studies are needed, what will be measured, how the measurement will be undertaken, and who the subjects of the assessment will be. But why is outcome research necessary? Although the answer to this question would seem obvious in some respects, the value of outcome data cannot be overemphasized. It has long been recognized that outcome data can " . . . serve the dual purpose of providing useful information to administrators and health care planners while contributing new knowledge to our understanding of the nature of illness and the effectiveness of treatment" (Schwartz et al. 1973). More recently, dramatic changes in regulatory and reimbursement policies have made outcome data even more important. Measurement of treatment outcome has become a part of quality of care monitoring (Council on Medical Service 1986; Joint Commission on Accreditation of Hospitals [JCAH] 1986), and the Joint Commission on Accreditation of Health Care Organizations (JCAHO) now has general policies for patient follow-up (JCAHO 1988). The magnitude of the impact of mental illness and our still-incomplete knowledge of natural history and treatment response in psychiatric disorders also speak to the need for continued research. For example, follow-up studies suggest that the long-term prognosis for patients with schizophrenia is more favorable than was formerly believed (Harding et al. 1987b; Shepherd et al. 1989), whereas the risk of chronic impairment in affective disorders is greater than previously expected (Keller et al. 1984, 1986).

The "what" and "how" questions have to do with methodological and implementation issues, the complexities of which have been well described elsewhere (Avison and Speechley 1987; Blotcky et al. 1984; Carpenter et al. 1981; Erickson 1972; Gossett 1989; McGlashan 1984a; Pfeiffer 1989; Schwartz et al.

1973; Shepard et al. 1989). As summarized by Avison and Speechley (1987), six variables for outcome are commonly used in psychiatric follow-up studies: 1) re-admission after discharge, 2) total time rehospitalized, 3) role performance (e.g., employment status), 4) social adjustment, 5) symptoms present at follow-up, and 6) global ratings. There is, however, no consensus on how to define improvement, how to measure community adjustment (Avison and Speechley 1987), or how best to utilize patient self-ratings in assessing outcome (Grob et al. 1978; McGlashan 1984a). These questions are even more complex when other variables are taken into account, such as practical constraints of funding ongoing patient assessments; tracking patients over a period of months or years following discharge; obtaining reliable and valid diagnoses in the clinical setting; and controlling for a multitude of treatment, demographic, and socioeconomic variables.

At present, there continue to be major questions about the procedures to be followed in outcome research. However, we can conclude that complete assessment of outcome must include *post-discharge* measurement of an array of factors. The post-discharge component is especially important in psychiatric studies, in contrast to medical or surgical intervention, which may be fairly evaluated at termination of the treatment if the condition is not expected to have an impact on the patient's subsequent ability to function. With many psychiatric conditions, however, impaired coping skills, family stability, and socioeconomic factors contribute to the ultimate outcome. For example, the determination can be made that a patient has recovered from an acute psychotic episode if the patient is symptom-free at discharge. But long-term follow-up is necessary to evaluate the effectiveness of the treatment in *maintaining* the improvement.

Who are the patients to be included in these studies? Most published reports focus on specific diagnostic groups, and other chapters in this volume provide detailed reviews of outcome studies in schizophrenia, depression, mania, substance abuse, borderline personality, narcissistic personality, and eating disorders. Other studies of outcome are limited to patients in particular age groups, and some investigators focus on specific factors such as predictors of rehospitalization (e.g., Rosen et al. 1971; Sandler and Jakoet 1985). Another approach is hospital-wide studies. Although a number of large-scale follow-up investigations have been described (Harding et al. 1987a; McGlashan 1984a, 1984b; Morrison et al. 1973; Winokur et al. 1972), few are prospective and incorporated into an institution's routine clinical functions. Grob and colleagues have reviewed their ongoing study of patients at the McLean Hospital (1978), and a recently implemented program at Butler Hospital (Stevenson et al. 1988) randomly selects admissions for independent evaluation and subsequent follow-up assessment.

Despite the absence of consensus as to what, how, and whom to "measure," it is clear that outcome studies are important for psychiatry. This chapter describes a model for patient evaluation that includes post-discharge assessment and incorporates the evaluation component into the routine clinical activities of the hospital. The application of the model is illustrated by data from two studies.

Post-Discharge Assessment as a Component of Clinical Care

The outcome assessment program of the Institute of Living, a private nonprofit psychiatric hospital, is designed to provide follow-up evaluation of any of the facility's inpatients. It allows for prospective study of any subset of patients regardless of clinical diagnosis, age, or assigned unit. The basic model can be expanded to provide follow-up on all consenting patients, and the program is part of the routine clinical activities of the hospital. Clinical interviewers routinely assess selected patients, and interrater reliability has been established. The interraters' work is blind to the clinicians' evaluations. Hospital staff are not required to complete additional research forms, but portions of the medical records were changed to facilitate computer entry of data to be used in outcome studies.

The clinical interviewers use standardized instruments (for example, the Diagnostic Interview Schedule [Robins et al. 1981] and the Yale-New Haven Hospital Depressive Symptom Inventory [Mazure and Nelson 1986]) as well as demographic questionnaires. For some studies clinician ratings on standardized instruments (for example, the Brief Psychiatric Rating Scale [BPRS]; Overall and Gorham 1962) are available, but no attempt has been made to establish interrater reliability among the approximately 100 staff physicians and clinical psychologists. Clinicians follow DSM-III-R (American Psychiatric Association 1987) criteria but do not routinely use standard diagnostic instruments such as the Structured Clinical Interview for DSM-III (SCID; Spitzer et al. 1985). (Symptom-specific information is available, however. Diagnostic checklists containing the criteria for each DSM-III-R diagnosis are part of the medical record.) Patient self-ratings can be obtained at admission, discharge, and follow-up, and the instruments currently used for this purpose are the Brief Symptom Inventory (BSI; Derogatis and Spencer 1982) and the Inventory to Diagnose Depression (IDD; Zimmerman et al. 1986). In some studies, follow-up data are also obtained from families and the treating clinicians.

This model has now been applied to studies of consecutive admissions to a long-term treatment service, to the evaluation of a newly organized short-term unit, to outcome determination in patients with a clinical diagnosis of major depression, and to the examination of the impact of various managed care arrangements on outcome. Preliminary data from two of these ongoing studies are presented in the following sections.

Outcome After Long-Term Hospitalization

Traditionally the Institute of Living has provided intermediate- to long-term inpatient care for severely impaired patients, many of whom have had multiple previous hospitalizations. In 1984, a follow-up study of this patient group was initiated. Inclusion criteria were all consenting patients who met the following criteria: 1) in their first Institute of Living hospitalization, 2) with a planned length of stay of 55 days or longer, and 3) ages 16–60. Findings were reported on 124 patients admitted between January 1984 and April 1986. Total admissions during this period were 2,067 (1,130 females, 937 males); 246 patients met the above criteria, but adequate follow-up data are currently available on only 124.

As shown on the accompanying tables, information was obtained from patients, families, and treating therapists at admission, discharge, and follow-up (1 year post-discharge). Patients completed the BSI and indicated level of stress and level of functioning using modified versions of DSM-III Axes IV and V. At follow-up, patients also completed a questionnaire to assess marital status, living arrangements, vocational/school activities, and current treatment, including subsequent hospitalizations. When permission was given by the patient, a similar questionnaire was sent to a family member. Family members also completed the level of stress and level of functioning scales on admission and at follow-up. The treating therapist completed a BPRS at admission, discharge, and follow-up.

Table 18–1 displays general descriptive data about the patients in the follow-up group compared to the patients lost to follow-up. The incidence of substance abuse in the latter group was significantly greater (X^2 = 6.631, df = 1, $P < .002$), and these patients were also less likely to have (or to acknowledge having) suicidal ideation, a history of a suicidal attempt (X^2 = 15.735, df = 1, $P < .001$), or a complaint of depression (X^2 = 6.956, df = 1, $P < .01$). Thus, the original sample (i.e., all patients enrolled) was not fully represented by the patients available at follow-up. The two groups were similar with respect to age, sex, marital status, previous hospitalizations, presence of psychotic symptoms (hallucinations, bizarre behavior), and reported age at onset of illness.

The patients meeting the inclusion criteria were relatively young (27.3 ± 10.6 years), and 85.2% had a history of previous inpatient treatment. Depression as a symptom (as distinct from a diagnosis of an affective disorder) was noted in the majority of patients, significantly more in the follow-up group (91.9%), but commonly among the remaining patients (80.3%) as well. The mean BSI scores at admission (Global Severity Index = 1.62 [females], 1.08 [males]) were comparable to the published norms (Derogatis and Spencer 1982) for psychiatric inpatients (1.15 [females], 0.78 [males]).

The patients can be characterized further by the diagnostic impression of the

TABLE 18–1.   Study I: patient characteristics

	Follow-up group (N = 124)		Lost to follow-up (N = 122)	
	n	(%)[a]	*n*	(%)
Sex (*N/%* female)	81	(65.3)	61	(50.0)
Married	23	(18.5)	21	(17.2)
Previous hospitalization(s)	92	(85.2)	80	(83.3)
Depression (symptom)[b]	114	(91.9)	98	(80.3)
Hallucinations	51	(41.1)	48	(39.3)
Bizarre behavior	23	(18.5)	28	(23.0)
History of				
Suicidal ideation or attempt[b]	91	(73.4)	60	(49.2)
Substance abuse[b]	58	(46.8)	77	(63.1)
Violence	36	(29.0)	33	(27.1)
Antisocial behavior	50	(40.7)	62	(50.8)
Occupation				
Housewife	7	(5.6)	7	(5.7)
Self-employed	2	(1.6)	3	(2.5)
Skilled[b]	40	(32.3)	19	(15.6)
Unskilled	4	(3.2)	3	(2.5)
Student[b]	40	(32.3)	55	(45.1)
Unemployed	30	(24.2)	33	(27.1)
Other	1	(0.8)	0	
Age	27.3 ± 10.6		26.1 ± 12.6	

[a] Not all measures are available on all patients; percentage represents percentage of sample for whom a given measure is available.
[b] Statistically significant differences between groups (*P* < .01).

treating clinician (Table 18–2), although the value of this information for comparative purposes is limited because diagnoses were not based on structured interviews.

Table 18–3 summarizes outcome measures available on patients at discharge, and the follow-up measures are shown in Table 18–4. By patient rating, 78.8% of the sample showed a superior to good level of functioning at discharge, whereas the clinicians' global rating on discharge indicated that 54% of patients had a good outcome and an additional 27.4% were moderately improved. At follow-up, 62.6% of patients considered themselves to be functioning in the superior to good range, whereas family ratings suggested that 51.9% were functioning at this level. Clinician ratings at follow-up, available on only 66 patients, indicated superior to good functioning in 34.9% of these patients. Of the 38 patients not in therapy at follow-up, 76.5% rated their level of functioning in the superior to good range, compared to 55.8% of the 86 patients still in

TABLE 18–2. Study I: primary discharge diagnoses

	n	(%)[a]
Major depression	30	(24.2)
Dysthymic disorder	20	(16.1)
Schizophrenia	14	(11.3)
Personality disorder	31	(25.0)
Bipolar disorder	8	(6.5)
Schizoaffective disorder	6	(4.8)
Substance abuse	2	(1.6)
Conduct disorder	4	(3.2)
Other[a]	9	(7.3)

[a] 2 or fewer patients in each of 7 diagnostic categories.

treatment ($r = .17$, df = 120, $P < .03$).

Figure 18–1 displays the BSI and BPRS global scales at admission, discharge, and follow-up. The change scores on the three BSI global scales between each of these time points are shown in Table 18–5. There was statistically significant improvement on all measures both at discharge and at follow-up compared to admission, although on some scales there was a worsening of symptoms from discharge to follow-up. The patients' global self-ratings were highly correlated with each of the BSI global scales ($r = .642$, df = 122, $P < .001$ for the GSI; $r = .565$, df = 122, $P < .001$ for the PSDI; $r = .598$, df = 122, $P < .001$ for the PST). Although this finding is not surprising, for purposes of outcome measurement it is useful to demonstrate that global assessment is highly correlated ($P < .001$) with a standardized inventory of specific symptoms. Patients' ratings were also correlated with therapists' ratings of functioning based on Axis V

TABLE 18–3. Study I: measures of outcome at discharge

	n	(%)[a]
Condition on discharge (clinician rated)		
Good	67	(54.0)
Moderate	34	(27.4)
Poor	23	(18.6)
Patient rated functioning		
Superior–good	98	(78.8)
Fair	16	(13.6)
Poor–grossly impaired	9	(7.6)
Mean BPRS (total score)	21.2 ± 12.6	
Mean GSI	0.771 ± 0.645	

[a] Not all measures are available on all patients; percentage represents percentage of sample for whom a given measure is available.

($r = .494$, df = 66, $P < .001$).

Table 18–6 summarizes patients' status at follow-up. Using these vocational/social measures of functioning, most patients appear to have adjusted at least reasonably well in the community, with 70% working full- or part-time, 74% indicating that they enjoy leisure time, and 83% indicating that they have friends.

These results show the characteristics and outcome, both at discharge and at 1-year follow-up, of patients treated in a highly specialized psychiatric setting. Therapy was multimodal, and the efficacy of any single type of treatment (e.g., medication versus intensive psychotherapy) cannot be assessed. However, the data indicate that as a group the patients were improved at discharge and that the improvement was sustained. Depending on the measure used, 35–74% had a "good" outcome at 1-year follow-up. "Poor," or at least suboptimal, outcome is suggested in at least 7.6% of the sample (based on patient rated functioning at discharge) and in a maximum of 28.8% (therapist rated functioning at follow-up). Twenty-five patients (20.2%) were rehospitalized during the year following discharge. Although they were not necessarily diagnostically similar to patients

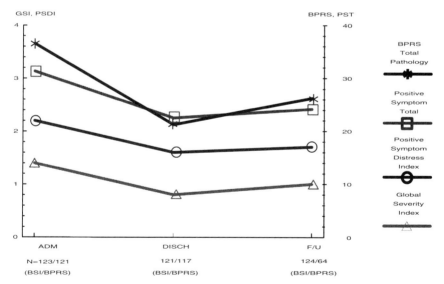

* All ADM vs DISCH and ADM vs follow-up (F/U) differences were significant at $P < .001$.
DISCH vs follow-up was significant at $P < .01$ for BPRS and GSI only.

FIGURE 18–1. Brief Symptom Inventory and Brief Psychiatric Rating Scale global scales at admission, discharge, and follow-up.

TABLE 18–4.   Study I: measures of outcome at follow-up

	n	(%)[a]
Global self-rating		
Good	86	(70.5)
Moderate	17	(13.9)
Poor	19	(15.6)
Global rating by family		
Good	62	(73.8)
Moderate	13	(15.5)
Poor	9	(10.7)
Patient rated functioning		
Superior–good	77	(62.6)
Fair	28	(22.8)
Poor–grossly impaired	18	(14.6)
Family rated functioning		
Superior–good	41	(51.9)
Fair	30	(38.0)
Poor–grossly impaired	8	(10.1)
Physician rated functioning		
Superior–good	23	(34.9)
Fair	24	(36.4)
Poor–grossly impaired	19	(28.8)
Mean BPRS (total score)	26.2 ± 15.6	
Mean Global Severity Index	0.969 ± 0.897	

[a] Not all measures are available on all patients; percentage represents percentage of sample for whom a given measure is available.

in other published reports, the proportion of patients in our sample who continue to be substantially impaired is consistent with results from other follow-up studies. Shepherd and colleagues (1989) found a readmission rate of 21% among schizophrenic patients, and McGlashan (1984b) reported "severe social impairment" in 19% of a mixed group of schizophrenic and affectively ill patients. Only 8% of patients in the latter study were symptom-free at follow-up.

TABLE 18–5.   Study I: change in BSI global scores

	Admission to discharge (df = 119)		Admission to follow-up (df = 122)		Discharge to follow-up (df = 120)	
	t	P	t	P	t	P
Global Severity Index	9.01	.001	5.43	.001	−2.79	.006
Positive Symptom Total (PST)	7.07	.001	4.97	.001	−1.22	.224
PST Index	9.11	.001	6.30	.001	−1.62	.109

TABLE 18–6. Study I: status at follow-up

	n	(%)[a]
Vocational status		
Full time	50	(42.0)
Part time	34	(28.6)
Not working outside home	35	(29.4)
Educational status		
Full time	23	(18.5)
Part time	13	(10.5)
Not in school	88	(71.0)
Neither work nor school	22	(18.6)
Have friends	103	(83.1)
Enjoy leisure time	92	(74.2)
Taking medications	71	(57.3)
In therapy	86	(69.4)
Rehospitalized	25	(20.2)

[a] Not all measures are available on all patients; percentage represents percentage of sample for whom a given measure is available.

Short-Term Hospitalization: Program Evaluation and Follow-up

In 1988, a 3-month study of consecutive admissions to a newly established short-term treatment service was undertaken to evaluate outcome after relatively brief inpatient treatment. All patients were interviewed at admission and discharge using a modified version of the Yale-New Haven Hospital Depressive Symptom Inventory, a semistructured interview that provides scores for the Hamilton Depression Rating Scale (HDRS; Hamilton 1960), Hamilton Anxiety Scale (HAS; Hamilton 1959), and the BPRS. The characteristics and symptom profiles of patients at admission and discharge are presented here; follow-up data are now being collected.

Ninety-seven patients were admitted to this service during the study period. Eighty-five of the 97 were interviewed within 3 days of admission, and 67 of these were also interviewed at discharge. The 12 patients not seen on admission refused to participate or were discharged within 48 hours. Eighteen patients initially evaluated withdrew consent or were discharged without notice.

As seen in Table 18–7, the group of patients evaluated at both admission and discharge (*n* = 67) appears to be a valid subsample of the larger group. The mean

TABLE 18–7. Study II: patient characteristics[a]

	Assessed at admission n = 85		Assessed at admission and discharge n = 67	
Age	36.5 ± 14.86		36.8 ± 15.0	
Sex (n/% female)	42	(49.4)	31	(46.3)
Married	37	(43.5)	28	(41.8)
Race (n/% white)	71	(83.5)	57	(85.1)
Education				
n/% attending or completed college	30	(35.3)	24	(35.8)
n/% < high school	26	(30.6)	20	(29.9)
Occupation				
Academic	8	(9.4)	4	(6.0)
Clergy	3	(3.5)	3	(4.5)
Health professional	2	(2.4)	1	(1.5)
Housewife	30	(35.3)	26	(38.8)
Management	9	(10.6)	6	(9.0)
Self-employed	16	(18.8)	13	(19.4)
Other, missing	17	(20.0)	14	(20.9)

[a] 67 of 85 patients interviewed at admission and discharge; 2 groups—not significantly different by t-tests, chi-squares on any variable.

age was 36.8 ± 15 years, and the numbers of males and females were approximately equal. The five clinicians working on this unit did not routinely use standardized means of assigning diagnoses, but diagnosis is a useful general descriptor of the population (Table 18–8). The primary diagnosis in 43.3% of the patients was a major affective disorder, with substance abuse diagnosed as primary in 26.8%. The frequencies and percentages of symptoms present based on the standardized ratings are shown in Tables 18–9, 18–10, and 18–11. These data also provide symptom profiles of the sample and a baseline from which

TABLE 18–8. Study II: primary discharge diagnoses

	n	(%)
Schizophrenia	2	(3.0)
Schizophreniform disorder	1	(1.5)
Schizoaffective	6	(9.0)
Major depression	22	(32.9)
Bipolar disorder	7	(10.4)
Other psychosis	3	(4.5)
Dysthymic disorder	5	(7.5)
Substance abuse or dependence	18	(26.8)
Adjustment disorder	1	(1.5)
Conduct disorders	1	(1.5)
Organic personality disorder	1	(1.5)

symptomatic change can be calculated.

The mean total score at admission on the HDRS was 19.18 ± 9.59, which suggests a moderate to severe level of illness. As noted by Endicott and colleagues (1981), a total score greater than 24 is consistent with severe depression in hospitalized patients, whereas scores less than 6 indicate essentially no depression. The mean HDRS score for our patients at discharge was 8.67 ± 6.18 (t = 9.04; P < .001), indicating that depressive symptoms remained but at a greatly reduced level.

The mean anxiety score at admission was 15.09 ± 8.09 and at discharge, 7.46 ± 5.30 (t = 8.20; P < .001). A score of 15 or greater on the HAS has been used to distinguish major from minor anxiety (Bech et al. 1986). As with the depression

TABLE 18–9.   Study II: symptoms present—Hamilton Depression Rating Scale[a]

Symptom	Admission		Discharge	
	n	(%)[b]	n	(%)
Psychic anxiety	55	(83.3)	39	(58.2)
Depressed mood	53	(79.1)	32	(47.8)
Somatic anxiety	52	(78.8)	35	(52.2)
Agitation	49	(73.1)	33	(50.0)
Guilt	47	(72.3)	27	(40.9)
Loss of interest	43	(66.2)	19	(28.4)
Worthlessness	39	(61.9)	23	(34.8)
Somatic general	39	(58.2)	26	(39.4)
Insomnia middle	36	(57.1)	19	(28.8)
Helplessness	35	(55.6)	21	(31.8)
Hopelessness	35	(53.8)	15	(23.1)
Hypochondriasis	33	(50.0)	28	(42.4)
Insomnia initial	33	(51.6)	18	(27.7)
Paranoid symptoms	31	(47.0)	16	(24.2)
Weight loss	28	(43.1)	13	(20.0)
Somatic gastrointestinal	27	(40.3)	10	(14.9)
Suicide	24	(36.9)	2	(3.0)
Insomnia delayed	22	(35.5)	10	(15.2)
Loss of insight	24	(35.8)	18	(26.9)
Decreased libido	12	(19.0)	3	(4.5)
Obsessional symptoms	11	(17.2)	3	(4.5)
Diurnal variation				
worse in a.m.	9	(14.5)	6	(9.4)
worse in p.m.	9	(14.5)	6	(14.1)
Retardation	8	(11.9)	3	(4.5)
Depersonalization	7	(10.9)	5	(7.7)

[a] Symptoms present, however slight.
[b] Not all measures are available on all patients; percentage represents percentage of sample for whom a given measure is available.

TABLE 18–10. Study II: symptoms present—Hamilton Anxiety Scale[a]

Symptom	Admission		Discharge	
	n	(%)[b]	n	(%)
Behavior at interview	58	(86.6)	45	(67.2)
Anxious mood	56	(83.6)	45	(67.2)
Depressed mood	53	(79.1)	32	(47.8)
Tension	52	(77.6)	27	(40.9)
Insomnia	48	(73.8)	30	(45.5)
Intellectual (cognitive)	40	(64.5)	19	(28.8)
Somatic (muscular)	36	(55.4)	23	(34.3)
Autonomic	35	(53.0)	24	(35.8)
Cardiovascular	29	(43.9)	11	(16.4)
Respiratory	27	(41.5)	6	(9.0)
Gastrointestinal	25	(39.1)	22	(33.8)
Somatic (sensory)	17	(26.2)	9	(13.6)
Fears	11	(16.9)	13	(20.0)
Genitourinary	7	(10.6)	1	(1.5)

[a] Symptoms present, however slight.
[b] Not all measures are available on all patients; percentage represents percentage of sample for whom a given measure is available.

TABLE 18–11. Study II: symptoms present—Brief Psychiatric Rating Scale[a]

Symptom	Admission		Discharge	
	n	(%)[b]	n	(%)
Anxiety	58	(86.6)	51	(76.1)
Tension	57	(85.1)	45	(67.2)
Depressive mood	54	(80.6)	37	(55.2)
Guilt feelings	49	(74.2)	30	(45.5)
Hostility	47	(70.1)	39	(58.2)
Somatic concern	40	(59.7)	37	(55.2)
Suspiciousness	31	(48.4)	13	(19.7)
Uncooperativeness	30	(44.8)	15	(22.4)
Emotional withdrawal	30	(44.8)	19	(28.4)
Blunted affect	23	(34.3)	7	(10.6)
Grandiosity	19	(29.7)	12	(17.9)
Excitement	19	(28.4)	14	(20.9)
Disorientation	12	(18.5)	4	(6.1)
Hallucinatory behavior	9	(13.8)	0	(0.0)
Unusual thought content	9	(13.8)	4	(6.0)
Conceptual disorganization	9	(13.4)	2	(3.0)
Motor retardation	8	(11.9)	2	(3.0)
Mannerisms	1	(1.5)	4	(6.0)

[a] Symptoms present, however slight.
[b] Not all measures are available on all patients; percentage represents percentage of sample for whom a given measure is available.

scores, minor symptoms persisted at discharge in these patients but were significantly decreased. Similarly, the BPRS mean score decreased from 16.05 ± 7.73 at admission to 8.27 ± 4.25 at discharge ($t = 8.30$; $P < .001$).

Three high-risk subgroups were of special interest: dual diagnosis patients, patients with suicidal ideation, and patients with severe depression. In the dual diagnosis subgroup, major depression was the most frequent concurrent disorder (12 of 21). Tables 18–12 and 18–13 compare patients with depression alone, with substance abuse alone, and with the two disorders concurrently. As postulated, the dual diagnosis patients were more symptomatic at admission, with significantly higher scores on the depression and anxiety scales (Table 18–12). At discharge, however, there were no differences between groups in any of the ratings (Table 18–13). Thus, outcome appears to be no less favorable for the patients with dual diagnoses, but this finding has not yet been validated in the post-discharge follow-up.

A similar analysis was conducted with patients having suicidal ideation (Table 18–14). Compared to all other patients in the sample, the suicidal group had significantly higher depression and anxiety scores at admission; but at discharge the mean ratings for the two groups were not significantly different. Longer-term follow-up is needed to determine the ultimate outcome of the suicidal patients, but the presence of suicidal ideation and higher mean scores at admission does not appear to predict status at discharge. There were no between-group differences in lengths of stay (27.04 versus 23.39 days, $t = .95$, NS), age (33.92 versus 38.88, $t = 1.33$, NS), or sex ($X^2 = .0885$, df = 1, NS).

In order to define a subgroup of depressed patients independent of clinician diagnosis, an admission HDRS score greater than 24 was used as an indicator of

TABLE 18–12. Study II: dual diagnosis patients mean ratings at admission

	Dual diagnosis $n = 12$ mean score	MDD[a] alone $n = 13$ mean score	Substance abuse $n = 13$ mean score	All patients $n = 67$ mean score
HDRS	30.50 ± 6.99^b	20.46 ± 10.64	18.00 ± 5.93	19.18 ± 9.59
HAS	23.83 ± 5.31^c	17.31 ± 7.45	12.77 ± 6.27	15.09 ± 8.09
BPRS	17.67 ± 6.05	13.92 ± 5.87	13.38 ± 4.68	16.05 ± 7.73

[a] MDD = major depressive disorder.
[b] Significantly different from major depression alone ($t = 2.81$; $P < .05$) and substance abuse alone ($t = 4.80$; $P < .000$) using t-tests.
[c] Significantly different from major depression alone ($t = 2.54$; $P < .05$) and substance abuse alone ($t = 4.77$; $P < .000$) using t-tests.
Note. Assessment instruments are the Hamilton Depression Rating Scale (HDRS), the Hamilton Anxiety Scale (HAS), and the Brief Psychiatric Rating Scale (BPRS).

TABLE 18–13. Study II: dual diagnosis patients mean ratings at discharge[a]

	Dual diagnosis $n = 12$ mean score	MDD[b] alone $n = 13$ mean score	Substance abuse $n = 13$ mean score	All patients $n = 67$ mean score
HDRS	11.75 ± 7.34	7.77 ± 5.45	10.46 ± 8.58	8.67 ± 6.18
HAS	10.42 ± 5.35	7.54 ± 6.79	8.00 ± 6.80	7.46 ± 5.30
BPRS	9.67 ± 4.19	6.77 ± 4.01	8.15 ± 4.38	8.27 ± 4.25

[a] No significant differences by *t*-tests.
[b] MDD = major depressive disorder.
Note. Assessment instruments are the Hamilton Depression Rating Scale (HDRS), the Hamilton Anxiety Scale (HAS), and the Brief Psychiatric Rating Scale (BPRS).

severe depression. These patients were significantly more anxious and had higher BPRS scores than the remaining patients (Table 18–15). The two groups did not differ in lengths of stay (28.79 versus 23.54, $t = 1.10$, NS), age (38.235 versus 36.26, $t = .52$, NS), or sex ($X^2 = .8469$, df = 1, NS). At discharge, there were no significant differences in any of the total scale scores, suggesting that outcome (i.e., number and severity of symptoms at discharge) is just as favorable for the more seriously depressed patients. Post-discharge assessment will determine if relapse is greater in the severe group.

These data indicate that patients admitted to this unit are moderately to severely ill, with elevated ratings on three scales of psychiatric symptomatology. As a group, the patients showed significant symptomatic improvement. Three subgroups at potentially greater risk for poor outcome were indistinguishable

TABLE 18–14. Study II: patients with suicidal ideation

	Present $n = 24$ mean score	Absent $n = 41$ mean score	*t*-value
HDRS			
admission	26.63 ± 9.72	15.07 ± 6.50	$t = 5.18; P < .000$
discharge	10.54 ± 8.26	7.63 ± 4.52	$t = 1.59$; NS
HAS			
admission	19.58 ± 7.93	12.61 ± 7.07	$t = 3.56; P < .001$
discharge	8.58 ± 5.89	6.83 ± 5.02	$t = 1.22$; NS
BPRS			
admission	17.08 ± 6.30	15.76 ± 8.54	$t = .72$; NS
discharge	8.92 ± 4.43	7.83 ± 4.22	$t = .97$; NS

Note. Assessment instruments are the Hamilton Depression Rating Scale (HDRS), the Hamilton Anxiety Scale (HAS), and the Brief Psychiatric Rating Scale (BPRS).

TABLE 18–15. Study II: patients with severe depression

	HDRS < 25 $n = 17$ mean score	HDRS < 25 $n = 50$ mean score	t-value
HDRS			
admission	32.41 ± 5.22	14.68 ± 5.79	$t = 11.76; P < .00$
discharge	10.41 ± 6.45	8.08 ± 6.03	$t = 1.31; NS$
HAS			
admission	23.82 ± 4.72	12.12 ± 6.75	$t = 7.85; P < .00$
discharge	8.88 ± 5.18	6.98 ± 5.31	$t = 1.30; NS$
BPRS			
admission	19.29 ± 6.19	14.94 ± 7.95	$t = 2.32; P < .05$
discharge	9.00 ± 3.45	8.02 ± 4.50	$t = .93; NS$

Note. Assessment instruments are the Hamilton Depression Rating Scale (HDRS), the Hamilton Anxiety Scale (HAS), and the Brief Psychiatric Rating Scale (BPRS).

from the remaining sample by the time of discharge.

This information about the distribution of patients by diagnosis, illness severity scores, and symptom profiles has been helpful in program planning and in determining treatment response. Additional clinical outcome data on these patients will be available when the follow-up component is complete.

Conclusion

The model presented is a practical approach to outcome assessment that has been successfully implemented in a large psychiatric hospital. Key features of the model are an evaluation component that has been incorporated into routine patient care, a clear definition of what symptom and sociodemographic data will be obtained, and delineation of how initial and follow-up assessments will be conducted. The model includes independent evaluations completed at several points in time, as well as patients' self-assessments. The basic model, illustrated in the studies we have discussed in this chapter, is easily expanded or modified. This program has evolved over several years and reflects a number of failed as well as successful data collection efforts. Subsequent experience and advances in the field can lead to further revisions in procedures and instruments used. In addition, greater utilization of computerized data is planned, including incorporating into the model an "expert system" component developed at the Institute of Living (Bronzino et al. 1989; Goethe et al. 1990; Morelli et al. 1989).

Some research questions cannot be addressed without control groups and more extensive patient assessment. However, studies such as those described provide important information for the field. As Schwartz and colleagues (1973) observed, "outcome research in nonexperimental situations can be a vital accompaniment to controlled studies of treatment outcome and has the potential for serving basic and applied research needs" (p. 102).

References

American Psychiatric Association: Diagnostic and Statistical Manual of Mental Disorders, 3rd Edition, Revised. Washington, DC, American Psychiatric Association, 1987

Avison WR, Speechley KN: The discharged psychiatric patient: A review of social, social-psychological, and psychiatric correlates of outcome. Am J Psychiatry 144:10–18, 1987

Bech P, Kastrup M, Rafaelson OJ: Mini-compendium of rating scales for states of anxiety, depression, mania, schizophrenia with corresponding DMS-III syndromes. Acta Psychiatr Scand Suppl 326:7–36, 1986

Blotcky MJ, Dimperio TL, Gossett JT: Follow-up of children treated in psychiatric hospitals. A review of the studies. Am J Psychiatry 141:1499–1507, 1984

Bronzino JD, Morelli RA, Goethe JW: Overseer: A prototype expert system for monitoring drug treatment in the psychiatric clinic. IEEE Trans Biomed Eng 36:533–540, 1989

Carpenter WE, Heinrichs DW, Hanlon TE: Methodologic standards for treatment outcome research in schizophrenia. Am J Psychiatry 138:465–471, 1981

Council on Medical Service: Quality of care. JAMA 256:1032–1034, 1986

Derogatis LR, Spencer PM: The Brief Symptom Inventory (BSI) Administration, Scoring & Procedures Manual I. Baltimore, MD, Clinical Psychometric Research, 1982

Endicott J, Cohen J, Nee J, et al: Hamilton Depression Rating Scale. Arch Gen Psychiatry 38:98–103, 1981

Erickson RC: Outcome studies in mental hospitals: A search for criteria. J Consult Clin Psychol 39:75–77, 1972

Goethe JW, Bronzino JD, Morelli RA: Clinical excellence in psychiatry: A computer model. Presented at the annual meeting of the American Psychiatric Association, New York, May 1990

Gossett JT: Hospital outcome studies in the 21st century. The Psychiatric Hospital 20:11–12, 1989

Grob MC, Eisen SV, Berman JS: Three years of follow-up monitoring: Perspectives of formerly hospitalized patients and their families. Compr Psychiatry 19:491–499, 1978

Hamilton M: The assessment of anxiety states by rating. Br J Med Psychol 32:50–55, 1959

Hamilton M: A rating scale for depression. J Neurol Neurosurg Psychiatry 23:56–62, 1960

Harding CM, Brooks GW, Ashikaga T, et al: The Vermont longitudinal study of persons with severe mental illness, I: Methodology, study sample, and overall status 32 years later. Am J Psychiatry 144:718–726, 1987a

Harding CM, Brooks GW, Ashikaga T, et al: The Vermont longitudinal study of persons with severe mental illness, II: Long-term outcome of subjects who retrospectively met DSM-III criteria for schizophrenia. Am J Psychiatry 144:727–735, 1987b

Joint Commission on Accreditation of Healthcare Organizations: Agenda for Change Update. Chicago, Joint Commission on Accreditation of Healthcare Organizations, June 1988

Joint Commission of Accreditation of Hospitals: JCAH catapults QA into a new era with shift to outcomes. Hospital Peer Review 11:121–125, 1986

Keller MB, Klerman GI, Lavori PW, et al: Long-term outcome of episodes of major depression. JAMA 252:788–792, 1984

Keller MB, Lavori PW, Rice J, et al: The persistent risk of chronicity in recurrent episodes of nonbipolar major depressive disorder: A prospective follow-up. Am J Psychiatry 143:24–28, 1986

Mazure C, Nelson JC, Price LH: Reliability and validity of the symptoms of major depressive illness. Arch Gen Psychiatry 43:451–456, 1986

McGlashan TH: The Chestnut Lodge follow-up study: I. Follow-up methodology and study sample. Arch Gen Psychiatry 41:573–585, 1984a

McGlashan TH: The Chestnut Lodge follow-up study: II. Long-term outcome of schizophrenia and the affective disorders. Arch Gen Psychiatry 41:586–601, 1984b

Morelli RA, Bronzino JD, Goethe JW, et al: Incorporating a language/action design perspective into a computer-based psychiatric alerting system. Proceedings of the 13th Annual Symposium on Computer Applications in Medical Care 129–132, 1989

Morrison J, Winokur G, Crowe R, et al: The Iowa 500: The first follow-up. Arch Gen Psychiatry 29:678–682, 1973

Overall JE, Gorham DR: The Brief Psychiatric Rating Scale. Psychol Rep 10:799–812, 1962

Pfeiffer SI: Follow-up of children and adolescents treated in psychiatric facilities: A methodology review. The Psychiatric Hospital 20:15–20, 1989

Robins LE, Helzer JE, Croughan J, et al: National Institutes of Mental Health Diagnostic Interview Schedule. Arch Gen Psychiatry 38:381–389, 1981

Rosen B, Klein DF, Gittleman-Klein R: The prediction of rehospitalization: The relationship between age of first psychiatric treatment contact, marital status and premorbid asocial adjustment. J Nerv Ment Dis 152:17–22, 1971

Sandler R, Jakoet A: Outcome after discharge from a psychiatric hospital. S Afr Med J 68:470–472, 1985

Schwartz CC, Myers JK, Astrachan BM: The outcome study in psychiatric evaluation research. Arch Gen Psychiatry 29:98–102, 1973

Shepherd M, Watt D, Falloon I, et al: The natural history of schizophrenia: A five-year follow-up. Psychol Med Monogr Suppl 15:1–46, 1989

Spitzer RL, Williams JBW, Gibbon M: Instruction manual for the Structured Clinical Interview for DSM-III-R (SCID, revision). Biometrics Research Department, New York State Psychiatric Institute, New York, 1985

Stevenson JF, Beattie MC, Alves RR, et al: An outcome monitoring system for psychiatric inpatient care. QRB 14:326–331, 1988

Winokur G, Morrison J, Clancy J, et al: The Iowa 500 II: A blind family history comparison of mania, depression, and schizophrenia. Arch Gen Psychiatry 27:462–464,1972

Zimmerman M, Coryell W, Corenthal C, et al: A self-report scale to diagnose major depressive disorder. Arch Gen Psychiatry 43:1076–1080, 1986

❖ 19 ❖

Assessing the Outcome of Managing Costs: An Exploratory Approach

Steven S. Sharfstein, M.D.

Reimbursement policy is having an increased role on reconfiguring the mental health service delivery system, especially the role of the psychiatric hospital. Benefit limits and managed care are shaping clinical decisions. An ongoing exploratory study on the outcome of economically-driven limitations on patient care is being conducted in one private psychiatric hospital, The Sheppard and Enoch Pratt Hospital. The major objective of this study is to examine the impact of health insurance benefit packages and managed care on inpatient treatment and patient outcome. The specific hypotheses to be tested are as follows:

1. Accelerated discharge planning required by limitations on benefits or concurrent utilization review makes the implementation of a discharge plan less effective, leads to less patient satisfaction, and is associated with poorer outcome, including a higher readmission rate as compared to cases where such constrictions are not operating.
2. With respect to these variables, the differences between patients whose inpatient episode has been shortened (either by an insurance benefit limitation or managed care), as compared to those patients not subject to premature discharge, will increase over time in the 15-, 65-, and 170-day follow-up periods.
3. These differences will hold even when researchers control for diagnosis, socioeconomic status of the patient, severity of condition, length of stay, or level of improvement achieved during the hospitalization.

The author would like to give special thanks to Carl I. Thistel, A.C.S.W., Gerald A. Whitmarsh, Ph.D., Jerod L. Scott, M.D., Norm Ringle, M.A., Rick Parente, Ph.D., Diane K. Brandt, B.S., Barbara A. Slusher, M.S.W., and Mark Geisler, B.A., who have contributed greatly to this study.

Background

Insurance for psychiatric hospitalization has been characterized by "inside limits," that is, benefit restrictions greater than those imposed for general medical hospitalization (Brady et al. 1986; Sharfstein 1984, 1985). There is evidence that additional lifetime, yearly, and day limits have been introduced in recent years. From 1983 to 1986, inside limits for psychiatric coverage increased. Beneficiaries with equal coverage for inpatient, psychiatric, and general medical treatment declined significantly during this 3-year period. Beneficiaries with equal coverage for inpatient care dropped from 53% in 1983 to only 37% in 1986. This drop in percentage of participants in employee health plans with equal coverage may represent a deterioration in the actual level of psychiatric coverage, such as additional copayments, day or visit limits, annual dollar limits, and/or lifetime limits (American Psychiatric Association, Office of Economic Affairs 1989). In addition to more limits, there has been more aggressive concurrent utilization review in managed care. It is estimated that more than half of the patients with indemnity insurance have a managed care program in which nurse and physician reviewers interact with clinical staff in an effort to shorten lengths of stay in the hospital. As lengths of stay have decreased because of these pressures, what has been the impact on patients and their families?

Providers are increasingly being put at financial risk when they admit patients with very limited benefits and/or who are under review by a managed care program. A particular concern centers on the treatment of the "catastrophic case": those patients who, due to clinical and social factors, are treatment-resistant and economically dependent and who present problems related to safety and social control. Many of these patients can now be found homeless in America (Sharfstein 1987, 1989). As patients are forced out of the hospital because of economic limitations or managed care pressure, has discharge planning become compromised? Is the rehospitalization rate going up? Are the outcomes of the hospital episode worse because of premature discharge as a result of these economic limitations? The study we are conducting at Sheppard Pratt focuses on the outcome of premature discharge necessitated by economic rather than clinical factors, utilizing a prospective, double-blind follow-up methodology.

Most studies have found no differences in the outcomes of short- and long-stay hospitalizations (Caton and Gralnick 1987). This is true whether studies are uncontrolled (Caton 1982; Gordon and Breakey 1983; Hibbard and Trimboli 1982) or controlled (Caffey et al. 1971; Glick et al. 1975; Hargreaves et al. 1977; Herz et al. 1979; Hirsch et al. 1979; Kennedy and Hird 1980; Mattes et al. 1977). Thus, the available studies indicate that the outcome of brief hospitalization is not necessarily better than that of long-term hospitalization, but neither is it worse, at least for some patients. Coupled with the economic advantage of short-term hospitalization, this has led to the widespread adoption of brief hospitalization policies and has fueled the managed care debate (Kirschner 1982; Mattes 1982). This study does not compare the outcome of brief versus longer stays in the hospital but will eventually control for length of stay. There is little work on the impact of economic constraints such as benefit limitations and managed care on patient outcome, regardless of length of stay.

The Study

In 1987, I circulated a memorandum to the clinical staff of Sheppard Pratt asking for instances of problems in clinical care due to insurance limitations or managed care denials. Over the next 6-month period, 30 anecdotal case reports were accumulated and results reported (Sharfstein et al. 1988).

In August 1988, the present study was launched when patients were routinely asked for their permission to have us contact them 15 days after discharge. The focus of this particular telephone survey was on the implementation of the discharge plan, an assessment having been made within a week of discharge by the social worker on the service as to the degree of influence of insurance limitations on discharge planning. We determined that longer follow-up periods of 65 and 170 days were practical as well, and that the available base of 1,300 adult admissions yearly would allow a large enough number of patients to be enrolled in a formal follow-up effort with adequate comparisons to test several hypotheses. The initial results of this ongoing investigation are presented in a later section of this chapter. I view them as suggestive rather than conclusive in light of the pilot status of the project.

Methodology

All adult inpatients are notified of a post-discharge contact procedure designed to help the hospital assess the quality of its work. All are asked to sign a consent form at the time of admission allowing for such follow-up. Within a week of the patient's discharge, the staff on each unit, specifically the unit social worker and service chief, are asked to evaluate the extent to which insurance or other related economic factors have had a disruptive or intrusive impact on the planning process. A disruptive insurance factor (DIF) is defined as any outside event or decision that has a disruptive impact on the care planning process in such a way that the patient's discharge is hastened. Specifically, we look for the following factors:

1. Benefit limits became more restrictive than was known at the time of initial care planning.
2. Managed care or recertification decisions during the course of treatment shortened the patient's length of stay.
3. A problematic concurrent review hastened discharge.
4. Mounting hospitalization costs to the patient and family hastened discharge.
5. Any combination of the above factors existed.

The initial rating by the social worker and service chief is used to form two groups, the first consisting of those with disruptive insurance factors significantly affecting discharge or treatment planning, and the second, those patients for whom factors did not affect discharge planning in a significant way. This rating is then put in a secure file. A social work student who is blind to the initial assessment calls the patients at 15, 65, and 170 days for a post-discharge contact. The follow-up phone call is made in order for the social work student to fill out a post-discharge contact report.

For purposes of this report, the workability of the discharge plan is ascertained as follows:

1. The patient's compliance with the plan;
2. The patient's own self-assessment as to how he or she is doing;
3. The patient's opinion as to whether the plan is working; and
4. The rater's overall assessment.

Positive responses in all four aspects are the basis for defining the discharge plan as working.

The Sample

The sample reported here (Post-Discharge Contact, PDC) consists of 332 patients, which represents 14.2% of the total adult discharges from Sheppard Pratt between August 1988 and February 1990. The patient population is profiled in Table 19–1. It *did not differ significantly* from the general population by age, gender, or primary admitting diagnosis.

At the 15-day contact point, 242 or 72.9% of the sample were contacted and responded; at the 65-day point, 172 or 51.8%; and at the 170-day point, 127 or 38.3%. As this is an ongoing study enrolling additional patients, the numbers will continue to grow, especially in the 65- and 170-day categories.

TABLE 19–1. Sample profile (N = 332)—sex, age, diagnoses

	n	*%*
Sex		
Male	183	55
Female	149	45
Age		
< 20	25	8
20–29	85	26
30–39	95	29
40–49	44	14
50–59	25	8
60–69	20	6
70+	33	9
Primary admitting diagnosis		
Depressive disorder	125	39
Schizophrenia	61	19
Bipolar	48	15
Substance abuse	24	8
Personality disorder	10	3
Adjustment disorder	8	3
Eating disorder	10	3
Anxiety disorder	3	1
Other	28	9

The Results

The results of the study are summarized in Figures 19–1 through 19–5.

All the results examine various parameters by whether or not there was a DIF. For purposes of this study, a *P* value of .05 or less is considered significant. Figure 19–1 shows that we had patients with and without disruptive insurance factors in all length of stay categories, including the longer lengths of stay of 46 or more days. In the longer length of stay periods, a greater proportion of patients had no DIF.

Figure 19–2 addresses the question of discharge plan working by disruptive insurance factor. The data are presented only for those patients for whom the plan was working. Thus, for example, plans were working for 82% of patients with no disruptive insurance factor at the 15-day contact interval, whereas only 62% of plans were working for the same contact interval for the DIF group. At each of the three time points—15, 65, and 170 days—discharge plans were working less well for patients with disruptive insurance factors (significant at all three levels, $P < .02$ for 15 days, and $P < .01$ for 65 and 170 days).

Satisfaction data are presented in Figure 19–3 for those who expressed a clear

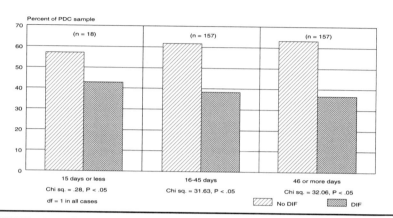

FIGURE 19–1. Patient length of stay by DIF.

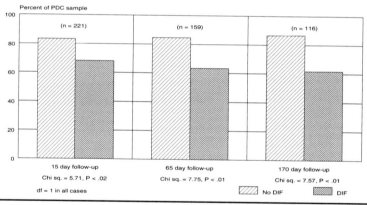

FIGURE 19–2. Discharge plans working by DIF.

statement of degree of satisfaction. In contrast to DIF patients, a significantly higher proportion of no disruptive insurance factor (non-DIF) patients stated they were very satisfied with the treatment. Figure 19–4 illustrates the global outcome assessment, or the patients' general well-being. Although equivalent at 15 days, at 65 and 170 days the patients' general well-being was one order of magnitude greater if there had been no disruptive insurance factor.

Figure 19–5 addresses the important question of readmissions by disruptive insurance factor. Although there were more readmissions as a percentage of the total sample among those with a disruptive insurance factor, the difference was not statistically significant.

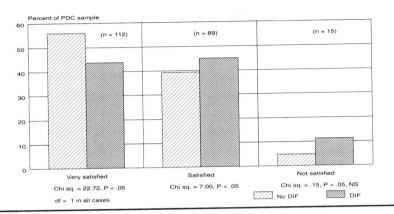

FIGURE 19–3. Patient satisfaction by DIF.

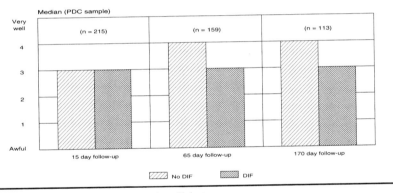

FIGURE 19–4. Patients' general well-being.

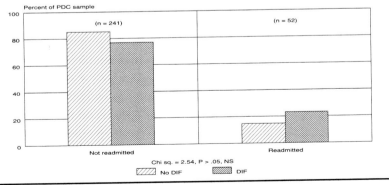

FIGURE 19–5. Readmissions by DIF.

Conclusion

In this early phase of the study, we have only considered the question of economic disruption through the categorization of disruptive insurance factors compromising treatment planning and discharge. Our initial results for those patients with disruptive insurance factors suggest poorer compliance, less positive outcome, and less satisfaction with discharge plans. There was no significant difference in readmission profiles for these patients for the period under review. We did not control for diagnosis, socioeconomic status, level of improvement in the hospital, global severity of illness, or length of stay. Controlling for these factors will be essential in order to more clearly delineate the relationship of economic pressure on outcome. The preliminary findings point to the need for further study utilizing multivariate techniques.

Providers are increasingly being put at financial risk when they admit patients with very limited benefits and/or patients who are being reviewed by a managed care program. Particular concerns center on the treatment of the "catastrophic case," as described previously. This study, albeit a preliminary report with many caveats and limitations, indicates a potential for less positive outcomes of premature discharge necessitated by economic rather than clinical factors. A prospective, double-blind follow-up method is one way to evaluate the impact on patients of hospital stays shortened by economic constraints.

As I have indicated, most studies on length of stay have found no differences in outcomes of short- and long-stay hospitalizations. Carried out primarily in the public sector, these studies reflect a point of view that length of stay may be decreased with outpatient alternatives and community services substituted. However, the studies often use sampling strategies that exclude certain kinds of patients, such as those who are actively suicidal or homicidal; the dually diagnosed (e.g., patients with chemical dependency problems and psychiatric diagnoses); and those with severe personality disorders. This is not a trivial critique, because these conditions are compelling reasons for hospitalizing patients as well as for continuing them in hospitals. Specific studies that look at diagnosis and severity of illness are lacking or incomplete. Also, the substitution of outpatient for inpatient care works only if there are adequate and accessible substitutes out of the hospital. The economic advantages of short-term hospitalization and outpatient care has led to the widespread adoption of insurance limits and has fueled the drive toward more aggressive utilization management. Without more specific understanding of the potential impact on patients and their families of changing economic or utilization management constraints, economic imperatives will tend to take precedence over concern for the quality of clinical care.

Although our results are preliminary and do not control for many relevant factors, including *longer* term effects, we are encouraged by the design and its potential for achieving our objectives. We are making efforts to refine the methodology so that we can be more confident about the meaningfulness of these and future findings.

An important source of bias is that the study is being conducted by a hospital that is itself having to cope with restrictions in benefits and managed care decisions. We are attempting to protect against this bias through the double-blind approach, but it should also be stated that this study should and could be done by a large insurance carrier and several hospitals, a utilization management company, or by independent researchers. Investigation of the potential "negative outcome" of managing costs must be pursued in this era of cost containment and also in relation to the possibility of universal health insurance, which is currently under consideration in the Congress of the United States.

One final comment is in order. The control of costs is often the overarching rationale for managed care and benefit restrictions. Managed care, ideally practiced, is, I believe, indistinguishable from excellent clinical care. Patients should be treated in the most effective and efficient settings, with the most effective and efficient modalities. In that process, when benefits are more readily made available to half- and quarter-way residential facilities, day treatment programs, and outpatient services, we may finally arrive at an era of sound integration of clinical and managed care.

References

American Psychiatric Association, Office of Economic Affairs: Insurance Coverage for Psychiatric Illness in the Private Sector, 1986: The Coverage Catalog, 2nd Edition. Edited by Scheidemandel P. Washington, DC, American Psychiatric Association, 1989, pp 3–26

Brady J, Sharfstein S, Muszynski I: Trends in private insurance coverage for mental illness. Am J Psychiatry 143:10, 1986

Caffey EM, Galbrecht CR, Klett CJ: Brief hospitalization and aftercare in the treatment of schizophrenia. Arch Gen Psychiatry 24:81–86, 1971

Caton CLM: Effect of length of inpatient treatment for chronic schizophrenia. Am J Psychiatry 139:856–861, 1982

Caton CLM, Gralnick A: A review of issues surrounding length of psychiatric hospitalization. Hosp Community Psychiatry 38:858–863, 1987

Glick ID, Hargreaves WA, Raskin M, et al: Short versus long hospitalization: a prospective controlled study: II, results for schizophrenic inpatients. Am J Psychiatry 132:385–390, 1975

Gordon T, Breakey WR: A comparison of the outcomes of short- and standard-stay patients at one-year follow-up. Hosp Community Psychiatry 34:1054–1056, 1983

Hargreaves WA, Glick IA, Drues J, et al: Short versus long hospitalization: a prospective controlled study. Arch Gen Psychiatry 34:305–311, 1977

Herz MI, Endicott J, Gibbon M: Brief hospitalization: two year follow-up. Arch Gen Psychiatry 36:701–705, 1979

Hibbard T, Trimboli F: Correlates of successful short-term psychiatric hospitalization. Hosp Community Psychiatry 33:829–833, 1982

Hirsch SR, Platt S, Knight A, et al: Shortening hospital stay for psychiatric care: effect on patients and their families. British Medical Journal 1:442–446, 1979

Kennedy T, Hird F: Description and evaluation of a short-stay admission ward. Br J Psychiatry 136:205–215, 1980

Kirschner LA: Length of stay of psychiatric patients. J Nerv Ment Dis 170:27–33, 1982

Mattes JA: The optimal length of hospitalization for psychiatric patients: a review of the literature. Hosp Community Psychiatry 33:824–828, 1982

Mattes JA, Rosen B, Klein DF: Comparison of the clinical effectiveness of "short" versus "long" stay psychiatric hospitalization: II, Results of a three-year posthospital follow-up. J Nerv Ment Dis 165:387–397, 1977

Sharfstein S: The impact of third party payer cutbacks on private practice of psychiatry: three surveys. Hosp Community Psychiatry 35:478–481, 1984

Sharfstein S: Financial incentive for alternatives to hospital care. Psychiatr Clin North Am 8:449–460, 1985

Sharfstein S: Reimbursement resistance to treatment and support for the long term mental patient. New Dir Ment Health Serv 33:75–85, 1987

Sharfstein S: The catastrophic case: a special problem for general hospital psychiatry in the era of managed care. Gen Hosp Psychiatry 11:268–270, 1989

Sharfstein S, Dunn L, Kent J: The clinical consequences of payment limitations: the experience of a private psychiatric hospital. The Psychiatric Hospital 19:63–66, 1988

Index

❖ A ❖

Accreditation of psychiatric
   facilities, 270–272
Achievement of Practitioner Goals
   Scale, 111
Affective disorder
   alcoholism, 149
   eating disorders, 171–173
   family intervention, 54
   treatment, 109
Aftercare programs, 24
Age of onset, 87
Alcoholics Anonymous, 147–148
Alcoholism
   affective disorder, 149
   outpatient studies, 145
   relapse, 149
   self assessment, 219–220
   subtypes, 144
Alcoholism treatment, 143–144
   brief interventions, 150
   cognitive-behavioral training, 153
   community reinforcement
      approach, 153
   marital and family therapy,
      151–152
   pharmacotherapy, 148–150
   psychotherapy, 147
   research, 144–145

residential, 146–147
self-help groups, 147–148
social skills training, 152
stress management training, 153
Anhedonia, 219
Anorexia nervosa
   mortality, 161, 167
   obsessive-compulsive disorder,
      173–174
   predictors, 165
   psychosocial functioning,
      164–165
   study design, 160–161
Anticonvulsants, 132
Antidepressants, 132
Antisocial personality disorder, 184,
      190–191
   borderline personality disorder
      comparison, 185
Assessment
   admission, 240, 242, 243–244
   environmental, 239
   method, 244
   nursing care, 280–281
   patient satisfaction, 245
   post-discharge, 295–308
   program evaluation, 240, 269–270
   psychiatric facilities, 271–272
   self-assessment, 215–230, 239
   serial, 241–242

training of raters, 238–239, 249,
    261–262
work, 245

❖ **B** ❖

BASIS-32, 224–226
Bellak Ego Function Scales, 261–262
Biological treatment resistance,
    87–88, 100
Bipolar disorder
    prediction of relapse, 133–135
Borderline personality disorder
    antisocial personality disorder
        comparison, 185
    course, 204
    long-term outcome, 186–192
    narcissistic personality disorder
        comparison, 202–209
    other personality disorders,
        185–186
    schizophrenia comorbidity,
        188–189
    short-term outcome, 181–186
    suicide, 192
Borderline Personality Scale, 184
Brief Psychiatric Rating Scale, 238
Bulimia nervosa, 163, 169–171

❖ **C** ❖

Case summaries
    nursing care, 284–285
    young adults, 40–42
Children, 21–28
    family functioning, 23–24, 26–27
    follow-up studies, 25–26
    follow-up study methodology,
        24–25

inpatient treatment, 22–24, 27
Chronicity of mania, 136–137, 138
Classification
    eating disorders, 171, 173
    mania, 136
    narcissistic personality disorder,
        195–198
    schizophrenia, 96–101
Client Satisfaction Questionnaire,
    228
Clinical significance of outcome
    studies, 251
Cognitive-behavioral training, 153
Community reinforcement approach
    for alcoholism treatment, 153
Comorbidity
    anorexia nervosa and other
        disorders, 164
    borderline personality disorder
        and other disorders, 184,
        188–189, 190–192
    narcissistic personality disorder
        and other disorders, 196–197
    predictor of relapse in bipolar
        disorder, 134
    schizophrenia and other
        disorders, 93–94, 101, 188–189
Compliance and quality treatment,
    121, 122–123
Confidentiality, 7, 16
Contraband, 288–290
Control groups, 8, 9, 144
Cost of health care
    cost-benefit ratios, 1–2
    cost control, 2
    effects of health insurance
        policies and managed care on
        outcome, 311–319
    risk-benefit analysis, 16
Criteria for Affective Disorder Form,
    110

Cross-national study, 107–123
    compliance, 121, 122–123
    data analysis strategies, 111–112
    family intervention, 117–118
    goals of treatment, 117–118, 120
    instruments, 110–111
    methodology, 108
    quality treatment equation,
        121–123
Cross-sectional analysis, 130

❖ **D** ❖

Deinstitutionalization, 32–36
Denver Community Mental Health
    Questionnaire, 221
Depression self-assessment, 217–219,
    222
Diagnosis
    narcissistic personality disorder,
        195–198
    schizophrenia, 96–101
Diagnosis practices, 121, 129
Diagnosis-Related Groups
    hospital length of stay, 1
    prognosis of mental disorders, 8
Diagnostic Interview for Narcissism,
    197
Dieting, 175
    See also Anorexia nervosa;
        Bulimia nervosa; Eating
        disorders
Disruptive insurance factors,
    313–314
Disulfiram, 148–149
Documentation, 268, 275
Double-blind placebo controlled
    studies, 130
Drug treatment studies, 131–132

DSM-III
    borderline personality disorder,
        183–184, 185
    discrimination of narcissistic
        personality disorder and
        borderline personality
        disorder, 201
    narcissistic personality disorder,
        195–196
    schizophrenia, 97
DSM-III-R
    assessment, 243
    narcissistic personality disorder,
        196, 197

❖ **E** ❖

Eating Attitudes Test, 174–175
Eating disorders
    affective disorders, 171–173
    anorexia nervosa, 160–169
    bulimia nervosa, 169–171
    classification, 171, 173
    pathogenesis, 174–175
Ethical issues
    control groups, 8, 9, 25
Explanatory trials, 130

❖ **F** ❖

Family Attitude Scale, 53
Family functioning, 23–24, 26–27
Family intervention
    affective disorder, 54
    alcoholism, 151–152
    assessment and statistical analysis
        procedures, 52–53
    compliance, 121, 122–123
    cross-national study, 117–118

efficacy, 58
goals, 48–49, 51
schizophrenia, 55–56
treatment design, 49–52
Family Treatment Variables, 257
Follow-up studies, 5, 90
anorexia nervosa, 161–165
benefits, 28
borderline personality disorder, 181–190
borderline personality disorder and narcissistic personality disorder comparison, 206
children, 22–24
long-term hospitalization, 296–300
methodology, 24–25, 38, 130, 237–251
schizophrenia, 62–91
short-term hospitalization, 301–308

❖ G ❖

Gender differences
narcissistic personality disorder, 197
schizophrenia, 92–93
General Health Questionnaire, 175
Global Assessment Scale, 53, 111, 185, 238
borderline patients, 189
borderline personality disorder and narcissistic personality disorder comparison, 205
Global Rating of Resolution of Index Episode, 111

Goals of treatment, 4
cross-national study, 117–118, 120
hospital length of stay, 260
patient perceptions, 214
risk-benefit analysis, 15–16

❖ H ❖

Health care providers
accountability, 266
Health care service overutilization, 17
Health Sickness Rating Scale, 188
Hospital discharge
against medical advice, 241
planning, 311
Hospital length of stay
optimal, 247–258, 262–263
prediction, 1, 258–260, 262–263
staff bias, 10
study design, 255–260
treatment program correlation, 256–257
young adults, 33–38

❖ I ❖

Idleness, 269
Incident reporting system, 269, 274
Individualized eclecticism unit, 37
Informed consent, 241
Inpatient treatment
acute and custodial care, 2
alcoholism, 155
children, 22–24, 27
evaluation, 222–223
family intervention, 47–58

long-term, 35–38
young adults, 31–38
Instrumental functioning of
  borderline patients, 188
Instruments, 176
  cross-national study, 110–111
  follow-up questionnaire, 38–39
  post-discharge assessment, 295
  See also specific instruments
Insurance
  disruptive factors, 313–314
  inpatient treatment of
    alcoholism, 155
Interpersonal therapy, 51–52
Interviews
  cross-national study, 109–110
  standardized, 176
  unstructured clinical interviews, 7
  See also specific interviews
Inventory to Diagnose Depression,
  218
Italy
  compliance, 122–123
  medical care, 120
  polypharmacy, 121–122

❖ **J** ❖

Japan
  compliance, 122–123
  medical care, 120
  polypharmacy, 121–122
Johnson Behavioral System Model,
  279–280
Joint Commission on Accreditation
  of Healthcare Organizations,
  270, 282, 293

❖ **L** ❖

Length of stay. *See* Hospital length
  of stay
Lithium, 131
Longitudinal analysis, 130
Long-term hospitalization, 296–300
  short-term hospitalization
    outcome comparison, 312–313

❖ **M** ❖

Major affective disorder, 190–191
Major depressive disorder, 107–123
Management trials, 130
Mania
  chronicity, 136–137
  classification, 136
  course, 128–130, 138, 139
  predictors of relapse, 133–135
  prevalence, 127–128
  psychosocial adjustment, 135–136
  recovery, 133
  suicide, 137
Marital therapy and alcoholism,
  151–152
Marriage and schizophrenia, 93
Medicare and Medicaid, 270
Medication
  alcoholism treatment, 148–150
  drug treatment studies, 131–132
  monitoring, 270, 275
  nursing care, 287–288
  polypharmacy in Japan and Italy,
    121–122
  risk-benefit analysis, 19
  schizophrenia treatment, 100
Methodology
  cross-national study, 108

follow-up research on treatment of children, 24–25
follow-up studies, 38, 130–131
health insurance study, 313–314
patient satisfaction, 227–229
patient selection, 7–8
survival analysis, 134–135
treatment program selection, 8–11
Misdiagnosis, 18
Mortality
anorexia nervosa, 161, 167
data, 176
mania, 137
schizophrenia, 84
Multivariate analysis, 248–249

❖ **N** ❖

Narcissistic personality disorder
borderline personality disorder, 196, 198, 202–209
classification, 195–198
course, 204–206
gender differences, 197
validity, 202–204
National Institute on Alcohol Abuse and Alcoholism, 144
Naturalistic studies, 130
Negative treatment outcome
risk-benefit analysis, 18–19
Neuroleptic drugs, 87
Nonresponders, 175–176, 228, 240, 242, 246–247
locating, 240–241
Nonsignificant results, 247
Nursing care
contraband, 288–290
medication incidents, 287–288
patient falls, 285–287

patient perceptions, 288
philosophy, 279–281

❖ **O** ❖

Obsessive-compulsive disorder and anorexia nervosa, 173–174
Outcome data
application to clinical practice, 138
impediments to collection, 6–7, 24, 175–76
Outcome measures, 71, 244–246
anorexia nervosa, 163–164
clinical status, 3, 136, 163–164
hospital length of stay, 261
length of medical illness, 85–86
level of functioning, 39–40, 136
long-term hospitalization outcome study, 297–300
nursing quality, 282, 283–284
patient satisfaction, 2–3, 227–230
post-discharge, 294
quality of life, 3
rehospitalization, 3, 39–40, 129
remission, 70
risk-benefit analysis, 15–19
Outpatient studies of alcoholism, 145

❖ **P** ❖

Paranoid and nonparanoid subtypes of schizophrenia, 93
Patient Entry Data and Treatment Data at Discharge database, 240
Patient perceptions
goals of treatment, 214
nursing care, 288

satisfaction, 227–230, 245
self-reports, 215–222
treatment design, 2
treatment selection, 9–10
Patient safety
falls, 285–287
Patient selection, 80, 130–131, 294
cross-national study, 112
long-term hospitalization
outcome study, 296
narcissistic personality disorder,
198–200
Patient-treatment matching, 7,
144–146, 152, 154–155
Peer review, 267–268
Pharmacotherapy. *See* Medication
Physical illness
schizophrenia, 84
Post-discharge assessment
instruments, 295
Predictors
anorexia nervosa, 165
baseline level, 250
borderline personality disorder,
190–192, 207–208
children's long-term adjustment,
27
hospital length of stay, 258–260,
262–263
mania, 133–135
narcissistic personality disorder,
208–209
schizophrenia, 92, 94
Private hospitals, 32–36
Prognosis
Diagnosis-Related Groups, 8
major depressive disorder, 114
mental disorders, 5
principles, 94–96
Prognostic scales, 94
Progress Evaluation Scale, 26

Prospective studies
borderline personality disorder,
186
children, 25–28
schizophrenia, 63, 70, 78–82
young adults, 42
Psychiatric Evaluation Form, 53
Psychiatric facilities
accreditation, 270–272
quality assurance, 269–270
Psychosocial functioning
anorexia nervosa, 164–165
Psychotherapy as alcoholism
treatment, 147

❖ Q ❖

Quality assurance, 120, 121
definition, 266–267
documentation, 268
evaluation process for psychiatric
facilities, 271–272
medical care, 265–276
nursing care, 281–290
peer review, 267–268
program description, 272–276,
282–283
psychiatric hospitals, 269–270
Quality Care Intervention
Checklist, 110
Quality of life, 3
Questionnaires. *See* Instruments

❖ R ❖

Rehabilitation programs, 80
Rehospitalization, 3, 39–40, 312, 316
length of stay effects, 35
mania, 129

Replication, 247–248
Residential treatment of alcoholism, 146–147
Retrospective studies
 borderline personality disorder, 196
 schizophrenia, 63, 70–83
Risk-benefit analysis, 15–19
 cost of health care, 16
 medication, 19
 misdiagnosis, 18
 negative treatment outcome, 18–19
 overutilization of health care services, 17
Risk management and quality assurance, 266
Role Performance and Treatment Scale, 53

❖ **S** ❖

Sample selection, 85, 100
Sample size, 246
Schedule for Affective Disorders and Schizophrenia, 42
Schizophrenia
 borderline personality disorder comorbidity, 188–89
 chronicity, 86–87
 classification, 96–101
 course, 84, 91, 92, 100
 family intervention, 55–56
 follow-up studies, 62–91
 gender differences, 92
 natural history, 83–91
 prognosis, 92–96
 prospective studies, 63, 70, 78–82
 retrospective studies, 63, 70–83
 subtypes, 93
 suicide, 84
Schizotypal personality disorder, 190–191
Seclusion and restraint, 274
Self-assessment
 clinical interview comparison, 218
 criteria for self-report measures, 223–224
 social functioning, 221
 value and limitations, 215–216
Self-Assessment Guide, 221
Self-help groups for alcoholism treatment, 147–148
Short-term and long-term hospitalization outcome comparison, 312–313
Social Adjustment Scale, 221
Social skills training, 37, 152
Sociocultural factors, 90–91
Statistical significance, 251
Statistical tests, 246
Stress management training as alcoholism treatment, 153
Structured clinical interviews, 7
Study design. See Methodology
Substance abuse, 190–192
 self-assessment, 220
 See also Alcoholism; Alcoholism treatment
Suicide
 anorexia nervosa, 167
 borderline personality disorder, 192
 mania, 137
 schizophrenia, 84, 100
 short-term hospitalization, 305
Survival analysis methodology, 134–135

❖ **T** ❖

Therapeutic Alliance Scale, 238–239
Therapeutic communities, 36
Thought disorder
  self-assessment, 220
Timberlawn Child Follow-Up
  Rating Scale, 26
Training of raters, 238–239, 249,
  261–262
Treatment design, 4, 5, 90, 273
  alcoholism, 143–144
  cross-national study, 120
  family intervention, 49–52
  inpatient, 37

Treatment dropouts, 10
  children, 25
Treatment programs
  assessment scales, 222–223
  evaluation, 213, 301–305
  length of stay correlation,
    256–257
Treatment Variables, 257

❖ **Y** ❖

Young adults
  case summaries, 40–42
  inpatient treatment, 32–38